INTERVENTIONAL PHYSIOLOGY ROUNDS

INTERVENTIONAL PHYSIOLOGY ROUNDS

CASE STUDIES IN CORONARY
PRESSURE AND FLOW FOR
CLINICAL PRACTICE

MORTON J. KERN, M.D.
J. Gerard Mudd Cardiac Catheterization Laboratory
St. Louis University Medical Center
St. Louis, Missouri

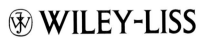

A JOHN WILEY & SONS, INC., PUBLICATION
New York · Chichester · Weinheim · Brisbane · Singapore · Toronto

Library of Congress Cataloging-in-Publication Data:

Kern, Morton J.
    Interventional physiology rounds : case studies in coronary
pressure and flow for clinical practice / Morton J. Kern.
        p. cm.
    Includes index.
    Compilation of articles published in Catheterization and
cardiovascular diagnosis.
    ISBN 0-471-25226-3 (pbk. : alk. paper)
    1. Cardiac catheterization—Case studies. 2. Coronary
circulation—Measurement—Case studies. 3. Coronary heart disease—
Diagnosis—Case studies. I. Catheterization and cardiovascular
diagnosis. II. Title.
    [DNLM: 1. Coronary Disease—physiopathology—collected works.
2. Coronary Circulation—physiology—collected works. 3. Blood Flow
Velocity—physiology—collected works. 4. Hemodynamics—physiology—
collected works. WG 300 K392i 1998]
    RC683.5.C25K47   1998
    616.1'23—dc21
DNLM/DLC
for Library of Congress   97-42364
                                                   CIP

Printed in the United States of America.

10 9 8 7 6 5 4 3 2 1

To Margaret and Anna Rose, merci bien.

The following chapters originally appeared in the *Journal of Catheterization and Cardiovascular Diagnosis.* The journal is the only appropriate literature citation for the articles printed on these pages.

Contents

Preface

The purpose of this book is to provide fundamental principles and clinical observations, using intracoronary flow and pressure both as an investigative tool to study the physiologic effects of various mechanical and pharmacologic interventions within the human diseased coronary circulation, and to assist in everyday clinical decision-making. The examination of human coronary physiology, at rest and during interventions, from locations previously available only to the experimental animal physiologist, can now be discussed in the context of direct observations.

The second purpose of this book is to provide a brief reference for the clinical use of coronary physiologic techniques in the catheterization laboratory. It is hoped that the material contained herein will support the case that coronary physiology can be a rational, alternative approach to decision-making beyond lumenology as well as a research tool of continuing importance in our understanding of cardiovascular disease.

Over the last six years new coronary physiologic observations have been made in patients during various balloon and nonballoon coronary interventions in catheterization laboratories around the world. As is always the case with unique, evolving information, these findings have produced many new questions, some challenging the classical concepts of coronary blood flow derived from years of experimental animal studies. The comparison of coronary flow responses in patients with advanced atherosclerotic arteries to those in normal canine vessels with occluders or mechanically induced thrombosis may not be valid, since analogous models for the clinical situations frequently encountered do not exist. Data from our laboratory and from others measuring blood flow in patients during angioplasty and other interventions is incorporated with both published and preliminary reports of interventional coronary physiology, placing each subject in perspective to assist interventional and noninvasively oriented cardiologists, physiologists, and students in extending their fundamental knowledge into the clinical realm.

The major areas that are emphasized include basic principles of flow and pressure measurements, coronary hemodynamics in the normal and diseased state, and blood flow alterations after coronary angioplasty, atherectomy, stents, and other interventional devices. The basic concepts are illustrated in a case presentation format with, hopefully, useful explanations of pathophysiology and the corresponding anatomy.

The inclusion of translesional pressure measurements is an integral component of coronary hemodynamics and is an indispensable aid in understanding coronary blood flow. However, as of this writing, the only clinically available pressure device in the United States is a 2.7F fluid-filled pressure catheter, too large for trustworthy hyperemic pressure measurements. Complete assessment of both the epicardial conduit and the microvascular flow status can only be obtained with simultaneous pressure-flow data.

The majority of the clinical observations in this book have been published in a series entitled "Interventional Physiology" in *Cardiac Catheterization and Cardiovascular Diagnosis*. I would like to thank Frank Hildner, MD, the editor, who has continued to support our efforts to bring active physiology into the catheterization laboratory in a clinically applicable fashion.

The magnificent collaboration of my colleagues, Frank V. Aguirre, Richard G. Bach, Eugene A. Caracciolo, Thomas J. Donohue, and Thomas L. Wolford, and of the interventional fellows-in-training, has made this work possible. Their input into the techniques, concepts, and data has greatly contributed to the delivery of physiology to patient care. The steadfast, diligent organization and productivity of Donna Sander are also greatly appreciated. I thank Dr. Coy Fitch, Chairman of the Department of Internal Medicine, St. Louis University, for supporting me in my career in our catheterization laboratory and during my sabbatical year abroad.

The support of Dr. Menahem Nassi, President of Cardiometrics, Inc., also contributed greatly to this work. His ability to ensure that only firm data and not opinion would be the guiding practice during the development and marketing of the Doppler guidewire allowed me to maintain complete scientific integrity while working closely with industry sponsors.

Finally, I thank Margaret and Anna Rose for their love and patience, especially on rue Lacordaire.

Morton J. Kern, MD

Contributors

Frank V. Aguirre, MD; Saint Louis University Health Sciences Center, St. Louis, MO

Bassam Al-Joundi, MD; Saint Louis University Health Sciences Center, St. Louis, MO

Richard G. Bach, MD; Saint Louis University Health Sciences Center, St. Louis, MO

Saad R. Bitar, MD; Saint Louis University Health Sciences Center, St. Louis, MO

Eugene A. Caracciolo, MD; Saint Louis University Health Sciences Center, St. Louis, MO

Scott Carollo, MD; Saint Louis University Health Sciences Center, St. Louis, MO

Bernard De Bruyne, MD; Cardiovascular Center Aalst, Aalst, Belgium

Danny Demoor, RN; Cardiovascular Center Aalst, Aalst, Belgium

Thomas J. Donohue, MD; Saint Louis University Health Sciences Center, St. Louis, MO

Michael S. Flynn, MD; Saint Louis University Health Sciences Center, St. Louis, MO

Guy Heyndrickx, MD, PHD; Cardiovascular Center Aalst, Aalst, Belgium

Alexander F. Khoury, MD; Saint Louis University Health Sciences Center, St. Louis, MO

Arthur J. Labovitz, MD; Saint Louis University Health Sciences Center, St. Louis, MO

Lawrence McBride, MD; Saint Louis University Health Sciences Center, St. Louis, MO

Courtland Monroe, MD; Saint Louis University Health Sciences Center, St. Louis, MO

Joseph A. Moore, MD; Saint Louis University Health Sciences Center, St. Louis, MO

Jan J. Piek, MD; Academic Medical Center, University of Amsterdam, Amsterdam, The Netherlands

Nico H.J. Pijls, MD; Catharina Ziekenhuis, Eindhoven, The Netherlands

Jan Stockbroeckx, RN; Cardiovascular Center Aalst, Aalst, Belgium

Christophe Tron, MD; Saint Louis University Health Sciences Center, St. Louis, MO

Thomas L. Wolford, MD; Saint Louis University Health Sciences Center, St. Louis, MO

Chapter 1

Introduction to Interventional Physiology Rounds: Case Studies in Coronary Pressure and Flow for Clinical Practice

Morton J. Kern, MD

INTRODUCTION TO INTERVENTIONAL CORONARY PHYSIOLOGY

The goal of coronary interventions in most patients is the relief of ischemic symptoms and myocardial dysfunction through the restoration of coronary blood flow. The search for suitable techniques to be used for both the diagnosis of flow-limiting coronary stenosis and the assessment of procedural endpoints beyond angiography has been principally confined to noninvasive methods due to inadequate direct means to measure coronary blood flow in awake subjects in the catheterization laboratory.

Miniaturization of sensors for catheter-based interventions has extended the applications of both vessel imaging and physiology (intracoronary pressure and flow) to the catheterization laboratory for the investigation and treatment of coronary artery disease. The development of an intracoronary Doppler-tipped angioplasty guidewire, an important technical advance over earlier Doppler catheter techniques, permits measurement of coronary blood flow velocity not only proximal, but also distal to coronary obstructions. Spectral velocity waveform analysis provides the additional advantage of a more accurate determination of velocity alterations.

Establishing objective indications for intervention is of critical importance for patient care. Particularly for questionable angiographic findings before or following angioplasty, the decisions for proceeding with treatment in the absence of other clinical data can now be augmented by objective physiologic data. Interventional physiology has provided new information about patient outcomes after cardiac catheterization and interventions. Table I lists current clinical applications of interventional physiology.

TABLE I. Clinical Applications of Interventional Physiology

Angioplasty
  Endpoint
  Monitoring complications
  Assessing additional lesions
  Collateral flow
  Stenting
  Atherectomy
Coronary vasodilatory reserve
  Chest pain, normal coronary arteries, syndrome X
  Transplant coronary arteriopathy
  Saphenous vein graft, internal mammary artery physiology
Coronary research
  Pharmacologic studies
  Intraaortic balloon pumping
  Coronary physiology of valvular disease
  Scintigraphic perfusion imaging correlation
  Endothelial function

RATIONALE

The rationale for using coronary physiology is mainly to overcome the limitations of angiography in determining the true effect of coronary artery disease and its impairment of blood flow through obstructive lesions. As a diagnostic technique, coronary angiography provides essential information regarding the presence, location, and extent of epicardial coronary lesions, but remains imperfect in determining their functional significance. Angiographic images visualize plaque indirectly (via the lumenogram) and are subject to large intra- and interobserver variability in interpretation. Uncertainty regarding lesional functional significance and, therefore, the need for intervention, can be especially problematic among stenoses with intermediate severity or complex morphology.

QUANTITATIVE CORONARY ANGIOGRAPHY AND PHYSIOLOGY

To address these limitations, adjunctive techniques have been developed, attempting to improve on conventional angiography. Computer-assisted quantitative angiographic analysis (QCA) and intravascular ultrasound enhance the ability to define lesion geometry [1–6]. While providing detailed analyses of coronary lesions, both techniques of lumenography remain confined to morphologic data. Physiologic consequences must be extrapolated using assumptions based on fluid dynamic principles that are difficult, if not impossible, to apply to the coronary arteries of patients [7,8]. The limits of angiography in accurately representing the luminal encroachment by plaque may be particularly important in cases of diffuse disease and eccentric lesions, and in the immediate postintervention period when disrupted plaque and intimal dissection may contribute to difficulty in estimating angiographic residual stenosis severity [9].

A reduction in the coronary luminal cross-sectional diameter, often estimated from the radiocontrast image during angiography, has been utilized to predict reductions in coronary blood flow of the associated clinical syndrome. This traditional angiographic approach, in clinical practice, is highly subjective. Although anatomic and physiologic lesion assessment methods are often complementary, contradictory results are not unusual. QCA approaches to the evaluation of coronary anatomy have narrowed the disparity between anatomy and physiology, but the physiologic significance of stenoses is still the predominant decision-making factor. QCA, currently required for nearly all sophisticated clinical investigations [10], was initially developed for post hoc, off-line analysis of cineangiographic film, but can now be applied to on-line digitized image information.

The instrumentation for quantitative angiography is relatively complex. Optical magnification of the cineangiographic image permits computer-assisted edge definition and quantitation of luminal narrowing. A substantial selection of computational hardware and software has been developed for commercial distribution. The most important component of the system is the computerized algorithm for boundary delineation within an area of interest. The operator first identifies the target arterial segment. A computer-assisted edge delineation of the segment-of-interest is then performed in an automated, semiautomated, or manual mode. Depending on the techniques, the operator interacts with the windows of interest [2], approximates borders [5], or points along the center line of the vascular segment [3]. More fully automated techniques compute the arterial center line after manual assignment of the visually-derived vessel center line [6]. Several approaches to edge detection utilize a manual mode wherein the operator traces the vessel edge [5,6]. More elaborate algorithms have first derivative, second derivative, and first semiderivative gray-scale edge-defining functions.

Quantitatively useful information also requires a calibration function. This function converts measured pixels to millimeters of vascular diameter, using reference standards derived from the (contrast-filled) catheter with known dimensions or known spacing distances between radioopaque markers on specially manufactured catheters. An internal calibration from geometric analysis of biplane images may avert the potential errors of differential magnification [4–6]. The validation of QCA documents the accuracy, precision, and reproducibility of the numerical estimates of coronary artery dimensions [5]. In radiographic "phantom studies," "stenoses" of known dimensions (typically 0.5–5.0 mm) are fashioned from nonbiologic materials, filled with radiocontrast agents, and imaged angiographically. Results of these studies generally predict an accuracy of 0.03 mm. Postmortem studies typically describe correlation coefficients of >0.9 between necropsy dimensions and the measured angiographic values. The observed relative absence of variability after serial quantitative analysis of a single coronary angiographic study is associated with mean differences in the predicted minimal stenosis diameter of 0.10 mm [11].

For in vivo clinical applications, serial assessment of changes in lumen diameter indicates a threshold for angiographic detectability of 0.44 mm [12]. A similar angiographic threshold for detectable true progression/regression (0.40 mm) has been described in a cohort of men followed prospectively after coronary bypass surgery [13]. The operator remains a key uncontrollable factor in the inter- and intraobserver variability, reported as between 5–20%.

QCA is less reliable when the vessel is diffusely diseased, a particularly important confounding effect when long segments of ectasia and atherosclerotic disease are present. Furthermore, the reference diameter, as well as the diameter of the diseased segment, may change in response to intervention. To minimize resultant variability and measurement error, the minimal lumen diameter can be employed for standard comparisons, in addition to the percent diameter stenosis [4,12].

CONSIDERATION OF ANGIOGRAPHICALLY-DERIVED PHYSIOLOGY

From data obtained with quantitative methodologies, the percent diameter stenosis, lesion length, area of obstruction, area of plaque, and minimal stenosis diameter are easily measured or calculated. Physiologic parameters, such as calculated resistance to flow and hypothetically-derived transluminal pressure gradients, can be obtained [7], but remain of questionable value relative to directly measured parameters in patients [8]. Enthusiasm for the accuracy and reproducibility of QCA must also be counterbalanced by an awareness of contradictory clinical evidence correlating anatomy with physiologic testing [14–23].

The greatest advantage of quantitative angiography lies in its theoretical freedom from observer influences and bias. In prospective studies, the potential for observer error in cinefilm analysis has been estimated to exceed 35% [24]. The extent of the variability rests, in part, upon the severity of the lesion under scrutiny: lesser degrees of variation are reported for stenoses which represent either <20% or >80% of the vessel diameter [25]; visual analysis generally leads to overestimation of severe stenoses, and to underestimation of more modest degrees of luminal narrowing [25]. Furthermore, there is significant discordance between the visual estimates of luminal narrowing and the physiologic significance of stenosis [26]. In standard cineangiography, the two-dimensional projection of the vessel onto the radiographic film poses an additional problem. Because of image foreshortening, certain segments of the coronary vessel (those which deviate from a plane which is parallel to the image intensifier) will be recorded in a distorted and qualitatively inaccurate manner. Foreshortening, lesional eccentricity, and overlap of vascular segments require examination of multiple angiographic projections, particularly for the more complex left coronary artery. A further difficulty is posed by the compensatory vasodilatation of the normal vessel surrounding a coronary stenosis. Quantitation of the normal reference diameter is therefore always problematic. Finally, the functional significance of coronary stenotic lesions is governed not only by the degree of stenosis, but also by such features as the shape, length, and eccentricity of the lesion, collateral routes of perfusion, and vasomotor tone, among others [27–29]. These physical properties and resultant flow characteristics contribute to the disparity between the angiographic and corresponding physiologic assessment of disease severity [30].

QCA has not translated effectively from the realm of clinical investigation to that of clinical application. The complex instrumentation, time, and angiographic technique required for quantitative angiography have limited its utility in the practice of interventional cardiology, particularly in acute or urgent situations [31]. The single greatest drawback of quantitative coronary angiography is the lack of correlation between the functional predictions of angiographic disease severity and directly measured physiologic variables, as they relate to coronary flow reserve. Although the hemodynamic predictions derived from quantitative angiography are well-supported in animal studies [32,33], in human coronary

artery disease, no similar useful relationship between quantitative angiographic findings (percent diameter stenosis and minimal luminal cross-sectional area) and coronary flow physiology, coronary flow reserve, and transstenotic pressure gradient exists [8,14–20].

In summary, while QCA has many actual and theoretical advantages, practical aspects and fundamental clinical studies continue to limit the applicability of the method. The propensity of angiographic predictions of clinical importance to deviate from physiologic measurements remains the greatest limitation. Since the results of quantitative angiography serve to under- or overpredict the functional significance of coronary stenoses, the expansion of adjunctive diagnostic modalities like translesional coronary physiology is more than justified.

CORONARY PHYSIOLOGY IN THE CATHETERIZATION LABORATORY[1]

The development of catheter-based Doppler ultrasound technology for quantitative measurement of blood flow has made physiologic coronary analyses clinically practical in patients. By sensor miniaturization and refinement of signal processing, the Doppler-tipped angioplasty guidewire has emerged as a significant advance, providing a clinically useful tool for the evaluation of coronary pathophysiology during cardiac catheterization and intervention. Information supporting clinical application of coronary physiologic measurements in patients is now available [22, 23, 34].

As currently practiced, an indirect physiologic approach to lesion assessment utilizes hospital facilities outside of the catheterization laboratory and requires additional time and costs. Moreover, some patients may not undergo physiologic evaluation before proceeding with angioplasty. Data from a large, insured population of 2,101 patients undergoing coronary angioplasty for the diagnoses of angina pectoris (69%), unstable angina (12%), or myocardial infarction (19%) showed that only 29% of all patients had prior stress testing [35]. The use of coronary physiologic data obtained in the catheterization laboratory following diagnostic angiography or prior to angioplasty provides an alternative to indirect testing and has facilitated clinical decision-making [36–38].

The hemodynamic significance of a given stenosis is determined by the pressure-flow relationship [32]. Coronary physiologic data have not been incorporated into clinical practice because of cumbersome catheter techniques [38,39] and questionable or conflicting results from patient studies related to coronary pressure or flow

[1]Portions of this section are reproduced in part from Kern MJ, De Bruyne B, Pijls NHJ: From research to clinical practice: Current role of intracoronary physiologically based decision making in the cardiac catheterization laboratory. J Am Coll Cardiol 1997;30:613–620.

[14–19]. Although predictable relationships between anatomic and physiologic parameters had been demonstrated in experimental studies, clinically useful relationships between angiography and myocardial perfusion scintigraphy, coronary flow reserve, or transstenotic pressure gradients were often not present in patients. The reasons for this weak relationship are not completely understood but include the limitations of coronary angiography as a standard of lesion severity, and complex, and at times, compromised physiologic measurement techniques. Recently, an additional reason for the poor correlation between coronary Doppler catheter studies and clinical testing has been identified. Flow velocity measured proximal to a stenosis may differ from post-stenotic flow data, a phenomenon related to lower pre-lesional branch resistance directing flow away from or around the stenosis [20, 40–42].

Coronary physiologic data can be acquired safely and rapidly using sensor-tipped angioplasty guidewires. The guidewire method has overcome catheter limitations, can be easily incorporated into routine procedures, and does not substantially interfere with blood flow across subcritical stenoses. In contrast to pressure measurements through angioplasty balloon catheters, pressure guidewires produce useful pressure signals without the artifact of a catheter shaft or balloon material in the artery lumen.

From guidewire pressure measurements during hyperemia, a new concept for the determination of coronary blood flow, i.e., the fractional flow reserve of the myocardium (FFRmyo), has emerged [43]. The FFRmyo is defined as the ratio of maximal hyperemic flow in the stenotic artery to the theoretic maximal hyperemic flow in the same artery without a stenosis. FFRmyo is computed as the ratio of distal mean coronary pressure and mean aortic pressure during maximal hyperemia and is a specific index to describe the influence of the coronary stenosis on maximal perfusion of the subtended myocardium.

The most confounding issue for decision-making using coronary vasodilatory reserve in patients within the catheterization laboratory is measurement variability. Biologic conditions impairing normal microvascular function exist in patients with diabetes mellitus, left ventricular hypertrophy, myocardial infarction, syndrome X, and various hematologic and rheologic abnormalities in the absence of obstructive atherosclerotic coronary disease. However, the incidence of impaired coronary vasodilatory reserve (<2.0) in 416 angiographically normal coronary arteries from 214 patients undergoing evaluation for chest pain or cardiac transplantation follow-up angiography is <12% [44]. To identify microvascular disease and lesion specificity of coronary vasodilatory reserve, an angiographically normal vessel may be inter-

rogated as a reference, since variation in coronary vasodilatory reserve among the coronary branch arteries is <10% [44,45]. The normal relative coronary vasodilatory reserve is 1.01 ± 0.2 [44].

It should be noted that hemodynamic changes will change coronary vasodilatory reserve [46], but the influence of systemic hemodynamics is negligible on pressure-derived fractional flow reserve because this index only uses hemodynamic responses during maximal hyperemia [47]. Fractional flow reserve is a specific index for epicardial stenosis, while coronary flow reserve addresses both the conduit and microvascular circulation. Since each current physiologic method individually reflects only one aspect of the pressure-flow relationship, borderline or ambiguous data, acquired by either pressure or flow velocity alone, can be theoretically confirmed using the complementary technique. A combined guidewire device with both pressure and flow sensors could eliminate questions related to borderline values. Despite limitations and given the subsequent correlations to ischemic stress testing, the variability of coronary vasodilatory reserve does not appear to represent a significant impediment to clinical use for stenosis assessment in vessels supplying the relatively normal myocardium.

The concepts of pressure and flow for determining coronary stenosis significance have not changed in over 20 years and are applicable to stable patients commonly encountered in the catheterization laboratory. The late Andreas Gruentzig used translesional pressure gradients to determine angioplasty endpoints when the angiogram could not be used with confidence. Unfortunately, pressure data were measured with inadequate devices under inadequate circumstances (i.e., not during maximal hyperemia) and were inadequately interpreted (i.e., resting gradients rather than FFR of the myocardium). With better angiographic systems and smaller angioplasty catheters, the physiologic approach to angioplasty was thought to be unimportant or unreliable, an extension of the now-known-to-be flawed concept that the angiogram is a precise reflection of the coronary lumen.

Coronary physiologic measurements are not an incentivized procedure. Rhetorically, would one want to perform a procedure that will potentially eliminate a patient in whom angioplasty would "ordinarily" be performed and also pay for the privilege from the catheterization laboratory budget without reimbursement? Nevertheless, the drive to perform intervention should not overwhelm a thoughtful, patient-directed approach. The expense of equipment for important decisions is trivial compared to the human expense of an unwarranted or complicated procedure.

Although technical improvements in equipment and more clinical studies are needed, in-laboratory coronary physiology correlates well with myocardial perfusion and ischemic stress studies. A physiologic approach complements lumenology and appears to have important clinical and economic implications for patients undergoing evaluation and treatment of coronary artery disease. Refinements in guidewire sensor technology will facilitate the physiologic approach. However, the more difficult task, which this book will hopefully make easier, is the conceptual development to incorporate the insight that physiologic, as much or more than anatomic, parameters ultimately determine the functional status and well-being of a patient.

REFERENCES

1. Reiber JHC, Kooijman CJ, Slager CJ, et al.: Computer-assisted analysis of the severity of obstructions from coronary cineangiograms. A methodological review. Automedica 5:219–225, 1984.
2. Nichols AB, Gabrieli CFO, Fenoglio JJ, Esser PD: Quantification of relative coronary arterial stenosis by cinevideodensitometric analysis of coronary arteriograms. Circulation 69:512–522, 1984.
3. Kirkeeide RL, Fung P, Smalling RW, Gould KL: Automated evaluation of vessel diameter from arteriograms. Comput Cardiol 5:215–224, 1982.
4. Reiber JHC, Koning G, Von Land CD, Van Der Zwet PMJ: Why and how should QCA systems be validated? In Reiber JHC, Serruys PW (eds): Progress in Quantitative Coronary Arteriography. Kluwer Academic Publishers, Dordrecht: 1994, 33–48.
5. Reiber JHC, Kooijman CJ, Slager CJ et al.: Coronary artery dimensions from cineangiograms: Methodology and validation of a computer-assisted analysis procedure. IEEE Trans Med Imaging 3:131–141, 1984.
6. Reiber JHC: Morphologic and densitometric quantitation of coronary stenoses: An overview of existing quantitation techniques. In Reiber JHC, Serruys PW (eds): "New Developments in Quantitative Coronary Arteriography." Dordrecht: Martinus Nijhoff, 1988, p 34.
7. Kirkeeide RL, Parsel L, Gould KL: Prediction of coronary flow reserve of stenotic coronary arteries by quantitative arteriography [abstract]. Circulation [Suppl] 70:250, 1984.
8. Tron C, Kern MJ, Donohue TJ, Bach RG, Aguirre FV, Caracciolo EA, Moore JA.: Comparison of quantitative angiographically-derived and measured translesion pressure and flow velocity in patients with coronary artery disease. Am J Cardiol 1995; 75:111–117.
9. Serruys PW, Reiber JHC, Wijns W, van den Brand M, Kooijman CJ, ten Katen HJ, Hugenholtz PG: Assessment of percutaneous transluminal coronary angioplasty by quantitative coronary angiography: Diameter versus densitometric area measurements. Am J Cardiol 54:482–488, 1984.
10. Ellis S, Sanders W, Goulet C, Miller R, Cain KC, Lesperance J, Bourassa MG, Alderman EL: Optimal detection of the progression of coronary artery disease: Comparison of methods suitable for risk factor intervention trials. Circulation 74:1235–1242, 1986.
11. Beatt KJ, Luijten HE, de Feyter PJ, van den Brand M, Reiber JHC, Serruys PW: Change in diameter of coronary artery segments adjacent to stenosis after percutaneous transluminal coronary angioplasty: Failure of percent diameter stenosis measurement to reflect morphologic changes induced by balloon dilation. J Am Coll Cardiol 12:315–323, 1988.
12. Reiber JHC, Serruys PW, Kooijman CJ, Wijns W, Slager CJ, Gerbrands JJ, Schuurbiers JCH, den Boer A, Hugenholz PG: Assessment of short-, medium-, and long-term variations in arterial dimensions from computer-assisted quantitation of coronary cineangiograms. Circulation 71:280–288, 1985.
13. Syvanne M, Nieminen MS, Frick MH: Accuracy and precision of quantitative arteriography in the evaluation of coronary artery disease after coronary bypass surgery. A validation study. Int J Card Imaging 10:243–252, 1994.
14. Wijns W, Serruys PW, Reiber JHC, van den Brand M, Simoons ML, Kooijman CJ, Balakumaran K, Hugenholtz PG: Quantitative angiography of the left anterior descending coronary artery: Correlations with pressure gradient and results of exercise thallium scintigraphy. Circulation 71:273–279, 1985.
15. Zijlstra F, van Ommeren J, Reiber JHC, Serruys PW: Does quantitative assessment of coronary artery dimensions predict the physiologic significance of a coronary stenosis? Circulation 75:1154–1161, 1987.
16. Goldberg RK, Kleiman NS, Minor ST, Abukhalil J, Raizner AE: Comparison of quantitative coronary angiography to visual estimates of lesion severity pre and post PTCA. Am Heart J: 119:178–184, 1990.
17. Wilson RF, Marcus MLO, White CW: Prediction of the physiological significance of coronary arterial lesions by quantitative lesion geometry in patients with limited coronary artery disease. Circulation 75:723–732, 1987.
18. Zijlstra F, Fioretti P, Reiber JHC, Serruys PW: Which cineangiographically assessed anatomic variable correlates best with functional measurements of stenosis severity? A comparison of quantitative analysis of the coronary cineangiogram with measured coronary flow reserve and exercise/redistribution thallium-201 scintigraphy. J Am Coll Cardiol 12:686–691, 1988.
19. Harrison DG, White CW, Hiratzka LF, Doty DB, Barnes DH, Eastham CL: The value of lesion cross-sectional area determined by quantitative coronary angiography in assessing the physiologic significance of proximal left anterior descending coronary arterial stenoses. Circulation 69:1111–1119, 1984.
20. Donohue TJ, Kern MJ, Aguirre FV, Bach RG, Wolford T, Bell CA, Segal J: Assessing the hemodynamic significance of coronary artery stenoses: Analysis of translesional pressure-flow velocity relationships in patients. J Am Coll Cardiol 22:449–458, 1993.
21. Miller DD, Donohue TJ, Younis LT, Bach RG, Aguirre FV, Wittry MD, Goodgold HM, Chaitman BR, Kern MJ: Correlation of pharmacologic 99mtc-sestamibi myocardial perfusion imaging with poststenotic coronary flow reserve in patients with angiographically intermediate coronary artery stenoses. Circulation 89:2150–2160, 1994.
22. Joye JD, Schulman DS, Lasorda D, Farah T, Donohue BC, Reichek N: Intracoronary Doppler guide wire versus stress single-photon emission computed tomographic thallium-201 imaging in assessment of intermediate coronary stenoses. J Am Coll Cardiol 24:940–947, 1994.
23. Deychak YA, Segal J, Reiner JS, Rohrbeck SC, Thompson MA, Lundergan CF, Ross AM, Wasserman AG: Doppler guide wire flow-velocity indexes measured distal to coronary stenoses associated with reversible thallium perfusion defects. Am Heart J 129:219–227, 1995.
24. De Rouen TA, Murray JA, Owen W. Variability in the analysis of coronary arteriograms. Circulation 55(2):324–328, 1977.
25. Fleming RM, Kirkeeide RL, Smalling RW, Gould KL: Patterns in visual interpretation of coronary angiograms as detected by quantitative coronary angiography. J Am Coll Cardiol 18:945–951, 1991.
26. White CW, Wright CB, Doty DB, Hiatza LF, Eastham CL, Harri-

son DG, Marcus ML: Does visual interpretation of the coronary arteriogram predict the physiological importance of a coronary stenosis? N Engl J Med 310:819–824, 1984.

27. Glagov S, Weisenberg E, Zarins CK, Stankunavicius R, Kolettis GJ: Compensatory enlargement of human atherosclerotic coronary arteries. N Engl J Med 316:1371–1375, 1987.

28. Epstein SE, Cannon RO III, Watson RM, Leon MB, Bonow RO, Rosing DR: Dynamic coronary obstruction as a cause of angina pectoris: Implications regarding therapy. Am J Cardiol 55:61B–68B, 1985.

29. Feldman RL, Nichols WW, Pepine CJ, Conti CR: Hemodynamic significance of the length of a coronary arterial narrowing. Am J Cardiol 41:865–871, 1978.

30. Gould KL. Percent coronary stenosis: Battered gold standard, pernicious relic or clinical practicality? J Am Coll Cardiol 7:775–789, 1986.

31. Gurley JC, Nissen SE, Booth DC, DeMaria AN: Influence of operator- and patient-dependent variables on the suitability of automated quantitative coronary arteriography for routine clinical use. J Am Coll Cardiol 19:1237–1243, 1992.

32. Gould KL, Kirkeeide RL, Buchi M: Coronary flow reserve as a physiologic measure of stenosis severity. J Am Coll Cardiol 15:459–474, 1990.

33. Gould KL, Kelley KO, Bolson EL: Experimental validation of quantitative arteriography for determining pressure flow characteristics of coronary stenosis. Circulation 66:930–937, 1982.

34. Heller LI, Cates C, Popma J, Deckelbaum LI, Joye JD, Dahlberg SST, Villegas BJ, Arnold A, Kipperman R, Grinstead C, Balcom S, Ma Y, Cleman M, Steingart RM, Loppo JA, for the FACTS Study Group: Intracoronary Doppler assessment of moderate coronary artery disease: Comparison with ²⁰¹Tl imaging and coronary angiography. Circulation 96:484–490, 1997.

35. Topol EJ, Ellis SG, Cosgrove DM, Bates ER, Muller DWM, Schork NJ, Schork MA, Loop FD: Analysis of coronary angioplasty practice in the United States with an insurance-claims data base. Circulation 87:1489–1497, 1993.

36. Kern MJ, Donohue TJ, Aguirre FV, Bach RG, Caracciolo EA, Wolford T, Mechem C, Flynn MS, Chaitman B: Clinical outcome of deferring angioplasty in patients with normal translesional pressure and flow velocity measurements. J Am Coll Cardiol 25:178–187, 1995.

37. Pijls NHJ, De Bruyne B, Peels K, van der Voort PH, Bonnier HJRM, Bartunek J, Koolen JJ: Measurement of myocardial fractional flow reserve to assess the functional severity of coronary-artery stenosis. N Engl J Med 334:1703–1708, 1996.

38. Wilson RF, Laughlin DE, Ackell PH, Chilian WM, Holida MD, Hartley CJ, Armstrong ML, Marcus ML, White CW: Transluminal subselective measurement of coronary artery blood flow velocity and vasodilator reserve in man. Circulation 72:82–92, 1985.

39. Peterson RJ, King SB III, Fajman WA, Douglas JS Jr, Gruentzig AR, Orias DW, Jones RH: Relation of coronary artery stenosis and pressure gradient to exercise-induced ischemia before and after coronary angioplasty. J Am Coll Cardiol 10:253–260, 1987.

40. Ofili EO, Kern MJ, Labovitz AJ, St. Vrain JA, Segal J, Aguirre F, Castello R: Analysis of coronary blood flow velocity dynamics in angiographically normal and stenosed arteries before and after endoluminal enlargement by angioplasty. J Am Coll Cardiol 21:308–316, 1993.

41. Geschwind HJ, Dupouy P, Dubois-Rande JL, Zelinsky R: Restoration of coronary blood flow in severely narrowed and chronically occluded coronary arteries before and after angioplasty: Implications regarding restenosis. Am Heart J 127:252–262, 1994.

42. Heller LI, Silver KH, Villegas BJ, Balcom SJ, Weiner BH: Blood flow velocity in the right coronary artery: Assessment before and after angioplasty. J Am Coll Cardiol 24:1012–1017, 1994.

43. Pijls NHJ, van Son AM, Kirkeeide RL, De Bruyne B, Gould KL: Experimental basis of determining maximum coronary, myocardial, and collateral blood flow by pressure measurements for assessing functional stenosis severity before and after percutaneous transluminal coronary angioplasty. Circulation 87:1354–1367, 1993.

44. Kern MJ, Bach RG, Mechem C, Caracciolo EA, Aguirre FV, Miller LW, Donohue TJ: Variations in normal coronary vasodilatory reserve stratified by artery, gender, heart transplantation and coronary artery disease. J Am Coll Cardiol 28:1154–1160, 1996.

45. Kern MJ, Tatineni S, Gudipati C, Aguirre F, Ring ME, Serota H, Deligonul U: Regional coronary blood flow velocity and vasodilatory reserve in patients with angiographically normal coronary arteries. Cor Art Dis 1:579–589, 1990.

46. McGinn AL, White CW, Wilson RF: Interstudy variability of coronary flow reserve: Influence of heart rate, arterial pressure, and ventricular preload. Circulation 81:1319–1330, 1990.

47. De Bruyne B, Bartuneck J, Sys SU, Heyndrickx GR, Pijls NHJ, Wijns W. Feasibility and hemodynamic dependency of invasive indexes of coronary stenoses. Circulation 92:I324, 1995.

Part I

Fundamentals of
Pressure and Flow
in Small Tubes

Chapter 2

Fundamentals of Translesional Pressure-Flow Velocity Measurements

Morton J. Kern, MD, Frank V. Aguirre, MD, Richard G. Bach, MD, Eugene A. Caracciolo, MD, Thomas J. Donohue, MD, and Arthur J. Labovitz, MD

INTRODUCTION

Fundamental to the application of physiologic measurements and data for interventional procedures is a basic understanding of flow and pressure in small tubes. This section of Interventional Physiology will briefly review the physical principles of pressure and flow in a simplified format. We would like to acknowledge the work of Dr. Yoganathan and his colleagues in the Cardiovascular Fluid Mechanics Laboratory [1] for the lucid discussion on which much of this section is based.

HYDRODYNAMIC LAWS OF FLOW

Doppler ultrasound flow velocity measurements may vary among and within the different flow conditions, characteristics, and forces which make up a flow field. The background of Doppler determined flow velocity is described in a later part of this Rounds.

Blood flow must follow three universal principles described by the laws of conservation of mass, momentum, and energy [2]. In brief, the volume and energy (pressure and velocity) of flow going into a conduit system always equals the volume, pressure (less pressure losses), and velocity (less velocity losses) exiting the conduit. From the law of conservation of mass is derived the continuity equation (volume flow in = flow out) and from the law of conservation of energy is derived the Bernouilli [3] and Poiseuille [4] equations for calculation of pressure and pressure loss across lesions.

Blood flow has two motion *conditions:* 1) steady state or constant flow, 2) unsteady state or pulsatile flow, with three dynamic field *characteristics:* a) laminar (smooth,

uniform), b) transitional (oscillations with some laminar flow) and, c) turbulent (oscillations and non-uniform flow).

Under steady state constant flow conditions, laminar flow in a tube produces a parabolic leading edge (Fig. 1). The parabolic flow profile is due to friction incrementally slowing concentric cylindrical shells of flow with the slowest flow at the wall caused by the boundary layer of friction along the vessel surface. Flow is slowest at the edge with the fastest moving flow shell in the vessel center. Each flow shell, from outside in, retards the flow of the next. This gradual change in flow across the artery results in a parabolic flow profile with an average velocity across the vessel which is constant. The energy loss of slowing flow is due to *viscous* forces. If there were no viscous forces acting at the boundary layer, then the flow profile would be uniformly blunt or flat. As flow enters a conduit, there is a minimum distance required for the development of laminar flow in a straight tube. This distance is determined by the Reynold's (Re) number, a measure of the degree of turbulent flow (vide infra). This concept is helpful when determining how distal to a stenosis should flow velocity be measured. For a 2–3 mm diameter vessel, laminar flow is usually reconstituted in 5–10 artery diameters ($\approx$2 cm) beyond a stenosis.

Whether flow is laminar or turbulent is dependent on the dynamic characteristics which are in turn determined by two flow field *forces:* 1) inertial forces and 2) viscous forces. Unlike most cardiovascular flow fields in large conduits and chambers, in small tubes like coronary arteries (>10 mm in length and <5 mm in diameter), inertial and viscous forces are not negligible and contrib-

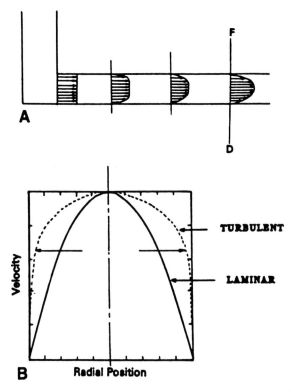

A

B   Radial Position

Fig. 1.   Demonstration of laminar and turbulent flow and developing velocity profile in a cylindrical tube. A: The profile becomes parabolic after originating as a blunt flat profile as the outer edges are slowed by viscous friction at the vessel wall. B: Shows relative flatness of turbulent velocity profile as compared with laminar flow velocity profile. With permission from ref. 1.

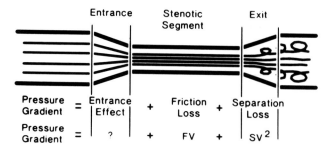

Fig. 2.   A schematic diagram of flow forces within a narrowing inside a small tube. The three segments are indicated as entrance, stenotic segment, and exit. Flow convergence occurs at the entrance to the stenosis, which may contribute to some pressure loss. Within the stenotic segment, pressure is lost owing to friction, and at the exit region, separation loss of re-acceleration and turbulent acceleration produces further pressure loss. The pressure is directly related to the velocity and volume of flow through this tube. With permission from Marcus ML: *The Coronary Circulation in Health and Disease*, McGraw-Hill, New York: 1983, p. 248.

ute to flow impairment and pressure loss across lesions. The degree to which flow is laminar is determined by the relationship of the inertial and viscous forces. This relationship is the Reynold's number. Inertial and viscous forces in steady state tubes are related by the Re number, which is computed by

$$Re = \frac{\text{inertial forces}}{\text{viscous forces}} =$$

$$\frac{(\text{fluid density}) (\text{spatial average velocity})}{\text{fluid viscosity}} = \frac{Vd}{\mu}$$

Laminar flow has a Re $<1,200$, transitional flow has a Re $1,200–2,300$, and turbulent flow has a Re $>2,300$ [1].

CONSIDERATIONS FOR PHASIC CORONARY BLOOD FLOW

Flow in coronary arteries is not in a steady state, but rather in an unsteady or pulsatile state. Two flow conditions exist for pulsatile flow, acceleration and deceler-

ation. Acceleration tends to stabilize turbulence and over consecutive cycles relaminarizes flow. Deceleration destabilizes flow promoting turbulence. Turbulent flow is most often found in the post-stenotic exit regions (Fig. 2).

Since a minimum time is required to develop turbulence, the pulse rate (frequency) also contributes to turbulent flow. Lower pulse rates permit time for flow deceleration to develop turbulence. Rapid rates reduce the potential for turbulence. Turbulence is related to pulse frequency by the Wormersley number (N_w), which is the same as the Re number for unsteady flow.

$$N_w = \frac{\text{diameter}}{2} * \frac{\text{density} * \text{circular frequency of HR}}{\text{viscosity}}$$

[N_w in human aorta (d$=2.5$ cm) at 60 beats/min $= 17.5$]

Fortunately, N_w is not generally required to assess Doppler flow in coronary arteries for clinical studies, but is responsible, in part, for questions regarding the leading edge flow profile in small coronary arteries.

GENERATION OF PRESSURE GRADIENTS FROM FLOW MEASUREMENTS

Pressure is produced by the energy of flow. Pressure across a tube is related to both volumetric flow and flow velocity. There are two formulas commonly used to compute pressure from flow: The Haagen-Poiseuille and simplified Bernouilli equations.

In small cylindrical tubes with fully developed laminar flow, the Haagen-Poiseuille equation can be used to de-

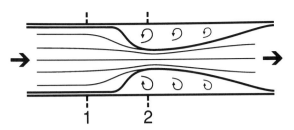

Fig. 3. Diagram of flow velocity accleration through a stenotic region in a tube. An increase in kinetic energy between points 1 and 2 results in decreased pressure between the two locations. This pressure loss in a tube >5 mm in diameter can be determined from the Bernouilli equation, but when the tube is <5 mm in diameter the Haagen-Poiseuille equation may apply. The vena contractra is at location 2. With permission from ref. 1.

termine the pressure gradient across a narrowing in a tube:

$$\frac{\text{Pressure } (P_1 - P_2)}{\text{Length}} =$$
$$\frac{128 \text{ (fluid viscosity, } \mu)}{\pi * \text{diameter}^4} * \text{(flow, Q)}$$

The second equation for pressure, the Bernouilli equation, is based on conservation of energy for pulsatile flow and includes terms of acceleration and friction (Fig. 2),

$$P_1 - P_2 = \text{(convective acceleration)} +$$
$$\left(\text{density} \cdot \frac{\Delta \text{ velocity}}{\Delta \text{ time} \cdot \text{ds}}\right) + \text{(viscous friction)}$$

where convective acceleration = ½ density [(peak maximal velocity$_2$)^2 − (reference velocity$_1$)^2], viscous friction between locations $P_1 - P_2$ = R (v), assumed to be zero at peak systolic or diastolic pressure. For large diameter tubes (>1 cm such as the aorta) acceleration at peak pressure is zero. Thus, the Bernouilli equation then becomes simplified:

$$(P_1 - P_2) = \text{½ density} * (V_2^2 - V_1^2),$$
[when corrected for mm Hg and density of blood],
$$(P_1 - P_2) = 4(V_2^2 - V_1^2); \text{ when } V_2 > V_1 \text{ then}$$
$$\blacktriangle P = 4V_2^2$$

Although it would be attractive to be able to use the jet of high velocity in a stenosis to compute a pressure gradient, the limitations of the Bernouilli equation apply to small conduits. It is important to note that viscous effects in the heart chambers and great vessels are much smaller than viscous and inertial forces in coronary arteries. Therefore, this relationship is *not* applicable for the *cor-*

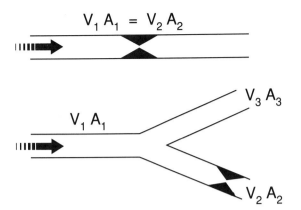

Fig. 4. Depiction of continuity equation when applied in a single non-branched tube model (top) and a branching tube model (bottom). The velocity (V) and area (A) product is equal to volume of flow. Within the single conduit, velocity/area product is equal to the velocity/area product at any other location. This relationship does not hold true when branching circuit may introduce resistance diverting flow to branches of lower resistance.

onary arteries where viscous forces act to produce more energy loss and hence greater pressure loss.

The simplified Bernouilli equation for pressure may not be accurate under four circumstances:

1. When proximal and distal velocity are similar.
2. When the distal pressure is not measured within the vena contracta of flow. The vena contracta (Fig. 3) is the site of the most rapid velocity of all flow streams pushed together just after going through a narrowing. Placing a catheter in the vena contracta may generate errors for translesional coronary measurements owing to relative catheter/stenosis sizes.
3. When stenoses are in series. Pressure drops are *not* additive due to pressure recovery and relaminarization of flow downstream from the vena contracta. The highest gradient will occur downstream from the most severe stenosis.
4. When viscous forces are considered significant. This condition exists for long (>10 mm) narrow (<5 mm) tubes at low flow rates. Coronary arteries and their stenoses meet these conditions. For coronary arteries, the Haagen-Poiseuille equation can be used to estimate pressure drop owing to viscous effects occurring in addition to convective acceleration.

CALCULATION OF VOLUME FLOW RATE FROM FLOW VELOCITY

For a flat velocity profile, volume flow rate (Q) = V_{peak} * cross-sectional area. V is the spatial average velocity. For a parabolic flow profile, 0.5 * V_{peak} has been used to correct for lower velocity at edges of the rounded parabolic profile. Alternatively, the volumetric flow rate, Q, can be derived from the following:

$$Q = \text{total flow velocity integral} * \text{heart rate} * \text{cross-sectional area [5]}$$

The flow velocity integral is the time × area product under the spectral flow velocity signal. The continuity principle equating flow entering and exiting a tube can be applied to assess lesions using angiographic and Doppler flow variables. Blood flow can be calculated at any point along the tube by the continuity equation (Fig. 4):

$$\text{Flow}_1 = \text{Flow}_2$$
$$\text{Area}_1 \cdot \text{velocity}_1 = \text{area}_2 \cdot \text{velocity}_2$$

However, the continuity equation will be modified when assessing flow in branching tubes. Total flow in the parent branch must equal the sum of sub-branch flow:

$$A_1V_1 = A_2V_2 + A_3V_3$$

where A_1, A_2, A_3 are the cross-sectional areas of parent and sub-branch$_2$ and sub-branch$_3$, respectively with V = velocity. In adherence with hydrodynamic laws of flow and resistance, when a resistance such as a stenosis appears in one of the sub-branches, flow will be diverted to the branch(es) of lower resistance [6] (Fig. 4). Validation of the classic hydrodynamic laws is easily demonstrated in plastic tubes with a roller pump delivering known flow volumes (Fig. 5A). Flow velocity in a single tube is the same proximal and distal to a narrowing regardless of the pressure gradient of the obstruction (Fig. 5B, bottom). However, in the branched tube model, as the sub-branch obstruction increases, as determined by the distal pressure loss, flow and velocity are increased in the non-obstructed branch while flow falls in the region distal to the obstruction (Fig. 5B, top). This relationship of flow velocity in proximal and distal regions appears to apply in the coronary circulation as shown in the cases presented in part I.

DOPPLER PRINCIPLES OF CORONARY FLOW VELOCITY

An observer moving toward a sound source will hear a tone with higher frequency than at rest. An observer moving away from the source will hear a lower frequency tone. This phenomenon also is true if the observer is stationary and the source is moving. This change in frequency is called the Doppler effect after Christian Johann Doppler (1803–1853), an Austrian physicist. In practice, a piezoelectric crystal on a catheter

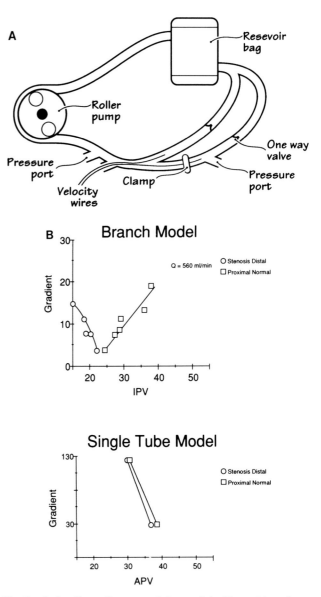

Fig. 5.   A: In vitro roller pump tube model of branching circulation in which simultaneous velocity was recorded proximal and distal to a variable lesion provided by the tube clamp. With flow constant, a pressure gradient was created across the clamp obstruction and flow velocity changes were measured. B: Relationship of pressure gradient and flow velocity proximal and distal to the stenosis in the branched model depicted in A. IPV = instantaneous peak velocity. As the gradient increases, velocity distal to the stenosis falls. At the same time, flow in the proximal region increases to maintain volume constant. In the single tube model (when one branch is completely clamped) velocity (APV) is the same proximally and distally, regardless of the pressure gradient produced in the tube.

or guidewire emits and receives high-frequency sound waves. Changes in the blood flow velocity alter the return frequency bouncing off the moving red cell targets, causing the Doppler shift (Fig. 6). Electronic circuits precisely determine velocity of the targets moving through a sound sampling zone. Flow velocity is calculated as the difference between the transmitted and returning frequency using the following Doppler equation:

$$V = \frac{(F_1 - F_0)\ (C)}{(2F_0)\ (Cos\ \phi)}$$

Where V = velocity of blood flow
F_0 = transmitting (transducer) frequency
F_1 = returning frequency
C = constant: speed of sound in blood
ϕ = angle of incidence

Maximum velocity can be recorded, provided the transducer beam is nearly parallel to blood flow and ϕ is zero so that the cosine ϕ is 1. A pulsed-wave Doppler permits determination of both magnitude and direction of the flow changes at a predetermined distance (a sample zone or volume range gate) from the transducer.

Intracoronary Doppler has several obvious advantages for interventional physiology. Doppler flow meters directly measure the red blood cell velocity so that flow

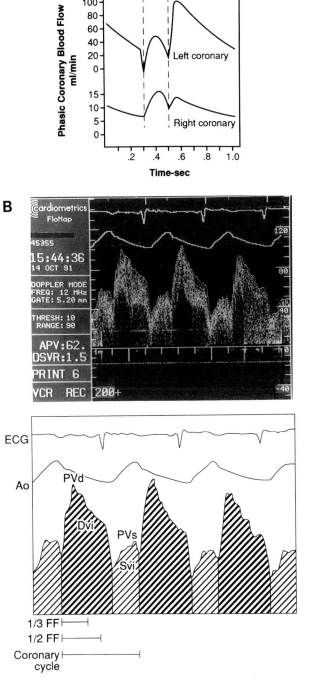

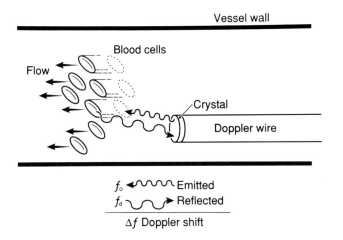

Fig. 6. Diagram of the Doppler principle. The frequency of emitted sound is reflected off the moving red cells producing a lower reflected frequency proportional to the velocity. This change in frequency is the Doppler shift and can be computed from the formula depicted in the text.

Fig. 7. A: Phasic patterns of coronary flow in animal models and corresponding aortic pressure. These waveforms are accurately reproduced by Doppler flow velocity (B) using a Doppler guidewire and spectral velocity analysis. The flow velocity signals have large diastolic components with smaller systolic components. The peak of systole and diastole (PVs, PVd) are easily noted. The flow integral, the area under the peak velocity curve, is noted for systole and diastole (DSi, DVi) as shaded areas. The means of the cycle and of individual portions of the cycle are easily quantitated when the velocity signal has well-defined spectra. Reprinted with permission from the American College of Cardiology (Journal of the American College of Cardiology 1993, Volume 21, pages 308–316.)

markers are not required. Doppler techniques allow a continuous assessment of flow. Since the Doppler catheter or guidewire can be selectively inserted in epicardial vessels, regional measurements are also possible in awake patients. The technical descriptions of the construction, validation, and methods of use have been described in detail previously [7–12].

NORMAL CORONARY FLOW VELOCITY PATTERNS

Normal coronary blood flow velocity, obtained by the intracoronary Doppler signals and analyzed in a spectral format, displays characteristic and classic physiologic features of the predominant diastolic velocity waveform coupled with the smaller systolic waveform (Fig. 7). This normal velocity pattern with diastolic predominance is routinely observed in the left and circumflex coronary arteries and, less commonly, in the normal right coronary artery. The diastolic/systolic flow velocity ratio >1.5 is maintained in both the proximal and distal segments in patients with normal left ventricles [7]. The average proximal left anterior descending and circumflex flow velocity values obtained in patients are approximately 30 cm/sec (mean diastolic velocity). Peak diastolic velocities are in the range of 40–80 cm/sec and peak systolic velocity is in the range of 10–20 cm/sec. Right coronary artery and distal locations may be reduced by 15–20%. The normal flow velocity characteristics are useful to establish baseline values in the proximal and distal segments for comparison in studies examining flow responses in patients with coronary lesions (Fig. 7).

Diseased arteries showed a reduction of distal diastolic flow velocity with relatively preserved systolic flow velocity. The systolic predominant pattern was seen in about 72% of diseased arteries and never in the normal arteries [7–9]. There was significant overlap of proximal normal and abnormal flow velocity parameters, thus limiting predictive accuracy. This alteration is probably due to the relative contributions of the stenotic resistance and the intramyocardial resistance in determining coronary perfusion. Thus, the stenotic resistance is a predominant determinant of coronary flow during diastole, whereas in systole the intramyocardial resistance appears more important. Systolic flow may, therefore, be maintained even in the presence of a significant stenosis.

The distal flow velocity parameters showed a more distinct pattern of abnormality with significantly lower mean velocity, peak diastolic velocity, and peak systolic velocity in the diseased arteries compared with the normal arteries; the blunted hyperemic response of the distal abnormal arteries compared with normal is one of several

features used to define an abnormal response of a hemodynamically significant lesion.

Of importance is the significant increase in the ratio of proximal-to-distal mean velocity in significantly narrowed arteries (2.4 ± 0.7 vs 1.1 ± 0.2 cm/sec in normal arteries, $p < .001$) [10]. This increase in the proximal/distal flow velocity ratio may be equated to a transstenotic gradient [11]. Doppler flow velocity data during angioplasty showed that the proximal-to-distal flow velocity ratio decreases significantly following relief of endoluminal obstruction [9,10].

These principles can be applied in the assessment of physiologic alterations of pressure and flow within the coronary circulation in patients with coronary artery disease [12–15]. A spectrum of applications and limitations of flow velocity, translesional pressure, and lesional morphology will be demonstrated in subsequent Interventional Physiology Rounds.

ACKNOWLEDGMENTS

The authors wish to thank the J.G. Mudd Cardiac Catheterization Team, Trina Stonner, RN, MSN, Marilyn Cauley, Carol Mechem, RN, Lisa Abbot, and Donna Sander for manuscript preparation.

REFERENCES

1. Yoganathan AP, Cape EG, Sung H, Williams FP, Jimoh A: Review of hydrodynamic principles for the cardiologist: applications to the study of blood flow and jets by imaging techniques. J Am Coll Cardiol 12:1344–1353, 1988.
2. Fung YC: ''Biodynamics: Circulation.'' New York: Springer-Verlag, 1984.
3. Nichols WW, O'Rourke MF (eds): ''McDonald's Blood Flow in Arteries: Theoretical, Experimental and Clinical Principles,'' 3rd Edition. Lea & Febiger, 1990, pp 21–22.
4. Poiseuille JM: Recherches experimentales sur le mouvemen des liquides dans les tubes de tres petits diametres. Comptes Rendus Acad Sci 11:961, 1041–1048, 1840.
5. Nichols WW, O'Rourke MF (eds): ''McDonald's Blood Flow in Arteries: Theoretical, Experimental and Clinical Principles,'' 3rd Edition. Lea & Febiger, 1990, p 24.
6. Nichols WW, O'Rourke MF (eds): ''McDonald's Blood Flow in Arteries: Theoretical, Experimental and Clinical Principles,'' 3rd Edition. Philadelphia, PA: Lea & Febiger, 1990, p 25.
7. Ofili EO, Labovitz AJ, Kern MJ: Coronary flow velocity dynamics in normal and diseased arteries. Am J Cardiol 71:3D–9D, 1993.
8. Doucette JW, Corl PD, Payne HM, Flynn AE, Goto M, Nassi M, Segal J: Validation of a Doppler guide wire for intravascular measurement of coronary artery flow velocity. Circulation 85:1899–1911, 1992.
9. Segal J, Kern MJ, Scott NA, King SB III, Doucette JW, Heuser RR, Ofili E, Siegel R: Alterations of phasic coronary artery flow velocity in man during percutaneous coronary angioplasty. J Am Coll Cardiol 20:276–286, 1992.
10. Ofili EO, Kern MJ, Labovitz AJ, St. Vrain JA, Segal J, Aguirre F, Castello R: Analysis of coronary blood flow velocity dynamics

in angiographically normal and stenosed arteries before and after endoluminal enlargement by angioplasty. J Am Coll Cardiol 21: 308–316, 1993.

11. Donohue TJ, Kern MJ, Aguirre FV, Bach RG, Wolford T, Bell CA, Segal J: Assessing the hemodynamic significance of coronary artery stenoses: analysis of translesional pressure-flow velocity relationships in patients. J Am Coll Cardiol 22:449–458, 1993.

12. Kern MJ, Anderson HV: A symposium: the clinical applications of the intracoronary Doppler guidewire flow velocity in patients: understanding blood flow beyond the coronary stenosis. Am J Cardiol 71:1D–86D, 1993.

13. Kern MJ, Flynn MS: Clinical applications of intracoronary coronary Doppler flow velocity in interventional cardiology. In White CJ (ed): ''Advances in Interventional Cardiology: New Technologies and Strategies for Diagnosis and Treatment.'' New York: Marcel Dekker, 1993, pp. 55–61.

14. White CW: Clinical applications of doppler coronary flow reserve measurements. Am J Cardiol 71:10D–16D, 1993.

15. Wilson RF, Laughlin DE, Holida MD, Hartley CJ, Marcus ML, White CW: Transluminal subselective measurement of coronary blood flow velocity and vasodilator reserve in man. Circulation 72:82–92, 1985.

Part II

Coronary Pressure
Gradient Measurements

Chapter 3

Role of Side Holes in Guide Catherters: Observations on Coronary Pressure and Flow

Bernard De Bruyne, MD, Jan Stockbroeckx, RN, Danny Demoor, RN, Gur R. Heyndrickx, MD, PHD, and Morton J. Kern, MD

INTRODUCTION

The cross-sectional area occupied by an angioplasty guide catheter advanced into the first millimeter of a coronary artery is often not negligible, as illustrated in Figure 1. Recently, Serruys et al. [1] pointed out the hemodynamic consequences of the presence of the guide catheter which become important during coronary hyperemia. When coronary angioplasty is to be performed in a vessel with a small or diseased ostium, it has been advocated to use a guide catheter with lateral side holes to provide sufficient blood flow to the distal coronary artery during selective intubation of the ostium with the tip of the guide catheter [2–4]. However, precise assessment of the dimensions of the coronary ostium is often difficult and, therefore, the selection of a guide catheter with side holes is most often prompted by an arterial pressure wave damping (''wedging'') observed at the time of cannulating the ostium with a standard guide catheter. The pressure tracing recorded with these guide catheters usually tracks the phasic pressure tracing recorded through the side arm of the femoral arterial sheath (one French size larger than the guide catheter) and, hence, gives the impression of a normal coronary pressure, considering peripheral pressure amplification and phase delay. The demonstration of guide catheter induced trans-ostial pressure gradients will be illustrated.

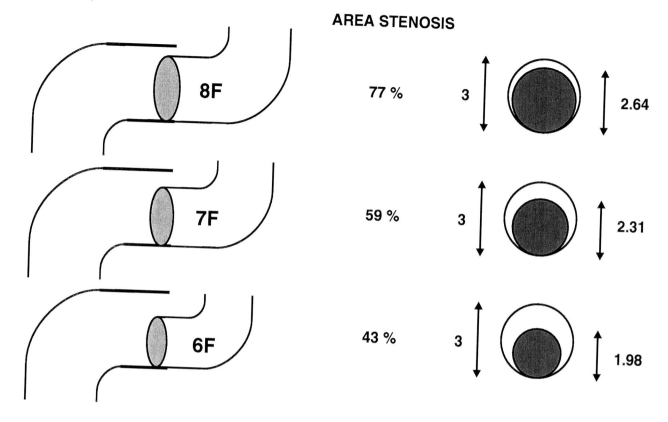

Fig. 1.   A scale drawing of the cross-sectional area occupied by different sized guide catheters in the coronary ostium of a 3 mm diameter vessel.

These findings suggest that in some circumstances, the pressure recorded through guide catheters with side holes does not reflect full coronary flow or true coronary perfusion pressure.

CASE REPORTS
Case 1

A 37-year-old man underwent coronary angioplasty of an 89% area stenosis (quantitative coronary angiography) in a large marginal branch of the circumflex coronary artery because of exertional anginal class II. The left main artery was slightly irregular and the left anterior descending coronary artery exhibited a 60% area stenosis. Global and regional left ventricular function were normal. When using a conventional 8F guide catheter, a "wedged" pressure tracing was obtained. Therefore, a guide catheter with side holes was selected. When cannulating the ostium of the left main stem, the pressure tracing obtained with the guide catheter with side holes was normal and the mean pressure recorded with this guide catheter was identical to the mean femoral artery pressure (Fig. 2). A 0.015 in. fluid-filled pressure mon-

itoring guidewire [5] (Premo Wire™, Advanced Cardiovascular Systems, Inc., Temeluca, CA) was advanced into the proximal circumflex coronary artery. When positioning the distal opening of the pressure monitoring guidewire 1 cm distal to the tip of the guide catheter (but still proximal to the stenosis), a mean gradient of 15 mm Hg was noted. When pulling back the pressure monitoring guidewire into the guide catheter, identical mean pressures were recorded. Hence, in this case, coronary pressure was lower than aortic pressure, although this could not be suspected on the basis of the pressure tracings recorded by the guide catheter with side holes.

Case 2

A 46-year-old patient suffered a non-Q wave myocardial infarction in July 1991. At that time, coronary angiography showed an occluded co-dominant right coronary artery and non-significant wall irregularities in the left anterior descending coronary artery. The patient remained asymptomatic for 18 months. In January 1993, he complained again of typical exertional angina. Repeat coronary angiography showed an 83% area stenosis in the

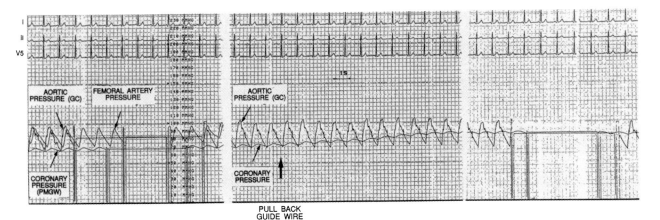

PULL BACK
GUIDE WIRE

Fig. 2. Recording of femoral pressure through the side arm of the sheath, aortic pressure through the guide catheter (GC), and coronary pressure through the pressure monitoring guide wire (PMGW). Left panel: The distal opening of the pressure monitoring guide wire is located in the proximal circumflex coronary artery and the tip of the guide catheter is advanced into the ostium of the left main stem. A pressure gradient of 15 mm Hg is noted between the guide catheter and the guide wire even though the mean pressures recorded by the guide catheter and the femoral sheath are identical. Middle and right panels: When pulling back the pressure monitoring guide wire into the guide catheter so that the distal opening of the wire is positioned in front of the side holes of the catheter, the pressure difference disappears, demonstrating that the pressure drop was located at the level of the tip of the guide catheter.

mid left anterior descending coronary artery. The left anterior descending and the circumflex coronary arteries had an independent ostium. Global and regional left ventricular function were normal at rest. A coronary angioplasty of the left anterior descending artery lesion was planned. At the start of the procedure, a guide catheter without side holes was used, but intubation of the ostium of the left anterior descending artery resulted in "wedging" of the catheter. In contrast, the pressure tracing obtained with a guide catheter with side holes was superimposable to the pressure tracing recorded through the side arm of the femoral introducer sheath. Coronary angioplasty was successfully performed with a monorail balloon catheter system advanced over a micromanometer-tipped pressure monitoring guidewire (Pressure-Guide™, Radi Medical Systems, Uppsala, Sweden). At the end of the procedure, the microtip pressure monitoring wire was pulled back in the proximal part of the left anterior descending artery so that the sensor was located exactly at the tip of the guide catheter. At that level, the pressure recorded both by the guide catheter and by the pressure monitoring guidewire, as well as the femoral artery pressure, were almost identical. However, 30 sec after intracoronary administration of 10 mg of papaverine, a decrease in coronary pressure occurred as recorded by the pressure monitoring guidewire, even though the pressure recorded by the guide catheter and by the side arm of the femoral introducer sheath remained unchanged. Three minutes after injection of papaverine, when hyperemic flow had subsided, no

significant difference persisted between the 3 pressure recordings (Fig. 3). This example shows that the side holes were not flow-limiting at rest, but that after maximal vasodilatation of the resistance vessels by papaverine, a decrease in coronary pressure occurred. This pressure drop in the proximal left anterior descending artery could not be suspected by the guide catheter pressure waveform.

Case 3

A 62-year-old man had a severe 90% diameter stenosis in the mid portion of the left anterior descending coronary artery. Coronary blood flow velocity and translesional pressure were measured before and after successful coronary angioplasty, reducing the stenosis to <20% diameter narrowing. Mean flow velocity in the proximal region near the lesion exceeded 70 cm/sec. Flow velocity 2 cm distal to the stenosis was 18 cm/sec with a reduced diastolic/systolic velocity ratio (Fig. 4A, upper panel). The translesional pressure was measured with a standard 8F guide catheter without side holes and a 2.7F Tracker™ catheter with fluid-filled transducers. The phasic quality of the distal pressure signal was satisfactory. The mean translesional pressure gradient was 80 mm Hg (Fig. 4A, lower panel). Successful dilatation of the artery restored distal flow velocity (39 cm/sec) (Fig. 4B). The final resting gradient was 14 mm Hg. Maximal hyperemic flow velocity was induced with 18 μg of adenosine. At the maximal flow increase (51 cm/sec), a translesional hyperemic gradient of 38 mm Hg could be

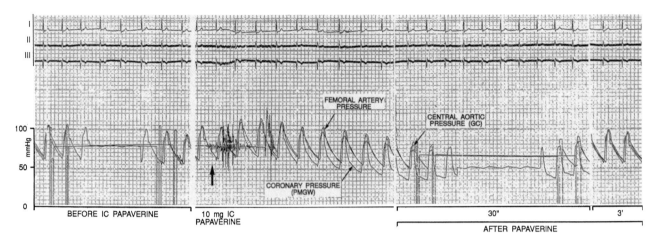

Fig. 3. Recording of femoral artery pressure through the side arm of the arterial introducer sheath, aortic pressure through the guide catheter (GC), and coronary pressure through the pressure monitoring guide wire (PMGW). Before intracoronary papaverine (left panel), the 3 mean pressures are identical. After administration of intracoronary papaverine (middle and right panels), a pressure difference progressively appears between the intracoronary and both the femoral and the aortic pressures. The pressure gradient reaches 16 mm Hg 30 sec after papaverine. By contrast, aortic and femoral pressures remain superimposable.

identified (Fig. 4B). The Tracker™ catheter was pulled back to the proximal normal segment of the left anterior descending artery and revealed an intrinsic gradient of 12 mm Hg. Coronary hyperemia now demonstrated a hyperemia gradient produced by the guide catheter (Fig. 4C). In the right coronary artery, which had a 50% lesion, the Tracker™ catheter was advanced outside the guide catheter without side holes proximal to the stenosis. There was a 10 mm Hg trans-ostial gradient at baseline across a normal section of the proximal right coronary artery (Fig. 4B, bottom). On injection of intracoronary adenosine, a hyperemic trans-ostial pressure gradient of approximately 30 mm Hg was recorded. Flow velocity in the right coronary artery achieved a mean velocity of 48 cm/sec. Advancing the tracking catheter and flowire across the 50% lesion in the proximal right coronary artery, a translesional gradient of 12 mm Hg was recorded which, again, increased to 38 mm Hg during a 2-fold increase in flow velocity (15 to 32 cm/sec) (Fig. 4D). Considering the intrinsic gradient and doubling of distal flow with a normal phasic pattern, this lesion was considered hemodynamically insignificant. The guide catheter in both the left anterior descending and right coronary artery ostia produced resting trans-ostial gradients in normal portions of the coronary artery. These small baseline gradients could be increased 3 to 4-fold during maximal hyperemic flow which doubled or tripled the flow (velocity). The simultaneous measurement of flow velocity and pressure indicates that at increased coronary flow, guide catheters can induce trans-ostial gradients. Interference with resting flow is unlikely in view of the preservation of mean and phasic flow velocity signals. In some cases, however, guide catheter obstruction may have significant impact on flow during the various interventional maneuvers which would be unappreciated by pressure waveforms alone.

In Vivo Flow Measurements

To measure blood flow through the side holes of guide catheters, 2 different sized commercially available guide catheters (7F and 8F) were tested in 10 patients at the end of a coronary angioplasty procedure. The distal opening of the guide catheter was occluded with a silicone plug. The guide catheters had 2 side holes with a diameter of 0.762 mm (7F) and 1.016 mm (8F). The sterile guide catheters were introduced into a 9F femoral sheath and the occluded tip was placed in the iliac artery. Blood flow through these guide catheters was exclusively dependent on the size of the side holes and on aortic pressure. Aortic pressure was continuously recorded via the side arm of the introduction sheath connected to a Spectranetics P23 Statham pressure transducer. The back flow of blood through the guide catheter was measured with a graduated cylinder over a 30-sec period and expressed in mL/min. The results are summarized in Figure 5. Blood flow through the side holes was proportional to mean aortic pressure. Since the side holes in 8F guide catheters were larger than in 7F guide catheters, the flow was larger at equal aortic pressure, and the increase in flow for the increase in aortic pressure (slope of the relationship) was larger in 8F than in 7F guide catheters. At the highest aortic pressures, the blood flow through the side holes did not exceed 80 and 60 mL/min for 8F and 7F guide catheters, respectively.

DISCUSSION

The cases discussed herein demonstrate that the pressure tracings recorded by guide catheters with side holes actually reflect aortic pressure rather than coronary pressure. In case 1, a gradient between the aortic pressure and the pressure in the proximal circumflex coronary artery was present under baseline flow conditions. In case 2, the size of the side holes was sufficient to avoid any pressure drop under baseline conditions, but when an increase in flow was induced by maximal coronary vasodilation, a significant pressure drop appeared between the aorta and the proximal left anterior descending coronary artery. In case 3, small resting trans-ostial gradients were present which could change dramatically with increasing flow. Interestingly, in all cases the decrease in coronary pressure could not be suspected from the pressure tracings recorded by the guide catheter with or without side holes.

The in vivo measurements of blood flow through side holes demonstrates that the flow allowed by the side holes at physiological pressure levels is limited. For the 8F guide catheter, the flow through the side holes reached approximately 80% of the resting blood flow commonly encountered in the left main coronary artery and approximately twice the resting blood flow through a right coronary artery [6,7]. In these in vivo experiments, no distal resistance was present at the proximal end of the guide catheter. Since myocardial resistance was neglected in our catheter model, the measured blood flow through the side holes represents the maximal achievable blood flow. Therefore, the limiting effects of the side holes on blood flow can only be underestimated by the experimental design.

Guide Catheter-Coronary Ostial Area Mismatch

In consideration of pressure gradients across guide catheters, a significant concern regarding unsuspected disease in the ostium of the artery always exists. This possibility commonly occurs, especially appreciated when damping is evident on engagement of a large diameter (8F) guide catheter. Evidence from intracoronary ultrasound has frequently indicated there is significant left main coronary artery disease which exceeds that appreciated angiographically. The presence of pressure damping, however, does not minimize the importance of side holes. Blood flow through this coronary segment may not perform as suggested by the normal pressure wave registered at the proximal end of the catheter.

Technical Limitations of Pressure Gradients

The Pressure Guide™ and the Tracker™ catheter produce excellent phasic signals. The Premo Wire™ (fluid-filled pressure monitoring guidewire) produces damped pressure tracings due to its tiny inner lumen. However, all 3 systems reliably reflect mean pressures. An artifactual pressure drop due to obstruction of the tip of the pressure catheter is highly unlikely when the catheter is aligned in a normal and relatively straight segment of a coronary artery. This occurrence is not evident from any of the tracings obtained. In contrast to the larger and stiffer angioplasty catheters, the pressure guidewires and Tracker™ catheter are not generally affected by tortuosity of a proximal artery segment.

Equivalent guide and coronary pressures or a minimal gradient at rest, which develops or is exaggerated during maximal hyperemia is consistent with the pressure-flow velocity relationships of any fluid tube with a region of limited cross-sectional area. Thus, the guide catheter filling the coronary ostium acts as a stenosis to the flow through the artery. This concept becomes clinically relevant under circumstances when coronary flow increases in association with tachycardia or hypertension. Myocardial ischemia may develop on the basis of impaired flow in which the guide catheter limits coronary perfusion without evidence of flow limitation on the resting pressure waveform. The in vitro flow measurements were of interest in that the side holes had a maximal flow rate for physiologic ranges of aortic pressure. By design, the experimental model was unphysiologic since no resistance to flow was established. Nonetheless, the blood flow data provided offer a range of side hole flow available to the coronary arteries. It is appreciated that normal flow through left coronary arteries may be between 100 and 150 mL/min on average, and that maximal flow through an 8F side hole catheter will not exceed 80 mL/min. The flow through normal right coronary arteries is highly variable, ranging from 50–150 mL/min depending on the artery size and bed perfused. Thus, side hole catheters may or may not provide a satisfactory flow range depending on the clinical circumstances. A comparison of guide catheter pressures to the femoral artery sheath side arm pressure must account for the phase delay and peripheral pressure amplification providing slightly higher and later arterial waveform. However, the femoral artery pressure is often used as an accurate approximation of proximal aortic pressure and, thus, a significant change in the waveform between the femoral artery sheath and the guide catheter can be appreciated as interference with the transmission of flow to the coronary artery. Measured coronary flow velocity in patients with guide catheter damping demonstrated that flow can increase 2 to 3-fold over basal levels and produces trans-ostial pressure gradients appropriate for the pressure-flow relationship across orifices with a fixed resistance.

LAD Lesion Gradient before PTCA

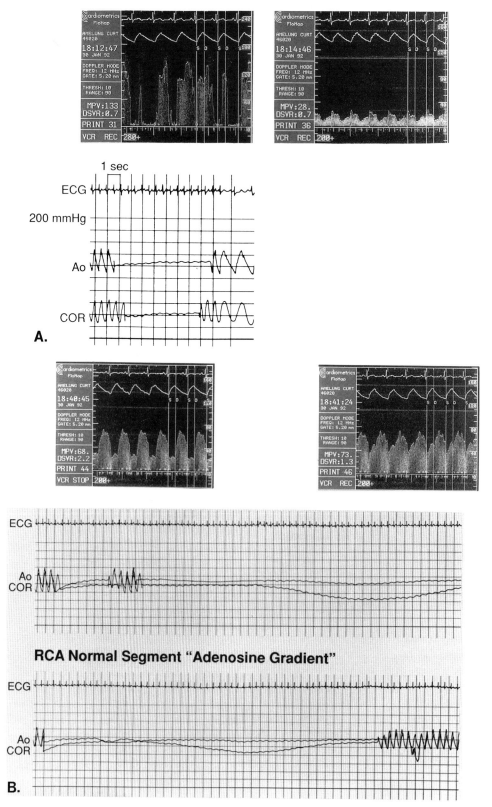

Fig. 4A–B.

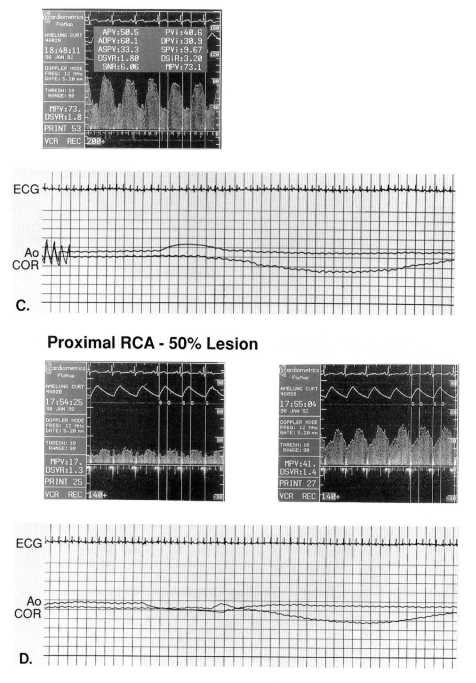

Proximal LAD - No Lesion

Proximal RCA - 50% Lesion

Fig. 4. A: Translesional flow velocity and pressure gradient in a patient with severe proximal left anterior descending (LAD) coronary artery. Top left: Proximal flow velocity is high (120 cm/sec) probably reflecting lesional jet velocity. Top right: Flow velocity 2 cm distal to the stenosis is low (18 cm/sec) and has an abnormal diastolic/systolic velocity ratio (DSVR, 1.3). Velocity scale is 0–200 cm/sec. Electrocardiography and aortic pressure signals are shown at the top of the panels (vertical lines). S, D represent systolic and diastolic periods based on electrocardiogram algorithm. Lower panel: Aortic (guide catheter, Ao) and distal coronary (COR) artery phasic and mean pressures. The mean pressure gradient is 80 mm Hg. B: Hyperemic flow velocity in the left anterior descending (LAD) artery after angioplasty (top left) and in the proximal normal segment of the right coronary artery (top right). Middle: Translesional pressure gradient after angioplasty of the left anterior descending steno-

sis at baseline and during maximal hyperemia. The gradient increases from 14 to 38 mm Hg with flow velocity increasing to 52 cm/sec. Lower panel: Trans-ostial pressure gradient in the right coronary artery (RCA) at baseline and maximal hyperemia (55 cm/sec). Format for velocity and pressure as in (A). C: Hyperemic flow velocity and trans-ostial pressure gradient measured after Tracker™ catheter pullback to the proximal left anterior descending (LAD) artery in a normal segment. The baseline gradient is 12 mm Hg which increased to 40 mm Hg during maximal hyperemia (57 cm/sec). Format as in (A). D: Baseline and hyperemic flow velocity (top panels) and translesional pressure (lower panels). Distal flow velocity increased from 15 to 32 cm/sec with the gradient increasing from 16 to 34 mm Hg. The trans-ostial gradient (B) was also 14 mm Hg, indicating no contribution of the 50% lesion to distal coronary pressure loss. Format as in (A).

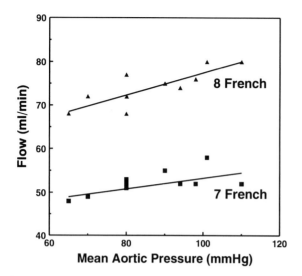

Fig. 5. Plot of the blood flow through the side holes of a 7F (squares) and 8F (triangles) guide catheter at varying mean aortic pressure levels.

Summary

Guide catheters with and without side holes may occasionally give a false impression of normal coronary perfusion pressure. In most instances, the side holes are large enough to maintain a normal flow without significant pressure drop, but during arteriolar vasodilation (e.g., after contrast medium injection, after injection of papaverine or adenosine, and during post-occlusion hyperemia) a significant pressure gradient may occur which is not always reflected by the pressure recorded through the guide catheter. These data should be taken into account when evaluating the functional severity of coronary lesions by means of intracoronary pressure measurements and Doppler velocimetry under different flow conditions. During these measurements, phasic femoral pressure monitoring might prove helpful since it is the only means to detect a pressure gradient related to the presence of the guide catheter in the ostium. Furthermore, the use of smaller sized guide catheters (rather than larger ones with side holes) might limit myocardial ischemia when performing angioplasty in arteries with narrowed ostium.

ACKNOWLEDGMENTS

The authors thank the teams of the catheterization laboratories of the Cardiovascular Center in Aaslt, Belgium, and of the J.G. Mudd Cardiac Catheterization Laboratory. They also acknowledge secretarial assistance of Josefa Cano and Donna Sander.

REFERENCES

1. Serruys PW, Di Mario C, Meneveau N, de Jaegere P, Strikwerda S, de Feyter PJ, Emanuelsson H: Intracoronary pressure and flow velocity with sensor-tip guidewires: A new methodologic approach for assessment of coronary hemodynamics before and after coronary interventions. Am J Cardiol 71(14):41D–43D, 1993.
2. Gruentzig AR, Meier B: Current status of dilatation catheters and guide systems. Am J Cardiol 43:92C–93C, 1984.
3. Harmjans D, Werner PC: Ein verbesserter Führungskatheter fur die PTCA. Z Kardiol 78:78–80, 1989.
4. Chua KG, Feldman T, Fromes B: Relief of pressure damping during coronary angioplasty: A device for creating side holes in PTCA guide catheters. Cathet Cardiovasc Diagn 11:331–333, 1985.
5. De Bruyne B, Pijls NHJ, Paulus WJ, Vantrimpont PJ, Sys SU, Heyndrickx GR: Transstenotic coronary pressure gradient measurement in humans: In vivo and in vitro evaluation of a new pressure monitoring angioplasty guide wire. J Am Coll Cardiol 22:119–126, 1993.
6. Ganz W, Tamura K, Marcus HS, Donoso R, Yoshida S, Swan H: Measurements of coronary sinus blood flow by continuous thermodilution in man. Circulation 44:181–198, 1971.
7. Serruys PW, Wijns W, van den Brand M, Meij S, Slager C, Schuurbiers JCH, Hugenholtz PG, Brower RW: Left ventricular performance, regional blood flow, wall motion, and lactate metabolism during translegional coronary angioplasty. Circulation 70:25–36, 1984.

Part III

Lesion Assessment

Chapter 4

Translesional Pressure-Flow Velocity Assessment in Patients

Morton J. Kern, MD, Frank V. Aguirre, MD, Richard G. Bach, MD,
Eugene A. Caracciolo, MD, and Thomas J. Donohue, MD

INTRODUCTION

The purpose of the first Interventional Rounds is to review current criteria of translesional flow velocity and pressure measurements. The correlation between translesional flow (velocity)-pressure gradient and the clinical demonstration of myocardial ischemia in patients has not been completely studied. The first case examples will also serve to illustrate the current status of lesion assessment.

TRANSLESIONAL PRESSURE-FLOW ASSESSMENT

In the Cardiac Catheterization Laboratory, there are three ways to assess a coronary stenosis: quantitative coronary angiography, translesional pressure, and flow velocity (Fig. 1). Quantitative angiography has been employed to improve the correlations between anatomy and physiology [1–3]. However, owing to well-known limitations of lumenography in predicting physiology, decisions regarding interventions are often supplemented by non-invasive, indirect ischemic stress testing with radionuclide perfusion imaging or pharmacologic hyperemic stress studies. Translesional pressure gradients have been rejected in clinical practice, in part, due to prior experience with large (>4F) catheters, poor signal quality, and a methodology too cumbersome and difficult to incorporate into diagnostic angiography [4,5]. This situation may be remedied by guidewire pressure systems [6,7].

Invasive methods using Doppler catheters to measure coronary vasodilatory reserve were thought to predict the significance of coronary stenoses, but have not been accepted by clinicians as reliable indicators of the physiologic impact of stenoses [3]. Intracoronary Doppler catheter methods in man are limited by catheter size and restriction to measurements made only in regions proximal to the coronary stenosis in question. Coronary flow reserve measured in regions with branches proximal to the lesion are diagnostically unreliable because flow is concurrently assessed for regions of varying vasodilatory reserve, therefore reflecting a weighted average of these potentially disparate zones. Use of a Doppler-tipped angioplasty guidewire 0.014–0.018″ in diameter (Flowire™, Cardiometrics, Inc., Mountain View, CA) (Fig. 1) permits measurement of blood flow velocity, both proximal and, more importantly, distal to a lesion [8,9]. With this information, translesional flow and distal myocardial hyperemic capacity can be easily characterized [10,11]. Directly measured basal and hyperemic blood flow distal to coronary stenoses thus provides an additional means of accurately assessing the physiologic impact of angiographic coronary narrowings [11,12].

With improvement in techniques to acquire translesional pressure and flow data, the hemodynamic criteria of lesion significance will require re-examination. What constitutes a clinically significant translesional pressure gradient and flow response in patients with coronary artery disease or infarction? Translesional pressure gradients of >30 mm Hg have been associated with myocardial ischemia on stress testing [2], and gradients of <20 mm Hg have been considered satisfactory end points after coronary angioplasty [12]. Whether all translesional pressure gradients of ≤20 mm Hg require angioplasty is under investigation.

Similarly, a significant lesion is characterized by impaired distal basal or hyperemic flow as established in normal canine models and awake patients measured with Doppler catheters. Most studies measured flow in relatively proximal regions with exclusion of any myocardial or systemic abnormality which might impair coronary flow reserve. Impaired coronary vasodilatory reserve (hyperemic/basal flow) can be due to microvascular and other myocardial abnormalities in the absence of epicardial luminal obstruction [13–15]. What constitutes a significant impairment of distal hyperemia is controversial. Should lesions that are not flow-limiting at rest or during hyperemia undergo mechanical intervention, regardless of a marginal pressure gradient? Before demonstrating these issues by case examples, several fundamentals of flow and velocity should be discussed. The limitations of translesional pressure gradients have been discussed elsewhere [16,17].

PRINCIPLES OF FLOW VELOCITY, VOLUMETRIC FLOW, AND BRANCHING ARTERIES FOR LESION ASSESSMENT

The use of translesional flow velocity for assessment of lesion significance is predicated on two major principles. First, volumetric coronary blood flow is the product of the velocity of the red cells moving through a conduit of a known cross-sectional area (Fig. 2) [18,19]. Thus, flow velocity accurately reflects blood flow volume when the cross-sectional area of a vessel remains constant. The volumetric translation of velocity is derived from the velocity (cm/sec) and cross-sectional area (cm^2) product yielding flow values in cm^3/sec. The second major concept involves the branching conduits of the human coronary circulation. The epicardial artery cross-sectional area diminishes in size as daughter branching arises across the myocardium (Fig. 2). Because of branching, both volumetric flow and cross-sectional vessel area diminish from the proximal to distal epicardial regions. Since both volume and cross-sectional area decrease proportionately, flow velocity is thus maintained from the proximal to the distal locations. A ratio of proximal to distal velocity approaching 1 is present in normal arteries [9,18]. Significant lesions produce resistance diverting blood flow to branches proximal to the lesion, reducing flow and, thus, velocity in the distal region.

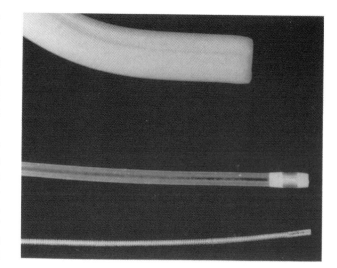

Fig. 1.   Catheterization laboratory methods to assess coronary flow. Top: An 8F angiographic (Doppler) catheter. Middle: A 2.2F pressure gradient catheter (Target Therapeutics). Bottom: Doppler Flowire 0.014″ diameter (Cardiometrics, Inc, Mountain View, CA).

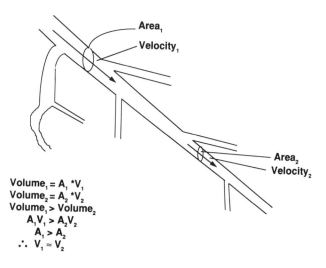

$Volume_1 = A_1 * V_1$
$Volume_2 = A_2 * V_2$
$Volume_1 > Volume_2$
$A_1 V_1 > A_2 V_2$
$A_1 > A_2$
$\therefore V_1 \approx V_2$

Fig. 2.   Volumetric flow is equal to [velocity * cross-sectional vessel area] at any point in the artery. Since the arteries are branched systems, flow volume is reduced as it is distributed by branches. The cross-sectional area is likewise reduced over the course of the vessel, resulting in proximal to distal velocity ratios approaching 1.

Initial studies in our laboratory [9,10,19,20] have demonstrated that flow velocity is maintained from the proximal to distal region in normal arteries and that loss of distal relative to proximal velocity (proximal/distal velocity integral ratios >1.7) is related to translesional pressure gradients >30 mm Hg in branching arteries [20] (Fig. 3).

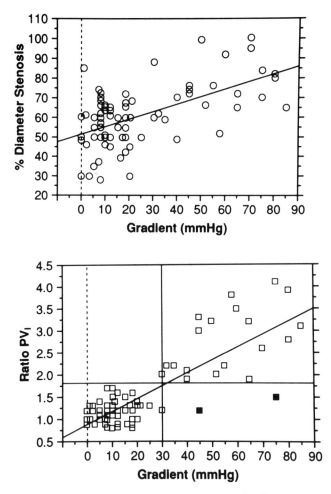

Fig. 3. Top: Correlation between angiography (% diameter stenosis) and translesional pressure gradients (mm Hg). Bottom: Correlation between the ratio of proximal to distal total velocity integral (ratio PVᵢ) and translesional pressure gradients (mm Hg). The two black boxes represent the proximal right coronary artery stenoses occurring prior to any branch points (see text for Discussion). Reprinted with permission from Wilson RF, Wyche K, Christensen BV, Zimmer S, Laxson DD: Effects of adenosine on human coronary arterial circulation. Circulation 82:1595–1606, 1990.

ASSESSMENT OF THREE CORONARY STENOSES

The translesional hemodynamic assessment of a single left anterior descending stenosis of equal angiographic severity in three patients will illustrate lesion specific flow and pressure findings. These data emphasize the physiology that cannot be differentiated by angiography alone.

Patient 1

Coronary angiography revealed a 60% diameter narrowing in the proximal left anterior descending coronary

artery in a 43 year old man after an acute anterior myocardial infarction (Fig. 4A) [23]. Low level exercise thallium-201 testing was also performed. Before angioplasty, translesional hemodynamic assessment of the stenosis was performed.

Basal and hyperemic flow velocity data were obtained 3–4 artery diameters or ≈1 cm proximal to the stenosis. The stenosis is traversed with the Doppler guidewire so that distal (at least 10 artery diameters, ≈2 cm) basal and hyperemic flow responses can be recorded. Maximal intracoronary hyperemia is produced by 12–18 μg of adenosine administered through the guiding catheter [24]. As previously described [9,25], the 0.018″ floppy angioplasty-style Doppler flowire is 175 cm long with a 12 mHz piezoelectric ultrasonic crystal at the tip. The Doppler signal is processed by fast Fourier transformation and displayed in gray scale spectral format. Automatic analysis provides phasic and mean, diastolic and systolic velocities, and flow velocity integrals (time-area of peak instantaneous flow velocity). These data are easily acquired without operator-dependent instrument adjustments. A 2.2F catheter (Tracker™, Target Therapeutics) connected through fluid-filled tubing and standard transducer is used to measure translesional pressure gradients.

Coronary lesion assessment.

Proximal flow velocity was normal in magnitude, phasic pattern, and coronary hyperemic capacity (Fig. 4B). Distal flow velocity was abnormal. The proximal average peak velocity was 32 cm/sec, distal was 17 cm/sec with a proximal/distal ratio of 32/17 = 1.9. In addition, the distal phasic diastolic/systolic velocity ratio was abnormally low (1.3; normal left coronary diastolic/systolic velocity ratio >1.5) [22]. Distal coronary reserve was also impaired [distal (hyperemic/basal flow = 1.42]. The basal translesional pressure gradient was 40 mm Hg, which increased to 48 mm Hg during maximal hyperemia. Coronary angioplasty was successfully performed. Distal flow velocity after angioplasty and the translesional pressure before and after angioplasty are illustrated on Figure 4C. The stenosis was improved to <30% diameter narrowing with restoration of the normal distal phasic flow velocity patterns (diastolic/systolic ratio = 1.6), improvement of basal flow (mean velocity = 33 cm/sec) and distal hyperemia (distal flow reserve = 1.96) (Fig. 4C, bottom panels). The final pressure gradient was 8 mm Hg at rest, which increased to 20 mm Hg during maximal hyperemia.

Patient 2

Coronary angiography in a 59 year old man with typical and atypical chest pain showed an eccentric severe

LAO

RAO

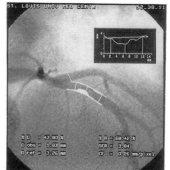

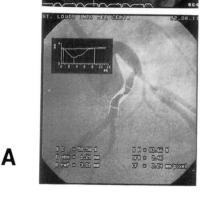

A

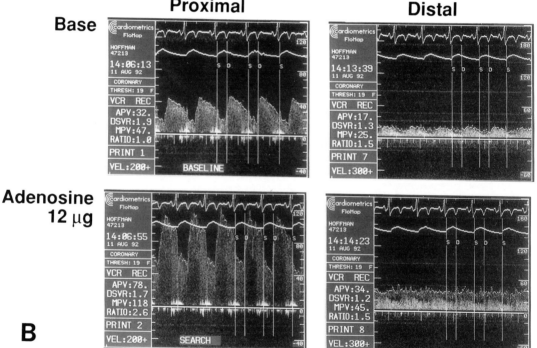

B

Proximal   Distal

Base

Adenosine 12 μg

Fig. 4. A: Frames from a coronary cineangiogram in the left anterior oblique projection (LAO) and right anterior oblique projection (RAO) of the left anterior descending artery demonstrating a 60% diameter narrowing (84% area) of the proximal segment by QCA in the ''worst'' projection. B: Coronary blood flow velocity proximal and distal to the left anterior descending stenosis at baseline and during maximal hyperemia with 12 μg of intracoronary adenosine (flow velocity scale = 0–200 cm/sec). Proximal flow is normal (mean velocity 32 cm/sec) with normal phasic pattern (DSVR 1.9). Proximal but not distal hyperemia is normal. The ratio of proximal to distal flow velocity is 1.9. Distal hyperemia was impaired with a flow reserve ratio of approximately 1.42. C: Top: Translesional gradient before and after angioplasty at baseline and during maximal hyperemia. Hemodynamic tracings show electrocardiogram, aortic pressure, and distal coronary pressure, both phasic and mean (from the top down, 0–200 mm Hg scale). Mean resting gradient is 40 mm Hg which widens to approximately 50 mm Hg at maximal hyperemia. Following angioplasty, mean baseline gradient is 8 mm Hg, which widens to approximately 20 mm Hg during maximal hyperemia. With permission from ref. 12. Bottom: The distal flow velocity after angioplasty demonstrated an increase of the distal velocity equivalent to proximal velocity with restoration of the phasic flow signal and hyperemia of 2.1 times basal flow. Reprinted with permission from Kern MJ, Flynn MS, Caracciolo EA, Bach RG, Donohue TJ, Aguirre FV: Use of translesional coronary flow velocity for interventional decisions in a patient with multiple intermediately severe coronary stenoses. Cathet Cardiovasc Diagn 29:148–153, 1993.

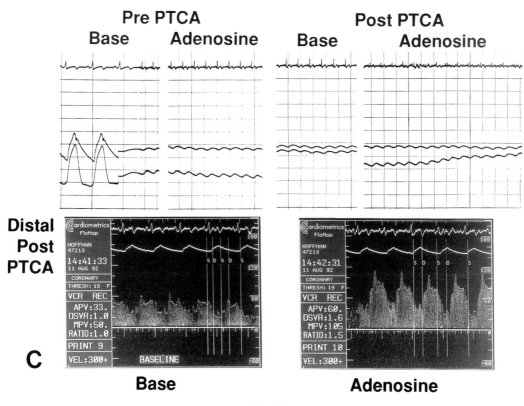

Fig. 4C.

lesion in the left anterior descending coronary artery [22]. The stress testing was non-diagnostic. In the left anterior oblique (LAO) view, the lesion is severe (>70%). In the right anterior oblique (RAO) view, the lesion is only moderate (<50%) (Fig. 5A). Translesional hemodynamics were measured before anticipated angioplasty (Fig. 5B). Translesional flow velocity spectra and pressure gradients were obtained at rest and during maximal hyperemia with adenosine. Proximal and distal flow velocity were similar (26 cm/sec) with a proximal/distal average velocity ratio of 1.05. The resting gradient is 0 mm Hg. Adenosine-induced hyperemia increases distal flow 2.7 × baseline and increases the pressure gradient to 10 mm Hg. Exercise thallium scintigraphy showed a minimal anterior-apical defect. No angioplasty was performed. The patient's symptoms abated and he was well at 14 month follow-up.

Patient 3

A 43 year old man who had a chest pain syndrome and an abnormal scintigraphic study with reversible defects in the anterior and anteroapical regions was scheduled for angioplasty. Coronary arteriography in the left anterior oblique projection revealed a 58% diameter stenosis of the left anterior descending coronary artery (Fig. 6A). Translesional flow velocity and pressure gradients dem-

onstrated that the proximal mean flow velocity was 30 cm/sec. The distal mean velocity was 25 cm/sec with a proximal to distal velocity ratio of 1.2 (Fig. 6B). The translesional pressure gradient was approximately 20 mm Hg. Distal hyperemic coronary flow velocity (after 18 μg of intracoronary adenosine) increased to 87 cm/sec with coronary reserve of 2.9. During hyperemia, the resting gradient of 20 mm Hg increased to 46 mm Hg (Fig. 6B, bottom right). Coronary angioplasty was successfully performed (Fig. 6A, bottom). The residual stenosis was 33% diameter by quantitative angiography. Distal flow velocity was recorded at 5 and 15 min after the procedure to assess immediate and delayed physiologic results (Fig. 6C). Five minutes after angioplasty, distal basal mean velocity was 27 cm/sec, unchanged from before the procedure. Distal hyperemia was 53 cm/ sec for a coronary vasodilatory reserve of 2.1. After 15 min, baseline flow velocity had fallen slightly to a mean value of 18 cm/sec and hyperemia remained unchanged at 52 cm/sec for a coronary reserve value of 2.7, nearly identical with that observed before angioplasty. The pressure gradient following the procedure was 3 mm Hg which increases to 25 mm Hg during maximal hyperemia. Several weeks later, exercise thallium scintigraphy was again abnormal. Clinically, the patient has done well.

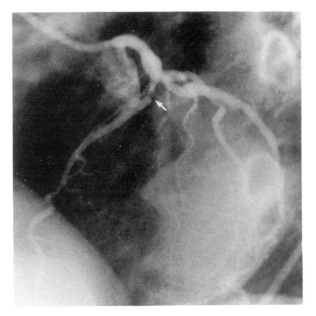 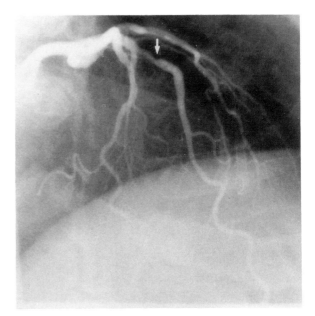

A   **LAO**   **RAO**

Baseline   ## Adenosine

Proximal Velocity   ### Distal Velocity   ### Distal Velocity

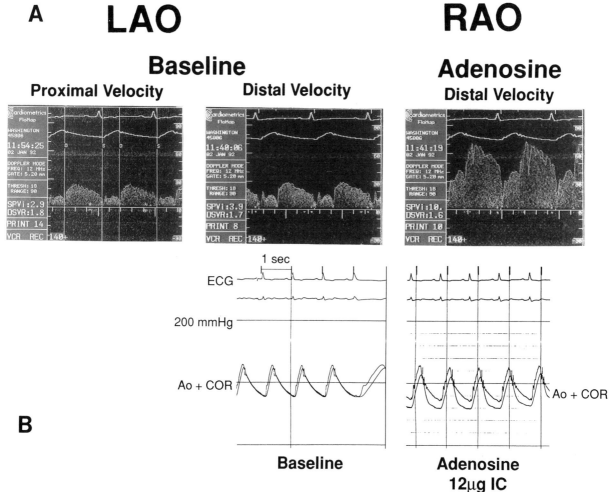

B

Baseline   Adenosine
12μg IC

Fig. 5. **A:** Angiographic views of eccentric lesion in the left anterior descending coronary artery in a 59 year old man with atypical chest pain. In the left anterior oblique (LAO) view, the lesion is severe (>70%). In the right anterior oblique (RAO) view, the lesion is moderate (<50%). **B:** Flow velocity spectra (top) and translesional gradients (lower) at rest and during maximal hyperemia with adenosine (12 μg intracoronary). Proximal and distal flow velocity are nearly identical with a ratio of 1.05. The mean resting gradient is zero. With adenosine, distal flow increases 2.5 × baseline and the mean hyperemic gradient is 10 mm Hg. A thallium scintigraphy exercise study showed a minimal apical defect and no angioplasty was performed. The patients symptoms abated spontaneously and he has been well at 8 month follow-up. Reprinted with permission from Donohue TJ, Kern MJ, Aguirre FV, Bach RG, Caracciolo EA, Ofili E, Labovitz AJ: Assessment of angiographically intermediate coronary artery stenosis using the Doppler flowire. Am J Cardiol 71:26D–33D, 1993.

DISCUSSION

These three case studies (summarized on Table I) highlight the important question of what limits for each major physiologic indicator should be accepted in determining clinical coronary lesion significance. The indications for angioplasty and the success after coronary interventions are also critical issues dependent on these criteria. Translesional pressure and flow velocity are two interdependent components describing lesion resistance (Fig. 7). Since simultaneous pressure-velocity systems are confined to technically demanding research studies, serial measurements of pressure and flow velocity must be made. It should be noted that the pressure-velocity relationship most accurately describes the severity of any given lesion (Fig. 7B), but the lower limits for pressure and flow requiring intervention remain to be defined. Across coronary lesions with pressure gradients >30 mm Hg in branching arteries, translesional flow velocity demonstrates three findings: 1) loss of distal flow velocity relative to proximal flow with an increased proximal to distal flow velocity ratio [20,21], 2) loss of the normal phasic diastolic predominant flow velocity pattern [23], and 3) impaired distal (but not necessarily proximal) hyperemic responses to vasodilators [20,23] (Table II).

Distal Flow Velocity

Distal flow velocity, a relatively new measure, was compared to the translesional pressure gradient. In 84 patients, a proximal to distal total flow velocity integral ratio of >1.7 is associated with translesional gradients of >30 mm Hg in branching artery systems (Fig. 3) [20]. A translesional velocity ratio value of ≥1.7 correctly identified 98% of stenoses with translesional gradients >30 mm Hg. In non-branched vessels, the proximal/distal velocity-pressure relationship cannot be used (see below). The proximal to distal ratio cannot be used in single unbranched conduits, ostial lesions, diffuse distal disease, or tandem or serial lesions where distal flow velocity may be accelerated. In acquiring a satisfactory proximal flow velocity signal, artifacts related to flow acceleration in the zone of lesional flow convergence should be identified. The lesional convergence zone accelerates flow on entering the stenosis. Proximal velocity in this location would be elevated relative to other regions in the proximal vessel, generating an abnormally high proximal to distal velocity ratio.

Distribution of Flow Velocity in Branching Arteries

The physiologic rationale for using a proximal to distal flow velocity ratio is based on classical hydrodynamic theory (described in Part II) and confirmed with directly measured translesional gradient data [20]. In unbranched

conduits, conservation of mass (flow) allows one to use the continuity equation stating that the velocity-cross-sectional area product at any point in the conduit will be the same [18] (Fig. 8). The continuity equation cannot be employed in branching arteries. Proximal arterial flow input can be diverted to the areas of lower vascular resistance owing to a moderate stenosis producing resistance to flow. Diversion of flow through branches proximal to the lesion diminishes distal flow (and velocity). In an artery with a significant stenosis, coronary hyperemia (and thus coronary flow reserve) can be normal when measured in the proximal artery segment owing to vasodilation of small and angiographically inconsequential branches (as shown in patient 1). Distal flow velocity is universally impaired beyond hemodynamically significant lesions.

Translesional Pressure Gradients

Translesional pressure gradients are not routinely used for several reasons. The technique is cumbersome and subject to signal artifact from catheter kinking and vessel tortuosity. The earlier studies used larger diameter 4F first generation angioplasty catheters to measure gradients. Pressure gradients, at times, conflicted with angiography and, thus, were considered unreliable. More important is the fact that a translesional pressure gradient reflects only half of the information needed to judge a lesion as significant. As shown in case examples during hyperemia, pressure gradients are directly related to the flow (Fig. 9). As flow increases, the gradient increases in a curvilinear relationship reflecting lesion resistance, as was described by Poiseuille over 100 years ago. A gradient of 25 mm Hg may be unimportant if distal flow can increase >3 × basal values. The ability to assess both relative pressure and flow with the distal flow velocity is a distinct advantage of flow velocity over the pressure gradient technique. Although pressure-flow criteria are clearly defined at the extremes of the spectrum as shown in cases 1 and 2, the criteria for decision making in case 3 are less straightforward.

Clinical Issues

Use of an isolated measurement in the absence of an appropriate clinical evaluation is contrary to good medical practice. Non-invasive stress testing or perfusion imaging is an important ancillary aid to decision making. However, the specificity of positive testing remains around 80% and specificity may be particularly limited after angioplasty [24–26]. As shown in case 3, a positive scan may persist even after the translesional gradient was relieved. A normal distal flow with a marginal (20–25 mm Hg) pressure gradient before angioplasty which is unchanged despite a reduced gradient (3 mm Hg) after angioplasty raises the question whether such a resting

43 yr old Male, LAD, Pre PTCA

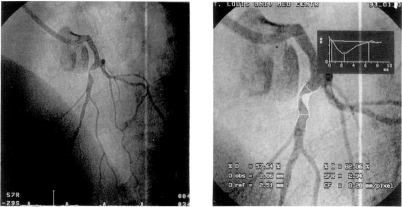

43 yr old Male, LAD, Post PTCA

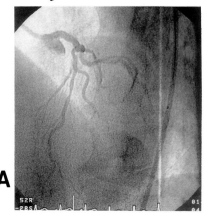
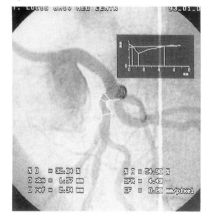

Fig. 6. A: Angiographic frames of a left anterior descending lesion (58% diameter narrowed) with an abnormal stress test. Before (top) and after (bottom) angioplasty. B: Translesional flow velocity and pressure gradient before angioplasty. Proximal and distal flow are nearly equivalent with a proximal/distal ratio of 1.2. Distal hyperemia is 2.9 × basal flow. The mean resting gradient of 20 mm Hg increases to 46 mm Hg during hyperemia. C: After angioplasty, distal flow is similar both at rest and during hyperemia. The resting gradient of 2 mm Hg increases to 20 mm Hg with 2.7 × basal flow increase. The thallium scan remained positive. Did angioplasty improve blood flow? See text. (MV = mean velocity, P = proximal, D = distal, CVR = coronary vasodilator reserve.)

gradient represents a flow-limiting lesion. Without improvement in distal flow or hyperemia, it is difficult to say that reduction of the translesional gradient was contributory to clinical improvement. Of interest, a hyperemic gradient of 45 mm Hg occurring with a 3-fold increase in distal flow was reduced to 25 mm Hg after angioplasty (Fig. 9). The physiologic significance of the large hyperemic gradient is unknown in this particular patient. Both the resting and hyperemia translesional pressure gradients are directly dependent on flow. The mechanical change in lesion geometry resulted in a parallel downward shift to the pressure-velocity curve without a change in the slope (resistance). Since augmenta-

tion of distal flow is the objective of anti-ischemic interventions, normalized flow velocity may be the most relevant indicator of lesion improvement.

Limitations of Coronary Flow Velocity Signal Acquisition

Occasionally it may be difficult to find the maximal distal flow velocity signals and falsely conclude that a significant flow reduction is present because of a significant lesion. Therefore, the Doppler guidewire tip in the distal region should be rotated in several different orientations in all patients to identify the maximal and most

43 yr old Male, Pre PTCA LAD

Proximal	Distal Base	Distal Hyperemia

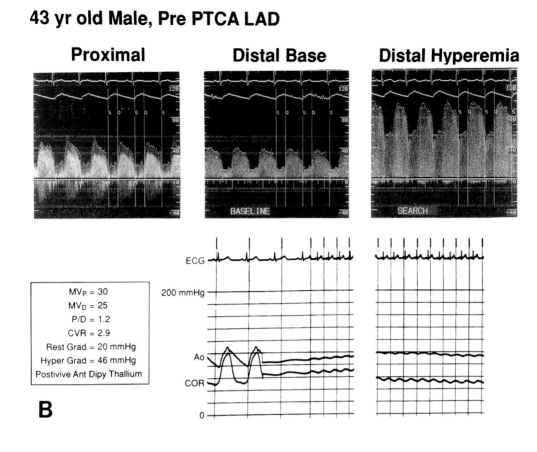

MV_P = 30
MV_D = 25
P/D = 1.2
CVR = 2.9
Rest Grad = 20 mmHg
Hyper Grad = 46 mmHg
Postivive Ant Dipy Thallium

B

43 yr old Male, Post PTCA LAD

Distal Base (5 min)	Hyperemia

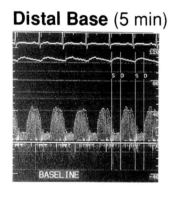

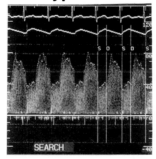

	MV		CVR
	5'	15'	
Base	27	18	2.1
Adenosine	53	52	2.7

Distal Base (15 min)	Distal Hyperemia

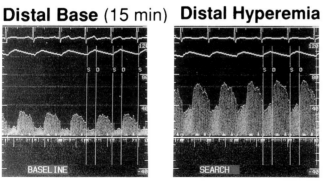

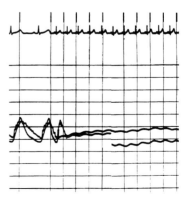

C

Fig. 6B, C.

TABLE I. Angiographic and Translesional Hemodynamic Data*

Patient	% DS	% area stenosis	MCSA	APV		P/D	CVR	Translesional pressure gradient		Procedure	Outcome
				Proximal	Distal			Baseline	Hyperemic		
1	44 (LAO)	68	1.83	32	17	1.9	1.1	40	48	PTCA	Flow and gradient improved
	59 (RAO)	83	1.21								
2	80	50	—	28	26	1.05	2.9	0	10	No PTCA	Clinically improved
3	58	82	1.06	30	25	1.2	2.9	20	45	PTCA	Flow unchanged, gradient improved

*APV = average peak velocity (cm/sec); CVR = coronary vasodilatory reserve (cm/sec); DS = diameter stenosis; MCSA = minimal cross-sectional area by QCA (mm^2); P/D = proximal/distal APV ratio.

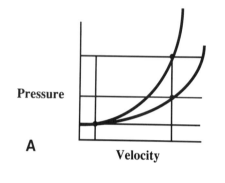

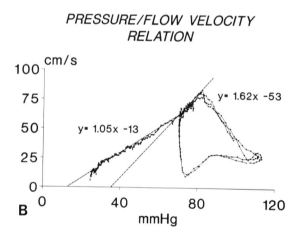

Fig. 7. A: Pressure-flow velocity relations of two coronary stenoses of similar angiographic severity but different resistances to blood flow. Both lesions have the same resting flow velocity and pressure. At high flow, the lesion characterized by the top curve has twice the pressure gradient as the lesion in the bottom curve. Which change is associated with ischemia? See text for Discussion. **B:** Flow velocity/pressure loops during maximal hyperemia in three consecutive sinus beats. During mid-late diastole, a linear relation is observed, with an extrapolated zero-flow pressure of 37 mm Hg. However, during a long diastolic pause (cardiac arrest induced by the intracoronary injection of 3 mg of adenosine), the pressure/flow velocity/pressure relation deviates considerably from the extrapolated curve. Reprinted with permission from Serruys PW, Di Mario C, Meneveau N, de Jaegere P, Strikwerda S, de Feyter PJ, Emanuelsson H: Intracoronary pressure and flow velocity with sensor-tip guide wires: A new methodologic approach for assessment of coronary hemodynamics before and after coronary interventions. Am J Cardiol 71:41D–53D, 1993.

intense spectral flow velocity signals that have a complete Doppler envelope. In tortuous segments, stable distal signals can usually be obtained. However, more guidewire manipulation is often needed to achieve satisfactory signals. In some patients, guidewire manipulation may not be suitable owing to tortuosity or lesion complexity. In these instances, the Doppler flowire can be exchanged for a finer, smaller, and softer guidewire. After the guidewire traverses the lesion, a tracking catheter is placed distally. The flowire can then be exchanged for the softer guidewire. Both pressure and flow velocity across the lesion can now be measured. An elevated distal flow velocity and falsely normalized proximal to distal flow velocity ratio, suggesting an insignificant lesion, might be seen if the distal measurements are made in a region with distal disease where there is flow acceleration secondary to distal luminal narrowing. In patients with serial lesions or diffuse distal disease, the proximal to distal flow ratio should not be used. In these cases, confirmation of lesion significance with coronary vasodilatory reserve and translesional pressure gradients may be needed.

Guide catheter obstruction to inflow at the ostium of the coronary artery may interfere with interpretation of both pressure and distal velocity signals. For this reason, intermediate lesions can be assessed at the time of diagnostic catheterization with 6F diagnostic or guiding catheters with outside diameters of <0.05" or with the guiding catheter disengaged from the ostium.

Finally, the translesional resting hemodynamics may not reflect ischemia producing conditions that could occur during coronary vasoconstriction and exacerbation of lesions as a result of increased myocardial demand during exercise or emotional stimulation [27]. Translesional pressure gradients will be increased to various degrees corresponding to lesion resistance as described by the pressure-velocity relationship. Whether clinical benefit would be conferred by dilating a lesion with a marginal resting pressure gradient and normal distal flow compared to medical therapy remains under investigation [28].

TABLE II. Translesional Flow Velocity Criteria for Hemodynamically Significant Lesions

1. Proximal to distal flow velocity integral ratio >1.7 = translesional pressure gradient >30 mm Hg (applies only in branching arteries: see below)[a]
2. Distal coronary vasodilatory reserve >2.0
3. Distal diastolic/systolic mean velocity ratio:

Location	Normal
Left anterior descending	>1.7
Circumflex	>1.5
Right coronary artery	>1.2 (proximal)
Right coronary artery	>1.4 (posterior descending, posterolateral branch)

[a]Proximal/distal ratio not applicable in 1) diffuse distal disease, 2) serial or tandem lesions, or 3) ostial lesions (no proximal location).

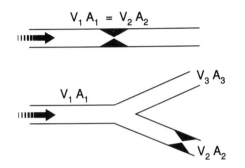

Fig. 8. Diagram of single (top) and branching tube (bottom) models. In the single tube, the continuity equation can be applied for proximal and distal flow. However, a resistance in the branching tube produces the diversion of flow to alter proximal and distal lesional flow values proportionally.

Clinically Significant Translesional Hemodynamics

Translesional gradients <20 mm Hg have been associated with reduced late restenosis rates and a lower incidence of post-angioplasty abrupt closure [12]. There is little data in patients to identify a translesional flow-pressure gradient that provides a reliable predictor of provokable myocardial ischemia. Although it is desirable to have a zero translesional gradient within the coronary tree, some lesions in patients may have pressure gradients without demonstrable evidence of exercise- or pharmacologic-induced myocardial ischemia. The translesional hemodynamic criteria correlating with inducible ischemia further depend on several additional factors, such as the size of the perfusion bed, coronary artery, aortic and left ventricular pressures, myocardial oxygen demand, and coronary vasomotor tone. Although the pressure-flow characteristics of a lesion should correlate with clinical findings and post-procedural outcomes, translesional pressure-velocity relationships have been difficult to obtain clinically. With miniaturization of sen-

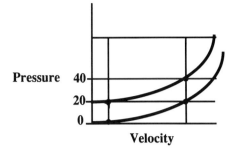

Fig. 9. Parallel shift of the pressure-velocity curves occurring in patient 3. Angioplasty reduced the angiographic left anterior descending stenosis from 75% to 20% diameter narrowing and the pressure gradients at baseline and hyperemia from 20 to 4 mm Hg and 45 to 20 mm Hg, respectively. However, baseline and hyperemic flow were unaffected. The abnormal perfusion imaging study was minimally changed after angioplasty. See text for details.

sor-tipped guidewires, this information will now be available to assess lesions before and after interventions. Since restoration of blood flow is the end point of an intervention, it remains questionable that dilating lesions with normal translesional blood flow will be helpful.

SUMMARY

Interventional physiology presents the operator with objective data to facilitate decision making. A thorough and validated understanding of the alterations of pressure and flow in the human coronary circulation is currently in progress. As illustrated in the case studies, some situations have data which may initially appear contradictory or unhelpful to clinical practice. These data should provide a framework to understand the dynamic physiology producing the clinical syndromes in patients undergoing coronary interventional procedures. Future Interventional Physiology Rounds will examine coronary pressure-flow responses during directional atherectomy, stents, and acute myocardial infarction.

ACKNOWLEDGMENTS

The author wishes to thank the J.G. Mudd Cardiac Catheterization Laboratory team, Trina Stonner, RN, MSN, Marilyn Cauley, Carol Mechem, RN, Lisa Abbott, and Donna Sander for manuscript preparation.

REFERENCES

1. Serruys PW, Zijlstra F, Juilliere Y, de Feyter PJ, van den Brand M: How to assess the immediate results of PTCA. Should we use pressure gradient, flow reserve or minimal luminal cross-sectional area? In Reiber JC, Serruys PW (eds): "New Develop-

ments in Quantitative Coronary Arteriography.'' Dordrecht: Kluwer Academic Publishers, 1988, pp 181–206.

2. Wijns W, Serruys PW, Reiber JHC, van den Brand M, Simoons ML, Kooijman CJ, Balakumaran K, Hugenholtz PG: Quantitative angiography of the left anterior descending coronary artery: correlations with pressure gradient and results of exercise thallium scintigraphy. Circulation 71:273–279, 1985.

3. White CW, Wright CB, Doty DB, Hiratza LF, Eastham CL, Harrison DG, Marcus ML: Does visual interpretation of the coronary arteriogram predict the physiologic importance of a coronary stenosis? N Engl J Med 310:819–824, 1984.

4. Peterson RJ, King SB III, Fajman WA, Douglas JS Jr, Grüntzig AR, Orias DW, Jones RH: Relation of coronary artery stenosis and pressure gradient to exercise-induced ischemia before and after coronary angioplasty. J Am Coll Cardiol 10:253–260, 1987.

5. MacIsaac HC, Knudtson ML, Robinson VJ, Manyari DE: Is the residual translesional pressure gradient useful to predict regional myocardial perfusion after percutaneous transluminal coronary angioplasty? Am Heart J 117:783–790, 1989.

6. DeBruyne B, Pijls NHJ, Paulus WJ, Vantrimpont PJ, Sys SU, Heyndrickx GR: Transstenotic coronary pressure gradient measurement in humans: in vitro and in vivo evaluation of a new pressure monitoring angioplasty guide wire. J Am Coll Cardiol 22:119–126, 1993.

7. Emanuelsson H, Dohnal M, Lamm C, Tenerz L: Initial experiences with a miniaturized pressure transducer during coronary angioplasty. Cathet Cardiovasc Diagn 24:137–143, 1991.

8. Doucette JW, Corl PD, Payne HM, et al.: Validation of a Doppler guidewire for intravascular measurement of coronary artery flow velocity. Circulation 85:1899–1911, 1992.

9. Ofili EO, Kern MJ, Labovitz AJ, St. Vrain JA, Segal J, Aguirre F, Castello R: Analysis of coronary blood flow velocity dynamics in angiographically normal and stenosed arteries before and after endoluminal enlargement by angioplasty. J Am Coll Cardiol 21: 308–316, 1993.

10. Kern MJ, Anderson HV (eds): A symposium: the clinical applications of the intracoronary Doppler guidewire flow velocity in patients: understanding blood flow beyond the coronary stenosis. Am J Cardiol 71:1D–86D, 1993.

11. Wilson RF, Laxson DD: Caveat emptor: a clinician's guide to assessing the physiologic significance of arterial stenoses. Cathet Cardiovasc Diagn 29:93–98, 1993.

12. Hodgson JM, Reinert S, Most AS, Williams DO: Prediction of long-term clinical outcome with final translesional pressure gradient during coronary angioplasty. Circulation 74:563–566, 1986.

13. White CW: Clinical applications of Doppler coronary flow reserve measurements. Am J Cardiol 71(14):10D–16D, 1993.

14. McGinn AL, White CW, Wilson RF: Interstudy variability in coronary flow reserve: the importance of heat rate, arterial pressure, and ventricular preload. Circulation 81:1319–1330, 1990.

15. Marcus ML, Mueller TM, Gascho JA, Kerber KE: Effects of cardiac hypertrophy secondary to hypertension on the coronary circulation. Am J Cardiol 44:747–753, 1979.

16. Anderson HV, Roubin GS, Leimgruber PP, et al.: Measurement of transstenotic pressure gradient during percutaneous transluminal coronary angioplasty. Circulation 73:1223–1230, 1986.

17. Serruys PW, Wijns W, Reiber JHC, de Feyter PJ, van den Brand M, Piscione F, Hugenholtz PG: Values and limitations of transstenotic pressure gradients measured during percutaneous coronary angioplasty. Herz 10:337–342, 1985.

18. Ofili EO, Labovitz AJ, Kern MJ: Coronary flow velocity dynamics in normal and diseased arteries. Am J Cardiol 71:3D–9D, 1993.

19. Kern MJ, Donohue TJ, Aguirre FV, Bach RG, Caracciolo EA, Ofili E, Labovitz AJ: Assessment of angiographically intermediate coronary artery stenosis using the Doppler flowire. Am J Cardiol 71:26D–33D, 1993.

20. Donohue TJ, Kern MJ, Aguirre FV, Bach RG, Wolford T, Bell CA, Segal J: Assessing the hemodynamic significance of coronary artery stenoses: analysis of translesional pressure-flow velocity relationships in patients. J Am Coll Cardiol 22:449–458, 1993.

21. Kern MJ, Flynn MS, Caracciolo EA, Bach RG, Donohue TJ, Aguirre FV: Use of translesional coronary flow velocity for interventional decisions in a patient with multiple intermediately severe coronary stenoses. Cathet Cardiovasc Diagn 29:148–153, 1993.

22. Wilson RF, Wyche K, Christensen BV, Zimmer S, Laxson DD: Effects of adenosine on human coronary arterial circulation. Circulation 82:1595–1606, 1990.

23. Segal J, Kern MJ, Scott NA, King SB III, Doucette JW, Heuser RR, Ofili E, Siegel R: Alterations of phasic coronary artery flow velocity in humans during percutaneous coronary angioplasty. J Am Coll Cardiol 20:276–286, 1992.

24. American College of Physicians: Efficacy of exercise thallium-201 scintigraphy in the diagnosis and prognosis of coronary artery disease. Ann Intern Med 113:703–704, 1990.

25. Ritchie JL, Trobaugh GB, Hamilton GW, Gould KL, Narahara KA, Murray JA, Williams DL: Myocardial imaging with thallium-201 at rest and during exercise: comparison with coronary arteriography and resting and stress electrocardiography. Circulation 56:66, 1977.

26. Bodenheimer MM, Banka VS, Helfant RH: Nuclear cardiology II. The role of myocardial perfusion imaging using thallium-201 in diagnosis of coronary artery disease. Am J Cardiol 45:674–684, 1980.

27. Ganz P, Abben RP, Barry WH: Dynamic variations in resistance of coronary arterial narrowings in angina pectoris at rest. Am J Cardiol 59:66–70, 1987.

28. Mechem CJ, Kern MJ, Aguirre F, Cauley M, Stonner T: Safety and outcome of angioplasty guidewire Doppler instrumentation in patients with normal or mildly diseased coronary arteries (Abstr). Circulation 86(4):I-323, 1992.

29. Serruys PW, Di Mario C, Meneveau N, de Jaegere P, Strikwerda S, de Feyter PJ, Emanuelsson H: Intracoronary pressure and flow velocity with sensor-tip guidewires: a new methodologic approach for assessment of coronary hemodynamics before and after coronary interventions. Am J Cardiol 71:41D–53D, 1993.

Chapter 5

Coronary Stenoses With Low Translesional Gradient and Abnormal Coronary Reserve:
Physiologic Results After Angioplasty

Morton J. Kern, MD, Richard G. Bach, MD, Thomas J. Donohue, MD,
Eugene A. Caracciolo, MD, and Frank V. Aguirre, MD

INTRODUCTION

The hemodynamic criteria for lesion significance generally involve narrowing of the arterial cross-sectional area such that translesional pressure gradients occur in ranges 15–20 mmHg [1,2]. In this setting, distal coronary flow, in response to exercise or pharmacologic stress, cannot increase in an adequate fashion to prevent ischemia. The significance of any single lesion is determined by the curvilinear pressure-flow velocity relationship describing the resistance to flow at any given pressure [3]. The physiologic nature of lesions cannot be determined from angiographic data alone, and thus the indirect measures of the ischemic potential by myocardial perfusion scintigraphy are commonly employed for more objective evidence to support intervention. Translesional flow and pressure data further improve the assessment of such lesions. However, the precise criteria of which lesions will benefit from epicardial luminal enlargement remains under study.

Coronary vasodilatory reserve can be easily assessed but has important limitations for clinical lesion significance. Distal flow hyperemia can be impaired from one of two mechanisms, epicardial flow restriction or distal microcirculatory dysfunction. Some epicardial lesions with low transstenotic pressure gradients have abnormal coronary vasodilatory reserve, which may be a function of abnormal distal microvasculature rather than significant flow impairment by epicardial stenosis. However, it is difficult to determine if such an epicardial stenosis may reduce flow due to resistance in series with the distal perfusion bed. Angioplasty in such a patient may provide benefit from mechanical enlargement of the epicardial lumen area despite only a minimal improvement in pressure-flow velocity measurements.

To illustrate the coronary physiology in such a patient, we examine the results of angioplasty of an angiographically moderate lesion with a low initial translesional pressure gradient and impaired distal hyperemic flow velocity. Functional pressure-flow velocity improvement of such lesions highlights the difficulties in establishing absolute criteria for translesional physiology in certain patient subsets.

CASE REPORT

A 41-year-old man with a history of chest pain at rest radiating to the left arm was admitted to the hospital 2 days prior to catheterization. Mild dyspnea was associated with the pain, which lasted 1½ hours, and was relieved with intravenous nitroglycerin and heparin in the Coronary Care Unit. Electrocardiography at the time of admission demonstrated inferior ST elevation, which re-

41 yr old Male, RCA, UA

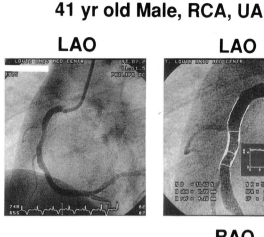

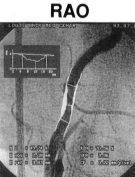

Fig. 1. Coronary angiography demonstrating proximal right coronary stenosis of 66% diameter in the left anterior oblique (LAO) view by quantitative angiography. RAO = right anterior oblique view.

solved with relief of the chest pain. Two-dimensional echocardiography revealed normal left ventricular and valvular function. The patient was transferred to the University Hospital for further evaluation and potential coronary revascularization with a diagnosis of unstable angina.

On physical examination, this young man had a blood pressure of 124/65 mmHg, pulse 62/min, with no jugular venous distension. The lungs were clear. Cardiac and peripheral arterial examination was unremarkable. Electrocardiogram demonstrated normal sinus rhythm with marked T-wave inversions in the inferior leads and peak T waves in leads V_2 and V_3. Coronary arteriography revealed normal left ventricular function with an ejection fraction of 74% without mitral regurgitation. The left coronary artery angiogram demonstrated only minimal 30 and 40% serial lesions involving the first large diagonal branch. The right coronary artery had a moderate (66% diameter) stenosis by quantitative angiography (Fig. 1).

With the symptoms and abnormal electrocardiograms as the presenting syndrome and the fact that this lesion was considered to be of intermediate severity by quantitative angiography, translesional pressure and flow velocity assessment were performed prior to angioplasty. Using a 0.018″ Doppler-tip guidewire (FloWire™, Cardiometrics, Mountain View, CA) and 2.2F tracking catheter, flow velocity and pressure were measured. Flow velocity at least 1 cm proximal to the lesion and again 3 cm distal to the lesion are shown on Figure 2. During intracoronary hyperemia (12 μg adenosine), proximal average flow velocity increased from 19 cm/sec to 38 cm/sec with a coronary vasodilatory reserve of 2.0. The phasic pattern of proximal flow was normal for the location with a diastolic/systolic velocity ratio of ~1.0. After crossing the coronary artery lesion, the distal flow velocity phasic pattern remained normal with a diastolic/systolic velocity ratio of 1.2. The average basal flow velocity was 21 cm/sec. Coronary hyperemia, again, increased distal flow to 38 cm/sec for a coronary reserve ratio of 1.8. Because of the difficulty in using a proximal to distal flow velocity ratio in proximal right coronary artery lesions where there may be minimal branching [4], a translesional pressure gradient was obtained (Fig. 3). The resting pressure gradient of 18 mmHg increased to 30 mmHg during peak coronary hyperemia. In view of the unstable symptoms, despite a low resting gradient, angioplasty was performed using a 4.0 mm balloon with 6 inflations to a maximal 9 ATM inflation pressure.

The postangioplasty angiographic result was satisfactory with a reduction in the percent diameter stenosis from 66 to 34% diameter narrowing (Fig. 4) with a zero resting translesional pressure gradient (Fig. 3, lower right panels) and maximal hyperemic gradient of 12 mmHg. Coronary flow velocity (Fig. 3, top panels) increased from 18 cm/sec at rest to 48 cm/sec during intracoronary adenosine, demonstrating an improvement in the distal coronary flow reserve (2.7 × basal flow).

The patient did well following coronary angioplasty. However, chest pain similar to his presenting symptoms recurred, which was not associated with new electrocardiographic changes. The pain was unrelieved despite a widely patent coronary artery after angioplasty with no translesional gradient or evidence of side branch or distal vessel occlusion. The continued chest pain was poorly responsive to intravenous nitroglycerin and narcotic analgesia. The patient was discharged on antacids with a minimally abnormal electrocardiogram.

DISCUSSION

This patient illustrates one of the more perplexing examples of translesional physiology undergoing intervention. It is clear that the active nature of the lesion, reflected by symptoms and electrocardiographic changes, may not always be identified by significantly abnormal

4l yr old Male, RCA, UA

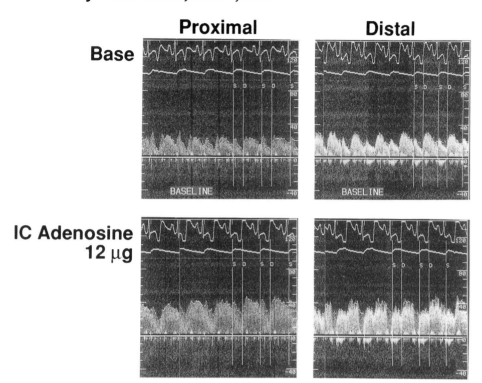

Fig. 2. Proximal and distal flow velocity data for the right coronary artery at baseline and during maximal hyperemia with intracoronary adenosine (12 μg). Flow velocity pattern proximal has a diastolic/systolic velocity ratio that is ~1.0. Intracoronary (IC) hyperemia with adenosine increases from 19 cm/sec to 38 cm/sec for a proximal reserve ratio of 2.0. Similar data are obtained distal to the lesion. Proximal to distal flow velocity ratio in the right coronary artery may be difficult to correlate with translesional gradients. Systolic (S) and diastolic (D) phasic periods are denoted by vertical lines.

pressure and flow relationships across a stenosis, especially when assessed at a later time in the setting of intravenous nitroglycerin, heparin, and other oral antianginal, antiplatelet, or antihypertensive medications. Coronary vasospasm or transient platelet aggregation with thrombus superimposed on the stenosis could have been responsible for the clinical problem. However, it is difficult to defer intervention when using the current angiographic and clinical criteria alone. Preliminary data in our laboratory suggest that in patients with significant angiographic stenoses with normal translesional hemodynamics, angioplasty can be safely deferred [5]. Only 6 of 65 patients with intermediately severe flow normal lesions had target lesion progression over 8±5 mo requiring later angioplasty or coronary artery bypass graft surgery. However, in the setting of an active and potentially vasospastic lesion, it is unknown when the current aggressive approach could be deferred.

The physiologic response to angioplasty of this lesion was also unusual in that the reduction of the low (18 mmHg) resting pressure gradient was associated with a striking improvement in coronary vasodilatory reserve. The improvement in coronary reserve after angioplasty was surprising, but not totally unexpected in that at least 50% of patients who undergo angioplasty can have an immediate improvement in coronary vasodilatory reserve assessed by Doppler flow velocity [6,7]. The more difficult issue to explain is how elimination of the minimal translesional gradient provides marked hyperemic flow improvement in this patient. It has been noted in other lesions that more severe resting pressure gradients may offer only minimal resistance to flow [3]. The contribution of postangioplasty endothelial mediators and vasomotor tone may play a role in control of postlesional flow. The precise mechanisms by which flow dynamics are altered by mechanical disruption of the proximal epicardial stenosis remains under study.

It is also interesting that the symptoms were unimproved despite a more than adequate angiographic and lesional hemodynamic result. The presence of continued symptoms with the elimination of epicardial flow reduction supports the notion that more precise and objective

4l yr old Male, RCA, UA

Post Distal Base

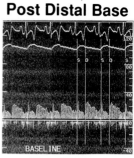

Pre-PTCA

Distal Adenosine

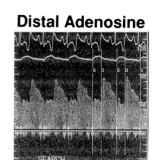

Post-PTCA

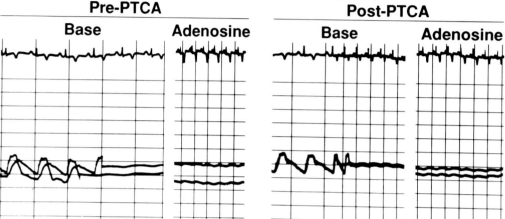

Fig. 3. Top: Postangioplasty distal flow at baseline (left) and during hyperemia with intracoronary adenosine (right). Mean velocity at rest is 18 cm/sec and 48 cm/sec during maximal hyperemia. Coronary reserve is 2.7. Flow velocity scale is 0–200 cm/sec. Bottom: Translesional pressure gradient at baseline and during peak adenosine responses before angioplasty (left) and again after angioplasty (right). The improvement in translesional gradient at rest from 18 mmHg to 0 mmHg is associated with flow velocity data shown on the top two panels. (Pressure scale is 0–200mmHg.)

measurements of bona fide ischemia may be required to assess the need for and results of various invasive coronary interventions.

Summary

Clinically active but angiographically moderate coronary stenoses present a difficult problem for intervention, especially when such lesions have a low translesional pressure gradient and impaired coronary reserve. Physiologic data suggest some lesions can be safely deferred, whereas others may benefit from immediate intervention.

ACKNOWLEDGMENTS

The authors thank the J.G. Mudd Cardiac Catheterization Laboratory Team and Donna Sander for manuscript preparation.

Fig. 4. Coronary angiography after angioplasty demonstrating proximal right coronary stenosis of 34% in the left anterior oblique (LAO) view by quantitative angiography. RAO = right anterior oblique view.

41 yr old Male, RCA, UA

LAO

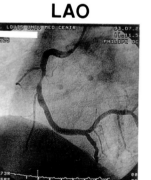

LAO

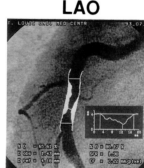

RAO

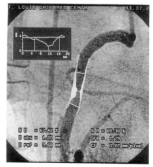

REFERENCES

1. Hodgson JM, Reinert S, Most AS, Williams DO: Prediction of long-term clinical outcome with final translesional pressure gradient during coronary angioplasty. Circulation 74:563–566, 1986.
2. Anderson HV, Roubin GS, Leimgruber PP, Cox WR, Douglas JS Jr, King SB III, Gruentzig AR: Measurement of transstenotic pressure gradient during percutaneous transluminal coronary angioplasty. Circulation 73:1223–1230, 1986.
3. Gould KL, Lipscomb K, Hamilton GW. Physiologic basis for assessing critical coronary stenosis: Instantaneous flow response and regional distribution during coronary hyperemia as measures of coronary flow reserve. Am J Cardiol 33:87–94, 1974.
4. Donohue TJ, Kern MJ, Aguirre FV, Bach RG, Wolford T, Bell CA, Segal J: Assessing the hemodynamic significance of coronary artery stenoses: analysis of translesional pressure-flow velocity relationships in patients. J Am Coll Cardiol 22:449–458, 1993.
5. Wilson RF, Johnson MR, Marcus ML, Aylward PEG, Skorton DJ, Collins S, White CW: The effect of coronary angioplasty on coronary flow reserve. Circulation 77:873–885, 1988.
6. Kern M, Donohue T, Bach R, Aguirre F, Caracciolo E, Mechem C, Cauley M, Flynn M, Chaitman B: Clinical outcome of deferred angioplasty in patients based on normal translesional pressure-flow velocity measurements (abstr). Circulation 88(4):I-204, 1993.
7. Kern MJ, Deligonul U, Vandormael M, Labovitz A, Gudipati R, Gabliani G, Bodet J. Shah Y, Kennedy HL: Impaired coronary vasodilatory reserve in the immediate post-coronary angioplasty period: analysis of coronary arterial velocity flow indices and regional cardiac venous efflux. J Am Coll Cardiol 860–872, 1989.

Chapter 6

Limitations of Translesional Pressure and Flow Velocity for Long Ostial Left Anterior Descending Stenoses

Morton J. Kern, MD, Thomas J. Donahue, MD, Michael S. Flynn, MD,
Frank V. Aguirre, MD, Richard G. Bach, MD, Eugene A. Caracciolo, MD

INTRODUCTION

The physiologic assessment of long (>10 mm) narrowings within coronary arteries is more difficult than shorter lesions due to the contribution of stenosis length to viscous friction and flow acceleration [1–3]. As noted by Poiseuille [2], the translesional pressure loss varies directly with the length of the stenosis [2]. The longer the stenosis for any given cross-sectional area, the greater the resistance to flow and thus the greater the pressure loss as demonstrated by a lower distal coronary pressure, provided the collateral supply to that zone is minimal [4]. The use of translesional coronary flow velocity for assessment of most coronary lesions involves three findings: (1) reduced distal flow velocity relative to that obtained proximal to the lesion in branching arteries [5], (2) an abnormal (systolic predominant) phasic flow signal distal to the lesion [6], and (3) impaired coronary vasodilatory reserve with a <2-fold augmentation of distal flow [5,7]. Correlations of the proximal to distal flow velocity ratio with translesional pressure gradients are dependent on the presence of proximal branching non-diseased arteries as previously discussed [4,8]. In a branching model with a lesion in one branch, flow is diverted to branches of lower resistance. Thus in a vessel with a gradient-producing lesion, flow velocity distal to the stenosis will be lower than flow proximal. In a non-tapered, cylindrical conduit without branches, flow will be equal at any point and since flow is calculated as the cross-sectional area-velocity product, the velocity proximal and distal to a stenosis should be equal provided the cross-sectional area is unchanged.

Ostial lesions present a particularly difficult situation

dient alone? Is it reasonable to rely on phasic flow patterns and distal (poststenotic) hyperemia to determine physiologic significance?

In this case example, we examine translesional pressure and flow velocity in an artery with a long, ostial left anterior descending coronary narrowing undergoing lesion assessment prior to angioplasty. The limitations of translesional flow velocity in this setting should be critically considered as to their utility. The issues regarding resistance to flow through a long, moderately narrowed ostial lesion, normal and abnormal distal flow velocity patterns, coronary hyperemia, and adequate flowire positioning are illustrated to facilitate decision making.

CASE REPORT

A 39-year-old man with renal failure maintained on chronic hemodialysis was referred for cardiac catheterization following an abnormal dipyridamole sestamibi perfusion imaging study obtained as part of his evaluation for renal transplantation. The patient had diabetes mellitus and long-standing hypertension. The dipyridamole sestamibi perfusion imaging study demonstrated a reversible anterior perfusion defect. Although the patient was asymptomatic, coronary arteriography was recommended. Medications at the time of evaluation included insulin, Minoxidil, Lasix, and Captopril. Physical examination demonstrated a blood pressure of 160/74 mmHg, for the evaluation of coronary pressure loss based on flow velocity. In the assessment of such a lesion, where should proximal velocity be measured? Should this measurement be abandoned for a translesional pressure gra-

39 yr old Male
Positive Anterior Thallium, DM, CRF
LAO   AP

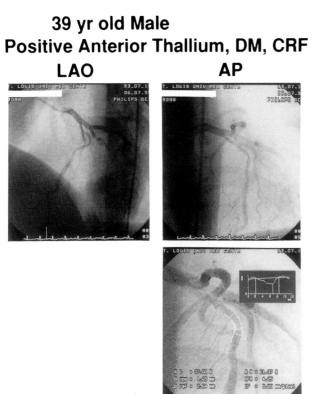

Fig. 1. Frames from coronary angiogram of a patient with a long left anterior descending stenosis (arrows) in the left anterior oblique (LAO) and AP cranial projections. By quantitative angiography, percent diameter stenosis was 38% with percent area stenosis of 61%.

pulse 96/min, and no jugular venous distension. There was a dialysis catheter in the right subclavian vein. The lungs were clear to auscultation and the heart sounds were normal. The peripheral arterial pulses were strong and equal throughout. The electrocardiogram showed left ventricular hypertrophy with early repolarization.

Cardiac catheterization revealed normal left ventricular function with an ejection fraction >70% without mitral regurgitation. Coronary arteriography revealed a diffuse 50% diameter narrowing, which was 8 mm long in the midright coronary artery. A proximal diffuse, long (>11 mm) narrowing (38% diameter) of the left anterior descending coronary artery extending from the ostium to beyond the large first diagonal branch was noted (Fig. 1). In view of the anterior perfusion defect, the left anterior descending lesion was thought to be physiologically significant. However, because of the angiographic appearance, the potentially flow-limiting nature of this lesion was evaluated prior to angioplasty.

Before angioplasty, translesional coronary flow velocity and pressure gradient data were obtained (Fig. 2). The methodology of measuring pressure and flow veloc-

ity has been previously described [5–7]. After heparin administration (10,000 units IV bolus and 1,000 units/hr infusion), a 0.018″ flowire (FloWire™, Cardiometrics, Mountain View, CA) was advanced into the left main where the average peak flow velocity was 95 cm/sec with a normal phasic diastolic pattern (Fig. 2, top left panel). The phasic pattern in this location had a diastolic/systolic velocity ratio of >2.0. The wire was then placed in the midcircumflex artery where the average peak flow velocity was 61 cm/sec with a normal diastolic/systolic velocity ratio of 1.6 (Fig. 2, top middle panel). Hyperemia obtained with intracoronary adenosine (18 μg) in the circumflex zone increased the circumflex flow velocity to 72 cm/sec (Fig. 2, top right panel). Coronary vasodilatory reserve in the circumflex region was impaired (coronary vasodilatory reserve = 1.2), perhaps secondary to the patient's long-standing hypertension. The flowire was withdrawn from the circumflex artery and on crossing from the left main to the left anterior descending artery, the flow velocity decreased to 46 cm/sec with an abnormal diastolic/systolic velocity ratio of 1.1 measured in the mid segment of the left anterior descending artery (Fig. 2, bottom middle panel). During coronary hyperemia produced by 18 μg intracoronary adenosine, distal left anterior descending flow velocity was unchanged (48 cm/sec), yielding a marked impairment of coronary vasodilatory reserve (~1.0). To gauge the variation in distal flow velocity, the wire was moved from 2 cm distal to the lesion to 4cm from the lesion. The phasic flow pattern remained impaired and relatively unchanged at 1.2 (Fig. 3). The average peak velocity decreased from 49 cm/sec to 37 cm/sec, a 24% decline. If the left main artery was assumed to be satisfactory for the proximal velocity relative to the ostial left anterior descending lesion, and the distal velocity values of 49 and 37 cm/sec are used, the proximal to distal velocity ratios would then be 1.9 (95/49) and 2.6 (95/37), consistent with previous empiric data indicating that the translesional pressure gradient generally is >30 mmHg when the proximal/distal ratio is >1.7 [4].

The left main/circumflex velocity ratio of 1.6 (95/61) would not be expected to have a pressure gradient. However, it is disturbing that the flow velocity in the circumflex segment was not closer to that of the left main since in normal arteries flow velocity usually declines by ≤15% from proximal to distal epicardial regions [7,9]. It should be noted that the very high left main velocity is unusual and could have been artifactually elevated if the Doppler wire was in the convergence zone of the ostial lesion and actually reading part of the left anterior descending jet flow velocity.

Because of the difficulty in assuring that the proximal to distal flow velocity ratio could be used in this case, a translesional pressure gradient was obtained with a 2.2F

39 yr old Male

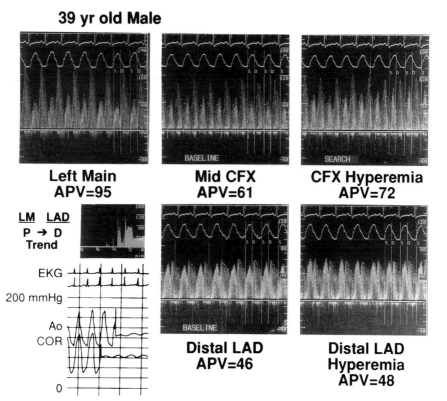

Fig. 2. Top 3 panels: Coronary flow velocity data in the left main and circumflex artery, and the circumflex artery during hyperemia, respectively. The scale factor for the left main flow (far left panel) is 0–400 cm/sec and for circumflex data (upper middle and right panels) 0–300 cm/sec. The lower panels from left to right show the trend velocity going from left main (LM)—proximal (P) to left anterior descending (LAD)—distal (D) locations. The trend plot scale is 0–200 cm/sec. Below the trend plot, the aortic (Ao) and distal coronary (COR) phasic and mean pressures demonstrate a 50 mmHg translesional gradient. Middle lower panel: Distal left anterior descending average peak velocity (APV) at rest and during normal hyperemia after intracoronary adenosine (far right lower panel). Note the impaired phasic pattern relative to the circumflex and left main stenoses. LAD velocity scale is 0–200 cm/sec.

tracking catheter (Tracker™, Target Therapeutics). The translesional pressure gradient was 50 mmHg (Fig. 2, bottom left panel).

Angioplasty was performed successfully with a reduction in the stenosis from 58% to 26% using a 2.5 mm balloon inflated to a maximum of 8 atmospheres for a total of 4 inflations. The postprocedure flow data was not obtained due to a technical problem with a wire connection. The posthospital course was unremarkable and the patient proceeded to renal transplantation.

DISCUSSION

The interventional physiology in this case illustrates several interesting features for long ostial lesions. Previous studies suggest that the use of the proximal to distal flow velocity ratio may be inaccurate or impractical for the ostial lesion due to an unreliable proximal velocity [5]. It should be noted that the left main velocity is generally an easily acquired reproducible signal, but the validation of the ratio using transostial flow to pressure gradients has not been performed. In this patient, the operators were justifiably reluctant to recommend this application without validation. To confirm the findings of the velocity signals, translesional pressure gradient measurements demonstrated significant lesion resistance with the knowledge that the tracking catheter itself may contribute to this gradient. Errors made with the 2.2F catheter would artifactually increase the pressure gradient favoring intervention. However, it was interesting to note that the left main/distal left anterior descending flow velocity ratio of >1.9 did indeed correlate with a pressure gradient of 50 mmHg. Further studies will be needed before ostial lesions and proximal/distal flow ratios can be used in place of pressure gradients. The proximal/distal velocity ratio notwithstanding, the lesion was further demonstrated to be significant by the impaired phasic (diastolic/systolic velocity ratio) nature of the distal flow signal and the inability to increase flow during hyperemia.

39 yr old Male

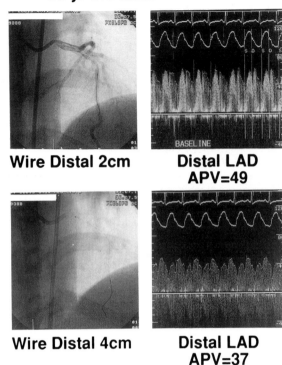

Wire Distal 2cm　　**Distal LAD APV=49**

Wire Distal 4cm　　**Distal LAD APV=37**

Fig. 3. Flowire positions (left panels) 2 cm and 4 cm distal to the lesion and flow velocity data obtained at the corresponding position. Velocity can normally decrease 15% from proximal to distal portions of a normal epicardial vessel. Flow velocity 2 cm and 4 cm beyond the lesion was 49 and 37 cm/sec, respectively. These data may impact on the proximal to distal flow velocity in some patients.

The use of coronary vasodilatory reserve has inherent limitations in patients with hypertension, infarction, or other systemic conditions (e.g., diabetes) affecting microcirculatory function, which can impair coronary vasodilatory reserve despite normal epicardial arteries [9,10]. Compared with the normal adjacent circumflex region, coronary flow reserve in the left anterior descending zone was also abnormally low. Regional reserve calculations would still be abnormal (0.8), but the data are less convincing with no "true normal" flow zone. Whether coronary artery disease alone in one region is associated with abnormal coronary flow reserve in multiple remote regions is unknown. In patients with angiographically normal arteries, regional coronary flow reserve is thought to be nearly equal [11,12].

Both the alterations in the phasic pattern and impaired reserve were compared to the same variables obtained in the circumflex zone. Relative coronary flow reserve thus may have limitations in the interpretation of epicardial lesion significance. The measurement of adjacent presumed normal regional coronary vasodilatory reserve re-

sponses to compute a relative flow reserve (coronary vasodilatory reserve, abnormal zone/coronary vasodilatory reserve, normal zone) has been suggested to be indicative of lesion severity, independent of myocardial and systemic factors [13]. This ratio has been proposed as an important predictor of lesion severity and of critical importance in ascertaining the significance of impaired flow responses distal to lesions under consideration.

Factors influencing abnormal coronary reserve in this individual would include small vessel disease of diabetes, severe hypertension, and a hyperdynamic state due to renal failure, all of which would impair coronary flow reserve [14]. The length of the lesions also contributes to both pressure loss and velocity abnormalities, which complicate the interpretation of flow in the assessment of such lesions.

Use of left main flow velocity to compare to either distal circumflex or left anterior descending flow velocity is under investigation to assess whether these values can be used to confirm translesional pressure loss across ostial narrowings. The confirmation of flow velocity data with a translesional pressure gradient is currently recommended for ostial lesions, as demonstrated here, since our understanding of the proximal/distal velocity ratio is not, as yet, adequately examined in this particular lesion subset.

Summary

Translesional pressure and flow velocity can be used to assess angiographically intermediate or indeterminate lesions. Ostial narrowings and long lesions represent situations that may require both pressure and flow velocity assessment. In patients with hypertension, diabetes mellitus, and chronic renal failure, distally measured absolute and regional coronary reserve values alone may not be helpful in selecting lesions requiring intervention.

ACKNOWLEDGMENTS

The authors thank the J.G. Mudd Cardiac Catheterization Laboratory Team and Donna Sander for manuscript preparation.

REFERENCES

1. Yoganathan AP, Cape EG, Sung H, Williams FP, Jimoh A: Review of hydrodynamic principles for the cardiologist: Applications to the study of blood flow and jets by imaging techniques. J Am Coll Cardiol 12:1344–1353, 1988.
2. Poiseuille JM: Recherches experimentales sur le mouvemen des liquides dans les tubes de tres petits diametres. Comptes Rendus Acad Sci 11:961;1041–1048, 1840.
3. Milnor WR: Steady flow. In: "Hemodynamics." Baltimore, Williams & Wilkins, 1983, pp 11–48.
4. Probst P, Zangl W, Pachinger O: Relation of coronary arterial

occlusion pressure during percutaneous transluminal coronary angioplasty to presence of collaterals. Am J Cardiol 55:1264–1269, 1985.

5. Donohue TJ, Kern MJ, Aguirre FV, Bach RG, Wolford T, Bell CA, Segal J: Assessing the hemodynamic significance of coronary artery stenoses: analysis of translesional pressure-flow velocity relationships in patients. J Am Coll Cardiol 22:449–458, 1993.

6. Segal J, Kern MJ, Scott NA, King SB III, Doucette JW, Heuser RR, Ofili E, Siegel R: Alterations of phasic coronary artery flow velocity in humans during percutaneous coronary angioplasty. J Am Coll Cardiol 20:276–286, 1992.

7. Ofili EO, Kern MJ, Labovitz AJ, St. Vrain JA, Segal J, Aguirre F, Castello R: Analysis of coronary blood flow velocity dynamics in angiographically normal and stenosed arteries before and after endolumen enlargement by angioplasty. J Am Coll Cardiol 21: 308–316, 1993.

8. Kern MJ, Aguirre FV, Bach RG, Caracciolo EA, Donohue TJ: Interventional physiology, part I: Translesional pressure-flow velocity assessment in patients. Cathet Cardiovasc Diagn 31:49–60, 1994.

9. Ofili EO, Kern MJ, St. Vrain JA, Al-Joundi B, Castello R, Labovitz AJ: Differences in spectral velocity and volumetric flow in proximal and distal normal human coronary arteries (abstr). J Am Coll Cardiol 21:75A, 1993.

10. Marcus ML, Gascho JA, Mueller TM, Eastham CH, Wright CB, Doty DB, Hiratzka LF. The effects of ventricular hypertrophy on the coronary circulation. Basic Res Cardiol 76:575–581, 1981.

11. Kern MJ, Tatineni S, Gudipati C, Aguirre F, Ring ME, Serota H, Deligonul U: Regional coronary blood flow velocity and vasodilatory reserve in patients with angiographically normal coronary arteries. Coro Artery Disease 1:579–589, 1990.

12. Goldstein R, Kirkeeide R, Demer L, Merhige M, Nishikona A, Smalling R, Mullani N, Gould KL: Relation between geometric dimensions of coronary artery stenoses and myocardial perfusion reserve in man. JCI 79:1473–1478, 1987.

13. Gould KL, Kirkeeide R, Buchi M: Coronary flow reserve as a physiologic measure of stenosis severity. Part I. Relative and absolute coronary flow reserve during changing aortic pressure. Part II. Determination from arteriographic stenosis dimensions under standardized conditions. J Am Coll Cardiol 15:459–474, 1990.

14. Marcus ML, Harrison DG, White CW, McPherson DD, Wilson RF, Kerber RE: Assessing the physiologic significance of coronary obstructions in patients: Importance of diffuse undetected atherosclerosis. Prog Cardiovasc 31:39–56, 1988.

Chapter 7

Angioplasty Decision Making Based on Abnormal Translesion Hemodynamics for an Intermediate Stenosis:
The Dilemma of a High Translesional Pressure Gradient and Normal Distal Flow Reserve

Scott Carollo, MD, and Morton J. Kern, MD

INTRODUCTION

The treatment of any ischemic syndrome requires the incorporation of objective data and clinical judgment. For patients currently presenting with an anginal-like symptom complex, there is a multiplicity of methods to identify the presence and physiologic significance of coronary artery disease. Despite the generally reliable data obtained from these methods, taken individually, each technique has well-appreciated limitations producing false positive and false negative results. The description and clinical value of presenting anginal symptoms can often be perplexing and vague. Exercise stress testing, especially in women, may have technical limitations. Both the visual and quantitative estimation of the severity of angiographically defined coronary stenoses is often imprecise. For these reasons, physicians apply clinical experience and make clinical decisions based upon the interpretations of the assembled results. Despite this approach, the available clinical information may be conflicting and will not provide a clear algorithmic treatment plan. To illustrate this point, we present a patient with an ischemic syndrome who posed a clinical dilemma regarding revascularization secondary to complicating objective data obtained in the catheterization laboratory.

HISTORY

A 38-year-old woman with a history of cocaine and tobacco abuse was admitted to another hospital with the acute onset of substernal pain for approximately 3 hr.

The chest pain was described as a heaviness which radiated to her neck and left upper extremity with varying levels of intensity without complete resolution. The initial electrocardiogram was reported as normal. Rapid symptom resolution was produced with the administration of intravenous nitroglycerin and heparin. Subsequent serial cardiac enzymes were consistent with a non-Q wave myocardial infarction (peak CPK 277 U, MB fraction 33.3 U). Two days later, she had a spontaneous recurrence of chest pain with new T wave inversions in the inferior and anterolateral electrocardiographic leads. The symptoms responded to a single sublingual nitroglycerin, however the electrocardiographic changes persisted. She was subsequently transferred to our institution for cardiac catheterization.

Coronary angiography demonstrated a 60% diameter stenosis of the mid left anterior descending artery with a 30% stenosis of the proximal right coronary artery (Fig. 1). The left main and left circumflex arteries were angiographically normal. The left ventriculogram was also normal. Before angioplasty, a translesional hemodynamic assessment of the left anterior descending lesion was performed using a 2.7F Tracker™ catheter and 0.014 inch intracoronary Doppler-tipped guidewire as previously described [1,2]. Coronary flow velocity proximal to the stenosis had an average peak velocity of 13 cm/sec, which increased to 53 cm/sec during intracoronary adenosine-induced hyperemia for a normal coronary flow reserve of 4.0 (Fig. 2). The flow velocity measured distal to the stenosis revealed a proximal-to-distal flow velocity ratio of 1.1 and a marginally adequate coronary flow reserve of 2.1 (Fig. 2). To confirm whether distal

Pre PTCA

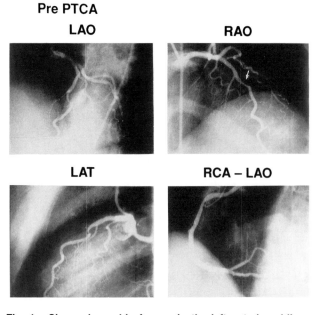

Fig. 1. Cineangiographic frames in the left anterior oblique (LAO), right anterior oblique (RAO), and lateral (LAT) projections of the left anterior descending artery demonstrating a 60% diameter stenosis (arrow). The right coronary artery (RCA) in the LAO projection (lower right panel) revealed a proximal 30% diameter stenosis.

flow was functionally satisfactory, a dobutamine stress echocardiogram was performed in the laboratory utilizing the standard incremental doses of intravenous dobutamine (Fig. 3) [3]. The patient achieved 85% of maximal predicted heart rate by the end of 30 μg of dobutamine (Table I). At peak dobutamine stress, there were no chest pain symptoms, no electrocardiographic abnormalities, and no regional left ventricular wall motion abnormalities identified.

At completion of this evaluation we had defined a relatively normal proximal-to-distal coronary flow ratio and post-stenotic coronary reserve with an entirely unremarkable maximal dobutamine stress echocardiogram. To complete the assessment and determine flow resistance, a translesional pressure gradient was measured (twice) with a 2.7F Tracker™ catheter and found to be 60 mm Hg (Fig. 2). Intracoronary nitroglycerin was given in the left anterior descending artery during the second measurements. This markedly abnormal translesional pressure gradient obtained in an angiographically intermediate stenosis conflicted with post-stenotic flow, flow reserve, and dobutamine stress echo left ventricular wall motion in a patient with a recent non-Q wave myocardial infarction whose course was complicated by post-infarction angina associated with new electrocardiographic changes. On which information should we base our decision to intervene with angioplasty?

Pre PTCA

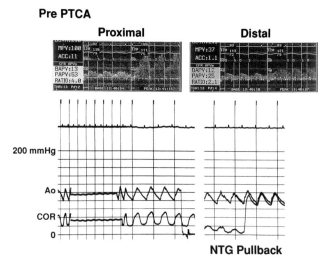

Fig. 2. Flow velocity spectra (top) and translesional gradient (bottom) before angioplasty. Flow velocity measurements were made at rest (Base, left side) and during maximal hyperemia (Peak, right side) with adenosine (18 μg intracoronary) proximal and distal to the left anterior descending (LAD) stenosis. The proximal and distal basal flow velocities (BAPV) are nearly identical with a normal phasic pattern and proximal/distal ratio of 1.1. During hyperemia, distal flow (PAPV) increased to 25 cm/sec with a coronary flow reserve ratio of 2.1. (Velocity scale 0–120 cm/sec. Heart rate and systolic and diastolic pressures are numbers in upper left corner of each flow tracing.) S,D = systolic and diastolic periods; BAPV = baseline average peak velocity; PAPV = peak average peak velocity ratio; Ratio = coronary flow reserve. Bottom: At rest (left) a 60 mm Hg translesional pressure gradient increases slightly following 150 μg of intracoronary nitroglycerin (NTG, lower right panel). Resolution of the gradient occurs as the intracoronary pressure catheter is pulled back across the left anterior descending stenosis to the proximal portion of the vessel. Ao = aortic pressure; COR = coronary pressure. Pressure scale = 0–200 mm Hg.

LAD

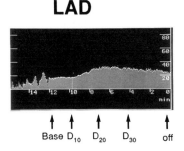

Fig. 3. A continuous trend of average peak velocities (APV) during dobutamine echocardiography. Flow velocities increase appropriately with incremental doses of dobutamine to a peak infusion of 30 μg. Velocity scale 0–100 cm/sec. Time marks are at 2 min intervals.

In light of her clinical course and the markedly abnormal translesional pressure gradient, we elected to proceed with coronary angioplasty of the mid left anterior descending artery stenosis. Angioplasty was successful,

TABLE I. Dobutamine Echo and Coronary Flow Measurements*

	Heart rate (bpm)	Blood pressure (mm Hg)	Average peak velocity (cm/sec)	Coronary flow reserve	DSVR
Baseline	81	118/78	12	—	3.5
Dobutamine (10 µg/min IV)	95	170/90	30	2.5	1.3
Dobutamine (20 µg/min IV)	117	168/91	33	2.8	1.4
Dobutamine (30 µg/min IV)	136	145/89	28	2.3	1.5
Recovery	74	127/84	16	—	3.5

*Hemodynamic and intracoronary flowire measurements obtained at baseline and at incremental doses of dobutamine infusion. DSVR = diastolic/systolic velocity ratio.

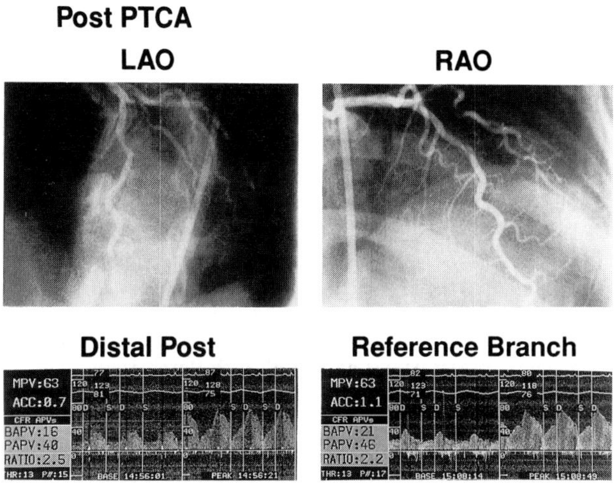

Post PTCA

LAO   **RAO**

Distal Post   **Reference Branch**

Fig. 4. Cineangiographic frames in the left anterior oblique (LAO) and right anterior oblique (RAO) projections (top) of the residual 20% left anterior descending (LAD) stenosis (arrow) following successful angioplasty. Flow velocity (bottom left) in the distal left anterior descending, demonstrating an increased average peak velocity of 16 cm/sec and peak average peak velocity of 40 cm/sec. Distal coronary reserve is 2.5. (Bottom right:) Flow velocity data obtained from a normal reference vessel (first obtuse marginal) shows a coronary flow reserve ratio of 2.2. Velocity format as in Figure 1.

reducing the diameter stenosis to 20% without any complications. Following angioplasty, the distal average peak velocity increased to 16 cm/sec, hyperemia was 40 cm/sec, and the distal coronary flow reserve increased to 2.5 (Fig. 4).

Shortly after completing the angioplasty and final flow velocity measurements, the patient complained of chest pain. An electrocardiogram was obtained and revealed new ST elevation in the inferior leads (not shown). Because the JL4 guide was still positioned, intracoronary nitroglycerin was given in the left anterior descending artery and repeat coronary arteriography was performed. The left anterior descending and circumflex coronary arteries were unchanged from the immediate post-angio-

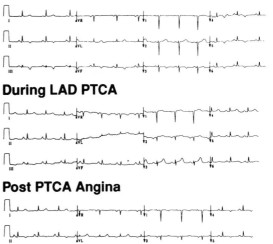

Pre LAD PTCA

During LAD PTCA

Post PTCA Angina

Fig. 5. Top: Admission electrocardiogram with T wave inversions present in the inferior (II, III, and aVF) and anterolateral leads (V₃-V₆). Middle: Electrocardiogram obtained during balloon inflation of the left anterior descending artery (LAD) associated with ST elevation in the anterior leads (V₁-V₅). Bottom: Electrocardiogram obtained following administration of intracoronary nitroglycerin (NTG) and resolution of post-angioplasty angina. The inferior ST elevation had resolved and the T wave abnormalities remain unchanged from the baseline tracing.

plasty study. The patient quickly became asymptomatic and the electrocardiographic changes resolved following the administration of nitroglycerin. The right coronary artery was then engaged and was also unchanged from the original angiogram. The chest pain and inferior electrocardiographic ST elevations were distinctly different from anterior ST elevation produced during left anterior descending balloon occlusion (Fig. 5). The patient was discharged from the laboratory in stable condition. The remainder of her hospital course was unremarkable. At 2 week follow-up she was well and denied any further chest pain on oral calcium channel blockers and long acting nitrates.

DISCUSSION

This case demonstrated an angioplasty decision based on an abnormal left anterior descending stenosis pressure gradient despite a normal post-stenotic flow reserve [2], flow velocity ratio, and maximal dobutamine echocardiographic stress test that may not have achieved the desired therapeutic result of alleviating angina, which may have been due to right coronary artery spasm. The presenting syndrome had atypical features for classic angina and non-specific T wave changes in an inferior and lateral distribution. Over the course of the intervention, inferior ST elevation with the presenting anginal symptoms appeared most likely due to vasospasm of the right coronary artery without involving the left anterior descending artery. The left anterior descending artery did not wrap around the apex to supply the inferior wall.

The large number of clinical parameters available to physicians to assess the presence and significance of coronary artery disease may yield conflicting results. When integrated, this information will assist in defining a particular treatment plan, a particularly important issue for the assessment of angiographically intermediate coronary artery stenoses [3,4]. The visual estimation of angiographically-defined stenoses is imperfect and often requires additive objective information to help define its hemodynamic importance. Of the five parameters acquired during in-laboratory adjunctive lesion assessment, only the pressure gradient suggested the presence of a hemodynamically significant coronary lesion. In general, gradients >20 mm Hg have been considered clinically significant [4,5]. Wijns et al. [5] noted a high sensitivity and specificity for gradients >30 mm Hg with thallium perfusion testing. On the other hand, poststenotic flow reserve was 2.1, a value which corresponds to negative thallium imaging [6]. Moreover, poststenotic flow velocity increased normally during a maximal dobutamine stress test which also failed to demonstrate a wall motion abnormality.

Was the gradient of 60 mm Hg accurate? The measurement was performed twice with a good fidelity signal and verified by the continuous demonstration of pressure during catheter pullback. A catheter kink at the lesion (which required 8 atmospheres to eliminate the angioplasty balloon waist) could contribute to an artifactually high gradient. Vasospasm at the lesion, or in the distal left anterior descending artery, was excluded by intracoronary nitroglycerin given during gradient measurement. The small (1.4 mm^2) cross-sectional area of the Tracker^{TM} catheter may have significantly contributed to the translesional gradient, especially in this relatively modestly sized left anterior descending artery.

The clinical history of a complicated non-Q wave myocardial infarction with a markedly abnormal translesional pressure gradient in the face of other normal data out-weighed a more conservative approach. In our experience, the normal dobutamine echocardiogram and normal coronary flow parameters alone would usually have been sufficient data to defer angioplasty as reported in a large series of stable anginal patients [9].

The technical limitations of each technique, coronary flow velocity [7], pressure gradients [8], and dobutamine stress echocardiogram [3] have been discussed in detail elsewhere. The decision in the laboratory was based on the clinical presentation and one of most objective pieces of data, the pressure gradient. Whether this piece of objective data is the most reliable for clinical decision making is in question. Prospective studies with patient follow-up based on various physiologic approaches to selection of lesions for intervention will be helpful to eliminate future dilemmas arising from such conflicting data.

ACKNOWLEDGMENTS

The authors thank the J.G. Mudd Cardiac Catheterization Laboratory team and Donna Sander for manuscript preparation.

REFERENCES

1. Kern MJ, Aguirre FV, Bach RG, Caracciolo EA, Donohue TJ: Translesional pressure-flow velocity assessment in patients. Cathet Cardiovasc Diagn 31:49–60, 1994.
2. Donohue TJ, Kern MJ, Aguirre FV, Bach RG, Wolford T, Bell CA, Segal J: Assessing the hemodynamic significance of coronary artery stenoses: Analysis of translesional pressure-flow velocity relations in patients. J Am Coll Cardiol 22:449–458, 1993.
3. Sawada SG, Segar DS, Ryan T, Brown SE, Dohan AM, Williams R, Fineberg NS, Armstrong WF, Feigenbaum H: Echocardiographic detection of coronary artery disease during dobutamine infusion. Circulation 83:1605–1614, 1991.
4. Hodgson JM, Reinert S, Most AS, Williams DO: Prediction of long-term clinical outcome with final translesional pressure gradient during coronary angioplasty. Circulation 74:563–566, 1986.
5. Wijns W, Serruys PW, Reiber JHC, van den Brand M, Simoons ML, Kooijman CJ, Balakumaran K, Hugenholtz PG: Quantitative angiography of the left anterior descending coronary artery: Correlations with pressure gradient and results of exercise thallium scintigraphy. Circulation 71:273–279, 1985.
6. Miller DD, Donohue TJ, Younis LT, Bach RG, Aguirre FV, Wittry MD, Goodgold HM, Chaitman BR, Kern MJ: Correlation of pharmacologic ^{99m}Tc-sestamibi myocardial perfusion imaging with poststenotic coronary flow reserve in patients with angiographically intermediate coronary artery stenoses. Circulation 89:2150–2160, 1994.
7. Kern MJ, Aguirre FV, Bach RG, Caracciolo EA, Donohue TJ, Labovitz AJ: Fundamentals of translesional pressure-flow velocity measurements. Cathet Cardiovasc Diagn 31:137–143, 1994.
8. DeBruyne B, Pijls NHJ, Paulus WJ, Vantrimpont PJ, Sys SU, Heyndrickx GR: Transstenotic coronary pressure gradient measurement in humans: In vitro and in vivo evaluation of a new pressure monitoring angioplasty guide wire. J Am Coll Cardiol 22:119–126, 1993.
9. Kern MJ, Donohue TJ, Aguirre FV, Bach RG, Caracciolo EA, Wolford T, Mechem C, Flynn MS, Chaitman B: Clinical outcome of deferring angioplasty in patients with normal translesional pressure and flow velocity measurements. J Am Coll Cardiol 25:178–187, 1995.

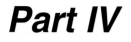

Part IV

Coronary Angioplasty

Chapter 8

Assessment of Circumflex Artery Stenoses Before High-Risk Coronary Angioplasty

Morton J. Kern, MD, Thomas J. Donohue, MD, Frank V. Aguirre, MD, Richard G. Bach, MD, and Eugene A. Caracciolo, MD

INTRODUCTION

Translesional pressure and flow velocity can characterize the hemodynamic significance of angiographically indeterminate or indistinct coronary lesions and may assist in decision making for high-risk interventions. An aggressive or conservative approach to the management of patients at risk of complications of coronary angioplasty would be a valuable adjunct, especially when the consequences of coronary dissection, transient ischemia, or closure might be life threatening [1,2]. The angiographic determination of circumflex artery lesion severity can, at times, be difficult because of the lesion location, vessel tortuosity, branch vessel overlap, and requirement of extreme cinefluoroscopic angulation for adequate lesion visualization. Interpretation of ill-defined angiographic features specific for circumflex lesion delineation is further compounded by vessel foreshortening and image deterioration due to the overlapping bony structures (i.e., spine).

Noninvasive physiologic assessment of circumflex stenoses, using myocardial perfusion stress studies or other ischemic risk stratification testing is also, at times, unhelpful due to indeterminate results involving imaging of the lateral left ventricular wall. In certain patients, noninvasive testing may not be reliable due to anatomic variations or electrocardiographically silent ischemic regions. In addition, clinical circumstances, such as unstable angina, recent myocardial infarction, or other conditions, may prohibit or complicate noninvasive physiologic evaluations.

An invasive approach to assessing translesional pressure during angioplasty across a circumflex coronary artery also represents a difficult technical challenge be-

cause of many of the anatomic features mentioned above, complicating angiographic image interpretation [3,4]. Additional objective measurements related to translesional flow restriction would be helpful. In this interventional physiology presentation, we discuss the approach to lesion assessment in two patients at high risk of angioplasty complications involving circumflex coronary stenoses of angiographically similar severity. Translesional physiology assisted the clinical decision making for each patient and contributed to the reduction of potential risk involved with coronary interventional procedures in these individuals.

CASES

Management of Recurrent Pulmonary Edema and a Circumflex Artery Stenosis

A 78-year-old woman was admitted to the coronary care unit for recurrent pulmonary edema. She had a history of severe coronary artery disease with prior extensive anterior and anterolateral myocardial infarctions. Despite vigorous medical management, dyspnea at rest with periodic episodes of pulmonary edema requiring hospitalization occurred. The electrocardiogram (ECG) showed a left bundle branch block with no new ECG changes during episodes of pulmonary edema. Cardiac catheterization was performed to evaluate whether coronary revascularization could be performed. Coronary arteriography demonstrated total left anterior descending coronary occlusion (Fig. 1, top), and severe narrowing of the proximal circumflex artery seen in only the left anterior oblique caudal projection. The right coronary artery was small and only minimally diseased. Because of vessel foreshortening and tortuosity, the right anterior oblique projection with extreme caudal angulation could not further delineate the circumflex artery lesion. Quantitative angiography showed that the lesion was 63% diameter narrowed and with 86% area reduction. The left ventricular ejection fraction was 25% with severe anterior, anterolateral, apical, inferoapical and inferior akinesis (Fig. 1, bottom left). The left ventricular end-diastolic pressure was approximately 32 mm Hg. The patient's family requested that intervention be performed. A cardiothoracic surgery consultation was obtained. The patient was declined for urgent coronary artery bypass surgery because of the severely depressed left ventricular function and the extensive and diffuse coronary artery disease. Dipyridamole stress perfusion imaging was equivocal for lateral wall ischemia with anterior, anteroapical, and inferior fixed defects. Increased oral and intravenous medical therapy for congestive heart failure was recommended due to the high-risk nature of percutaneous intervention. However, because of recurrent episodes of pulmonary edema, presumably related to silent lateral wall myocardial ischemia despite the inconclusive ECG and noninvasive stress testing results, angioplasty was scheduled.

The high-risk nature of the procedure was explained to the patient and family. In the catheterization laboratory, both femoral arteries were cannulated; the right femoral artery with an 8F long angioplasty sheath and the left femoral artery with a 5F sheath for rapid vascular access for intra-aortic balloon pump support, if necessary. Prior to the introduction of the coronary angioplasty balloon catheter, translesional flow velocity and pressure data were measured as previously described [5,6]. Using standard angioplasty technique, a 2.7F tracking catheter (Tracker, Target Therapeutics) was loaded with a 0.018-inch Doppler flowire (FloWire, Cardiometrics, Mountain View, CA). Heparin, 10,000 units intravenous bolus, was given and the flowire/tracker catheter system advanced into the vessel. Flow velocity data obtained in the circumflex artery proximal to the lesion demonstrated a normal phasic pattern with a mean velocity of approximately 20 cm/sec (Fig. 2, top). After traversing a tortuous segment and crossing the lesion, the distal circumflex artery flow velocity was similar to the proximal velocity in both phasic pattern and mean velocity of approximately 29 cm/sec. Intracoronary adenosine (12 μg) was administered producing a twofold increase in distal flow velocity. The average peak velocity increased to 44 cm/sec during hyperemia. The proximal/distal velocity ratio was approximately 1, suggesting a gradient of <30 mm Hg [6]. Translesional pressure was measured, confirming the flow velocity data. A resting pressure gradient of 8 mm Hg increased to 12 mm Hg during maximal hyperemia (Fig. 2, bottom). On the basis of the minimal

translesional pressure gradient, normal phasic pattern and near normal distal hyperemia, coronary angioplasty of this lesion was deferred. The patient was returned to the coronary care unit and was continued on vigorous medical therapy for symptomatic left ventricular dysfunction. She was discharged from the intensive care unit on an optimal medical regimen for ischemic cardiomyopathy. The patient did well for approximately 5 months after which time the patient succumbed to refractory congestive failure.

Atypical Chest Pain, Left Ventricular Dysfunction, and a Circumflex Stenosis

A 68-year-old woman complaining of dyspnea at rest and exertion with an atypical anginal chest pain syndrome was evaluated for coronary revascularization. The patient was also being treated for longstanding hypertension and insulin-dependent diabetes. Myocardial perfusion stress imaging was equivocal for lateral wall perfusion redistribution. Coronary angiography demonstrated a highly tortuous and convoluted circumflex artery, which contained an eccentric, moderately severe (63%) stenosis in the proximal portion of the circumflex artery (Fig. 3, top). The remaining coronary arteries were only minimally involved with atherosclerotic irregularities. The left ventricular ejection fraction was 39% with global hypokinesis. Because of the symptomatic but nonspecific ischemic presentation with a potentially causative circumflex stenosis, angioplasty was recommended. However, before angioplasty was to be performed, the physiologic significance of the coronary stenosis was determined after diagnostic coronary angiography. Translesional velocity and pressure were measured as described for the first patient using a 0.014-inch Doppler flowire and 2.7F pressure catheter. Proximal coronary flow velocity was normal in its phasic pattern with a mean velocity of approximately 32 cm/sec (Fig. 3, bottom). The flowire was passed distal to the lesion negotiating the tortuous proximal segment. Distal flow velocity was similar to proximal values with a mean velocity of approximately 29 cm/sec. The proximal/distal flow velocity ratio was 1.2. The translesional pressure gradient measured at rest was 10 mm Hg. Distal hyperemia was not induced in this individual. Angioplasty of this lesion was therefore deferred. The patient was discharged on antihypertensive afterload reduction therapy and has remained minimally symptomatic 12 months after the evaluation.

DISCUSSION

The angiographic assessment of circumflex lesions can be particularly difficult, complicating decision making which is critically important for high risk angio-

78 yr old Woman - High Risk; PTCA?
LAD 100%   CFX 65%
RCA 30%   LVEF 30%

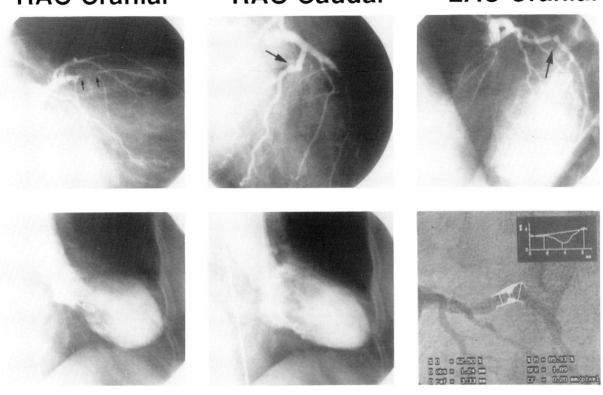

RAO Cranial   RAO Caudal   LAO Cranial

Systole   Diastole   QCA

30° RAO LV

Fig. 1. Top, left to right: Coronary cineangiographic frames of the totally occluded left anterior descending artery (double arrows), the circumflex artery stenosis (single arrow) in the right anterior oblique projection with cranial angulation. Bottom, left, middle: Left ventriculogram in systole and diastole demonstrating severely impaired ejection fraction. Right: Quantitative angiography of circumflex artery stenosis in the left anterior oblique projection alone showing stenosis is 63% diameter narrowed.

plasty. As demonstrated in the two cases, lesions in circumflex arteries are often obscured angiographically because of highly tortuous segments, vessel foreshortening, lesion eccentricity, and overlapping structures.

The application of translesional flow velocity is a relatively new method to assess the physiologic impact of coronary stenosis. Donohue et al. [6] indicate a proximal to distal flow velocity ratio of >1.7 in a branching artery

is associated with translesional pressure gradients >30 mm Hg in 90% of studies. It should be recognized, however, that although the proximal to distal ratio is sensitive for important gradients, the specificity for precise gradients is poor. In addition, the circumflex artery often does not have branches originating before the first obtuse marginal, limiting the application of a proximal/distal velocity ratio. Whether a hyperemic gradient of >20 mm Hg

78 yr old Woman - High Risk; PTCA?
CFX 65%

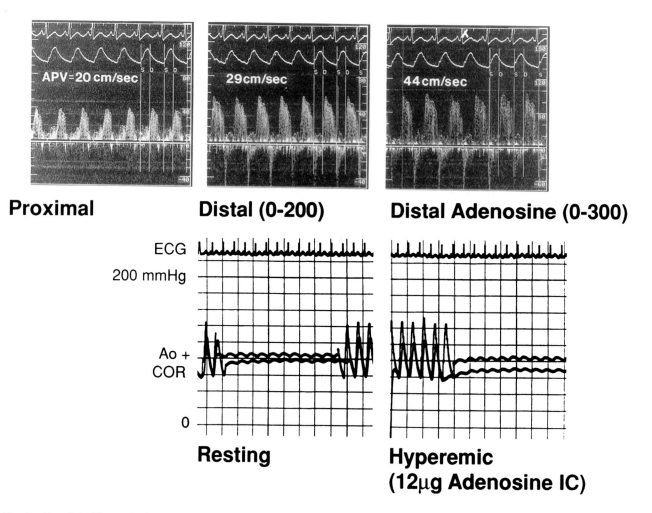

| Proximal | Distal (0-200) | Distal Adenosine (0-300) |

Resting   **Hyperemic (12μg Adenosine IC)**

Fig. 2. Top, left: Flow velocity signal proximal to the circum-flex artery stenosis. Mean (average peak) velocity (APV) is 20 cm/sec. Middle: Flow velocity distal to the stenosis is 29 cm/sec with a normal phasic diastolic predominant pattern. Velocity scale for basal proximal and distal flow velocity is 0–160 cm/sec. Right: Distal hyperemic velocity is 44 cm/sec (scale was increased to 0–240 cm/sec). The proximal/distal ratio was 0.95 with coronary vasodilatory reserve of 2.0. Bottom: Translesional pressure gradient at rest (left) and during maximal hyperemic (right) with adenosine. Gradient increased from 8 to 12 mm Hg. Angioplasty was deferred. (AO = aortic pressure; COR = distal coronary artery pressure)

but <30 mm Hg would be clinically tolerable in patients as described here is unknown. Because of the low gradient specificity of the proximal–distal ratio, the question of an adequate location to measure proximal flow velocity, and impaired distal hyperemia, the lesion significance can be further evaluated with a translesional pressure measurement confirming the flow data. In high-risk studies or cases in which the proximal–distal ratio may be questioned, direct translesional pressure gradient measurements are needed.

Translesional pressure gradients are subject to artifact by catheter size, catheter kinking, and poor pressure transmission through fluid-filled transducer systems. However, most, if not all, artifacts associated with this methodology would produce increased pressure gradients and not artifactually low-pressure gradients. Errors induced by the catheter contributing to stenosis narrowing would also favor intervention. Thus, a non-flow-limiting stenosis can likely be confirmed with a low translesional pressure gradient.

Flow velocity data suggesting clinically satisfactory lesional physiology included a normal distal flow phasic

Intermediate CFX (68 yr old Female Diabetes)
0.014" Flowire

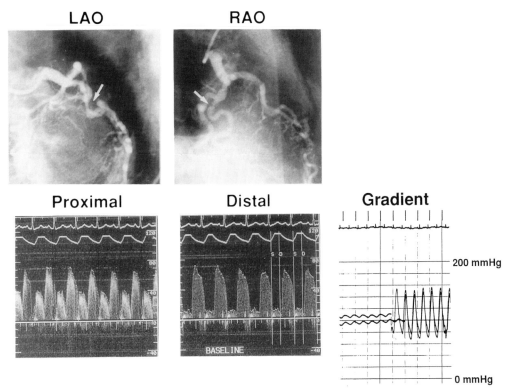

Fig. 3. Top: Cineangiographic frames of a moderate circumflex artery lesion in the left (LAO) and right anterior oblique (RAO) projections. Bottom, left, middle: Proximal and distal flow velocity demonstrate normal phasic patterns with a proximal–distal flow velocity ratio of 1.2. The resting translesional gradient was 10 mm Hg. Angioplasty was also deferred.

pattern, proximal–distal ratio of <1.7 [6], and distal hyperemia of >2 times basal average peak velocity [7]. Coronary flow velocity data in the circumflex artery had demonstrated that the phasic velocity pattern has a diastolic–systolic velocity ratio of >1.5, which is often lower than the diastolic–systolic velocity ratio observed in the left anterior descending coronary artery [7]. For the circumflex and right coronary arteries, the peak and mean flow velocity values also are on average lower than the left anterior descending value, a finding with unknown clinical significance.

Coronary vasodilatory reserve, the ratio of hyperemic to baseline mean flow, in normal coronary circulations is similar among left anterior descending and circumflex regions [7]. An estimate of impaired regional reserve can be obtained by comparing coronary vasodilatory reserve in an angiographically normal zone to the coronary vasodilatory reserve measured in the region supplied by the stenosed artery in question (e.g., distal circumflex). An impaired global coronary flow reserve thus suggests that impaired distal target artery reserve is not entirely due to

the influence of epicardial narrowing. Assessing regional coronary flow reserve for lesion severity is currently under evaluation. Lesion-specific hemodynamics should be measured with distal hyperemia whenever possible.

Complications of coronary angioplasty in patients with depressed left ventricular function may be life threatening. Decisions as to the benefit of coronary revascularization for improving left ventricular dysfunction in such patients can be difficult, whether recommending complete revascularization with coronary artery bypass for all involved vessels, or incomplete revascularization with culprit lesion coronary angioplasty. Whether a single-vessel angioplasty would provide benefit for symptomatic left ventricular dysfunction cannot be determined in advance in some patients. From the data available, the benefit of mechanical lumen enlargement providing increased or normalized translesional pressure and flow velocity in the arteries of the two cases described herein would likely have been negligible due to the near-normal findings on initial evaluation. Deferred angioplasty based on normal translesional physiology in patients with stable ischemic syndromes is a departure from routine clinical decision making. A pilot study has been reported demonstrating translesional measurements are a safe and feasible method with <10% lesion progression in a 2-year follow-up study [8]. The objective data obtained by translesional physiology can support a conservative approach to high-risk angioplasty decision making in selected patients. Prospective studies to confirm a physiologic approach to assist decision making for interventional procedures are under way.

ACKNOWLEDGMENTS

The authors thank the J.G. Mudd Cardiac Catheterization Laboratory team and Donna Sander for manuscript preparation.

REFERENCES

1. Hibbard MD, Holmes DR Jr, Bailey KR, Reeder GS, Bresnahan FJ, Gersh BJ: Percutaneous transluminal coronary angioplasty in patients with cardiogenic shock. J Am Coll Cardiol 19:639–646, 1992.
2. Gacioch GM, Ellis SG, Lee L, Bates ER, Kirsh M, Walton JA, Topol EJ: Cardiogenic shock complicating acute myocardial infarction: The use of coronary angioplasty and the integration of the new support devices in patient management. J Am Coll Cardiol 19:647–653, 1992.
3. Anderson HV, Roubin GS, Leimgruber PP, Cox WR, Douglas JS Jr, King SB III, Gruentzig AR: Measurement of transstenotic pressure gradient during percutaneous transluminal coronary angioplasty. Circulation 73:1223–1230, 1986.
4. MacIsaac HC, Knudtson ML, Robinson VJ, Manyari DE: Is the residual translesional pressure gradient useful to predict regional myocardial perfusion after percutaneous transluminal coronary angioplasty? Am Heart J 117:783–790, 1989.
5. Segal J, Kern MJ, Scott NA, King SB III, Doucette JW, Heuser RR, Ofili E, Siegel R: Alterations of phasic coronary artery flow velocity in humans during percutaneous coronary angioplasty. J Am Coll Cardiol 20:276–286, 1992.
6. Donohue TJ, Kern MJ, Aguirre FV, Bach RG, Wolford T, Bell CA, Segal J: Assessing the hemodynamic significance of coronary artery stenoses: analysis of translesional pressure-flow velocity relationships in patients. J Am Coll Cardiol 22:449–458, 1993.
7. Ofili EO, Kern MJ, Labovitz AJ, St Vrain JA, Segal J, Aguirre F, Castello R: Analysis of coronary blood flow velocity dynamics in angiographically normal and stenosed arteries before and after endolumen enlargement by angioplasty. J Am Coll Cardiol 21:308–316, 1993.
8. Kern M, Donohue T, Bach R, Aguirre F, Caracciolo E, Mechem C, Cauley M, Flynn M, Chaitman B: Clinical outcome of deferred angioplasty in patients based on normal translesional pressure-flow velocity measurements. Circulation 88:I-204, 1993.

Chapter 9

Application of Translesional Pressure and Flow Velocity Assessment in a Severely Calcified Coronary Narrowing in a Patient With Unstable Angina

Joseph A. Moore, MD, Richard G. Bach, MD, and Morton J. Kern, MD

INTRODUCTION

Decisions to proceed with coronary interventions are generally based on the clinical presentation and angiographic anatomy. Coronary arteriography is the accepted clinical standard used to estimate stenosis severity. In symptomatic patients, the angiographic findings frequently suggest an obviously severe lesion(s) for which the need for intervention is considered unequivocal. However, in the presence of equivocally severe or high-risk intermediate lesions, hemodynamic assessment may aid in determining the need for intervention. Balloon angioplasty of coronary narrowings in severely calcified vessels carries an increased potential for dissection and abrupt closure [1]. In this ''Interventional Physiology'' we discuss a patient with unstable angina and a highly calcified severe lesion with unusual hemodynamic and coronary flow velocity findings that influenced our management decision.

CASE REPORT

A 70-year-old man with a history of coronary artery disease hypertension, chronic pulmonary disease, prostate carcinoma, mild renal insufficiency, and adult-onset diabetes mellitus was transferred for treatment of an unstable chest pain syndrome. The patient reported hospitalizations for two myocardial infarctions and angioplasty of ''multiple (unknown) sites'' 8 years prior to this admission. He recently experienced episodes of nocturnal angina, which were usually relieved by two sublingual nitroglycerin tablets. While hospitalized at another institution, the patient had a 1-hour long episode of typical angina, which was finally relieved by intrave-

nous nitroglycerin and heparin. The electrocardiogram showed mild T-wave abnormalities in leads II, III, and aVF, and evidence of an old septal infarction. No enzymatic evidence of acute myocardial infarction was found.

Diagnostic catheterization at the referring hospital revealed a severe (>80%) lesion in the distal right coronary artery which was diffusely and severely calcified. A moderate lesion (50%) was also noted in the mid left anterior descending coronary artery. Left ventriculography revealed no focal wall motion abnormalities. Medications at the time of transfer included intravenous heparin, amlodipine, metoprolol, hydralazine, aspirin, nitroglycerin patch, furosemide, NPH insulin, and albuterol and ipratropium bromide inhalers.

Right Coronary Artery Lesion Assessment

Before angioplasty, repeat coronary arteriography revealed a diffusely, heavily calcified right coronary artery with a hazy distal narrowing that was severe by the ''worst-view'' visual estimate. Quantitative coronary angiography (QCA) using the guide catheter tip diameter as a reference revealed a diameter stenosis of 83% at the distal site in the most severe view (left anterior oblique projection; Fig. 1). In orthogonal views, the lesion appeared less severe (50–70% diameter stenosis range by visual estimate) but hazy. A moderate lesion was also noted in the proximal right coronary artery at the guide catheter tip. Because of an increased risk of complication associated with angioplasty in this calcified vessel, the lesion was assessed with a 0.018 in. Doppler angioplasty guidewire (FloWire™, Cardiometrics, Inc., Mountain View, CA) through a 2.7F Tracker 18™ end-hole catheter (Target Therapeutics, Freemont, CA).

70 yr old Male, RCA

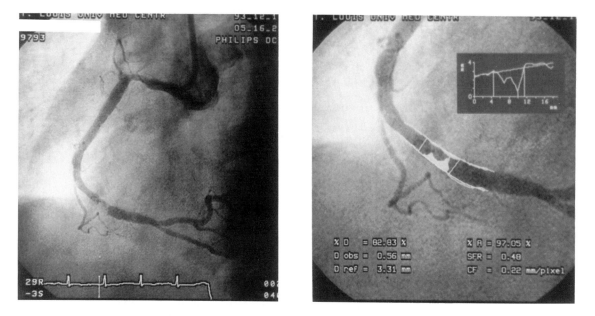

Fig. 1. Right coronary artery (RCA) angiogram in the left anterior oblique projection demonstrating a severe lesion prior to the posterior descending artery. A moderate lesion is also seen proximally.

Coronary flow velocities recorded in the proximal right coronary artery revealed a resting average peak velocity (APV) of 14 cm/sec with a normal phasic pattern (Fig. 2, top left) (Table I). Following intracoronary adenosine administration (6 μg), the peak velocity increased to 45 cm/sec, yielding a coronary flow reserve of 3.3 (Fig. 2, top right). The guidewire was then advanced across the lesion without difficulty. Flow velocity distal to the lesion in an area of mild diffuse narrowing had an accelerated resting APV of 31 cm/sec with a normal diastolic predominant pattern (Fig. 2, middle left). The peak flow velocity after intracoronary adenosine was 51 cm/sec, yielding a coronary vasodilatory reserve of 1.7 (Fig. 2, middle right). The Tracker catheter was then advanced across the lesion and the guidewire removed. The resting translesional pressure gradient was 10 mm Hg and increased to 25 mm Hg following intracoronary adenosine (Fig. 2, bottom). Based on these translesional flow and pressure measurements, which suggested impairment of distal vasodilatory reserve, but which did not clearly demonstrate critical obstruction to coronary blood flow by pressure gradient, angioplasty was deferred.

Left Anterior Descending Artery
Lesion Assessment

Translesional physiologic assessment of the left coronary artery was then performed. Angiography demon-

TABLE I. Hemodynamic and Angiographic Measurements from the Right, Left Anterior Descending, and Left Circumflex Coronary Arteries*

Artery	QCA stenosis	Proximal		Distal		Gradient
		APV	CVR	APV	CVR	
RCA						
Resting	83	14	—	31	—	10
Hyperemic		45	3.3	51	1.7	25
LAD						
Resting	49	23	—	23	—	10
Hyperemic		38	1.7	38	1.7	15
CFX						
Resting	—	23	—	12	—	—
Hyperemic		36	1.7	19	1.5	—

*APV = average peak velocity (cm/sec); CFX = circumflex coronary artery; CVR = coronary vasodilatory reserve; LAD = left anterior descending coronary artery; RCA = right coronary artery; QCA = quantitative coronary angiography.

strated a moderate lesion in the midportion of the left anterior descending artery with a QCA diameter stenosis of 49% (Fig. 3). Translesional flow velocities and pressure gradients were measured as described earlier for the right coronary artery. In the proximal left anterior descending, near an area of mild narrowing, resting APV was accelerated at 44 cm/sec with a normal phasic pattern of 1.7 (Fig. 4, top). As the Doppler guidewire was

70 yr old Male, RCA

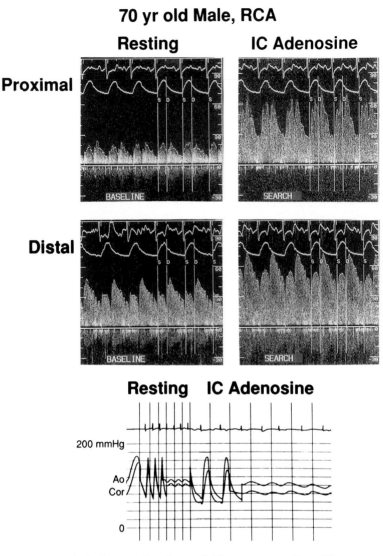

Fig. 2. Flow velocity measurements recorded in the proximal (top) and distal (middle) right coronary artery (RCA) at rest and after intracoronary (IC) adenosine (6–8 μg bolus). S = systole; D = diastole. The velocity scale is 0–120 cm/sec. Bottom: Translesional pressure gradient across the severe angiographic lesion. Ao = pressure in the guide catheter; Cor = pressure in the tracker catheter.

advanced into an angiographically normal portion of the mid vessel, proximal to the stenosis, resting APV was 23 cm/sec and increased to 38 cm/sec after intracoronary adenosine (Fig. 4, middle), yielding a coronary vasodilatory reserve of 1.7. Distal to the lesion of interest, the resting APV was 23 cm/sec with a hyperemic APV of 38 cm/sec, again yielding a coronary vasodilatory reserve of 1.7 (Fig. 4, bottom). Throughout the study, the phasic pattern of flow showed a normal diastolic predominance. The resting translesional pressure gradient measured us-

ing a Tracker catheter was 10 mm Hg and increased to 15 mm Hg after intracoronary adenosine (Fig. 5).

Circumflex Artery Assessment

After left anterior descending coronary lesion assessment, flow velocities were then measured in the proximal circumflex artery and distally in a large obtuse marginal branch, where there was mild diffuse disease. Proximal resting APV was 14 cm/sec and peak hyperemic APV was 27 cm/sec, yielding a coronary vasodila-

70 yr old Male, LAD

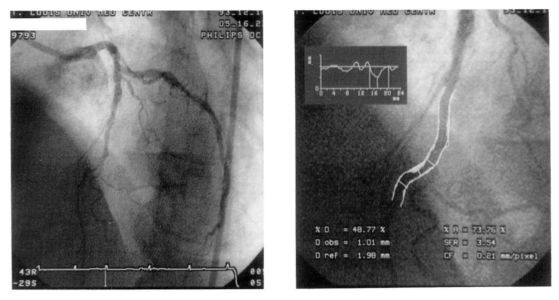

Fig. 3. Left: Coronary angiography of the lesion in the mid left anterior descending (LAD) artery demonstrating a moderate stenosis. **Right:** Diameter stenosis is 49% by quantitative coronary angiography.

tory reserve of 1.4 (Fig. 6, top). Distal resting average peak velocity was accelerated at 31 cm/sec in an area of mild narrowing within the obtuse marginal branch. The peak hyperemic flow velocity was 52 cm/sec, again yielding a coronary vasodilatory reserve of 1.6 (Fig. 6, bottom).

Clinical Course

After cardiac catheterization to correlate noninvasive assessment of regional ischemia measured with translesional physiology, the patient underwent pharmacologic stress radionuclide perfusion imaging using dipyridamole and thallium-201. Hyperemic imaging demonstrated a small defect in the inferobasilar segment with some reversibility on re-injection of thallium. Of note, 4 days after the physiologic lesion assessment, while being treated with calcium channel blockers, aspirin, and oral nitrates, the patient developed recurrent symptoms associated with inferior T-wave inversion and slight ST depression. Angioplasty of the right coronary artery lesion was then performed using multiple dilatations with a 3.5 mm Predator (Cordis, Corp., Miami, FL) and a 4.0 mm RX Perfusion (ACS, Inc., Santa Clara, CA) balloon catheter, resulting in a residual stenosis of 32% by QCA without angiographic evidence of dissection. Following angioplasty, translesional pressure gradient and flow velocity data were not reacquired. The patient did well

following angioplasty and was discharged without complications.

DISCUSSION

A significant lesion in a heavily calcified vessel with an unstable presentation suggests compromise of distal myocardial blood flow delivery. In the case presented, the stenosis of interest appeared most severe in the left anterior oblique view. In the right anterior oblique and right lateral views (not shown), the lesion appeared less severe but hazy. These findings have been previously associated with lesional eccentricity, complexity, and/or superimposed luminal thrombus. As has been discussed previously in "Interventional Physiology" [2], QCA diameter stenosis does not predictably correlate with direct flow velocity measurements, nor does the angiographic appearance of complex lesions always accurately predict their hemodynamic severity. Given the known risks associated with coronary intervention and reduced success rates in extensively calcified vessels, an evaluation of the physiologic significance of such lesions might help avoid unnecessary procedures and potential complications.

Translesional Pressure Gradient Assessment

Translesional pressure gradients have been advocated as a means of determining lesion severity and as a guide

70 yr old Male, LAD

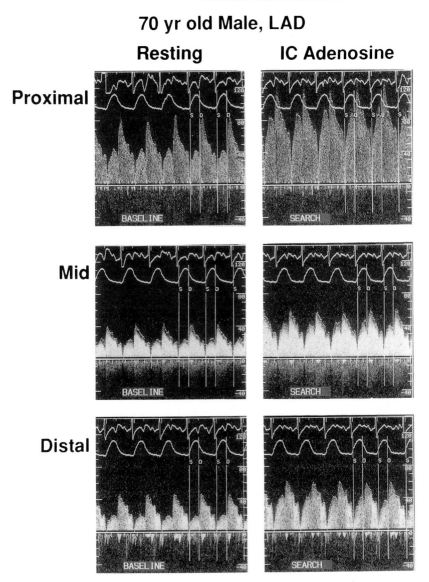

Resting   IC Adenosine

Proximal

Mid

Distal

Fig. 4.   Flow velocity measurements in the left anterior descending (LAD) artery. Top: Proximal, before first diagonal branch. Middle: In the midportion of the left anterior descending proximal to the lesion. Bottom: Distal to the lesion. Peak hyperemia recorded after 18 μg intracoronary (IC) adenosine. S = systole; D = diastole. Velocity scale is 0–160 cm/sec.

to intervention [3–7] and have been discussed earlier in this series [2]. Interventions on lesions with a mean translesional pressure gradient >10 mm Hg at rest or >20 mm Hg during peak hyperemia have been reported, as well as successful dilatation of such lesions associated with relief of ischemia on objective testing and a relief of ischemic symptoms [3]. Residual resting translesional pressure gradients of <20 mm Hg, measured through angioplasty balloon catheters, have also been associated with successful early and late results after coronary angioplasty and a final angiographic diameter stenosis ≤30% [4,5]. The precise level of resting translesional pressure gradient that produces provokable myocardial

ischemia remains to be determined. Surprisingly, in this patient, despite the angiographic appearance of the right coronary artery lesion both in severity (diameter stenosis = 83%) and complexity, the resting translesional gradient was only 10 mm Hg, with a peak hyperemic gradient of 25 mm Hg, findings of borderline hemodynamic significance. Preserved resting distal flow velocity values were confirmed by the Doppler velocity measurements.

Intra-Arterial Variance of Coronary Vasodilatory Reserve

Coronary vasodilatory reserve is influenced by a variety of factors and is dependent on the balance between

70 yr old Male
Resting IC Aden

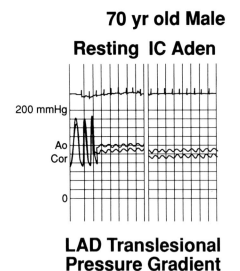

LAD Translesional
Pressure Gradient

Fig. 5.   Pressure gradient at rest and hyperemia across the left anterior descending (LAD) artery lesion. Ao = pressure in the guide catheter; Cor = pressure in the perfusion catheter.

flow within the epicardial conductance vessel and the vasoreactivity of the resistance microcirculation. Coronary vasodilatory reserve measured proximal to stenoses in branching coronary arteries is affected by both the contribution of hyperemia in proximal branches, as well as flow restriction due to lesion severity. Coronary vasodilatory reserve may be abnormally low due to altered microvascular vasoreactivity in the absence of severe epicardial narrowings in the presence of left ventricular hypertrophy, hypertension, diabetes, cigarette smoking, and infarcted myocardium [7]. In patients with significant coronary stenoses with resting translesional pressure gradients ≥20 mm Hg, coronary vasodilatory reserve was shown to decrease from 2.1 ± 0.7 proximally to 1.4 ± 0.6 distally [7]. Thus, characteristics of the lesion, the microcirculatory vasoreactivity, and distal myocardium must be taken into account when using coronary vasodilatory reserve to evaluate coronary stenoses.

In this patient, coronary vasodilatory reserve recorded in the proximal right coronary artery was higher than that recorded distally (Table I), with similar peak hyperemic flow values. This disparity is likely due to a contribution of proximal branch hyperemic responses. Proximal and distal flow velocity phasic patterns in the right coronary artery differed in a typical fashion (Fig. 2). Proximal right coronary artery flow had nearly equal systolic and diastolic components, with low peak velocities consistent with the flow pattern typically observed in the proximal and mid right coronary artery, again probably due, in part, to the contribution of right ventricular myocardial flow [9]. In the distal right coronary artery, which supplies predominantly the inferior left ventricular myo-

cardium, the flow velocity pattern evolved to a diastolic predominant pattern, more closely matching the flow pattern recorded in the left coronary circulation (Figs. 2 and 4). The phasic flow data suggest the coronary vasodilatory reserve recorded in the proximal right coronary artery was elevated, in part, due to a low resting flow velocity and the vasoreactivity in the right heart vessels, and that the distal right coronary vasodilatory reserve may more accurately reflect the microvascular vasoreactivity of the inferior left ventricle supplied via the right coronary artery. Furthermore, peak average flow velocities were maintained across the lesion and matched those in the left coronary artery (Table I).

Lesion Instability

Because distal flow velocity was maintained and the translesional pressure gradient was not consistent with a critically flow-limiting stenosis, angioplasty in this patient was deferred at the time of the initial evaluation, despite the angiographic appearance of the lesion. Current studies evaluating *stable* lesions with noncritical hemodynamic and flow velocity characteristics indicate these patients can be safely managed medically without intervention [10]. This patient, however, had been admitted with crescendo angina consistent with an *unstable* lesion, and on later stress testing was found to have a small reversible defect inferiorly suggestive of provokable ischemia. The recurrence of the patient's symptoms while in the hospital prompted angioplasty, which was subsequently performed without complication. Although the lesion was not flow limiting on initial evaluation, the presence of thrombus with intermittent flow interruption due to variable luminal narrowing or superimposed vasoreactivity, characteristic of unstable angina, cannot be excluded and likely contributed to the patient's subsequent clinical course.

SUMMARY

While the angiographic appearance of coronary stenoses commonly directs interventional decisions, it may correlate imprecisely with hemodynamic or physiologic lesional significance. Previous data would suggest that direct measures of translesional physiology can be helpful in assessing the hemodynamic significance of stable coronary stenoses. In unstable ischemic syndromes, however, the hemodynamic severity of lesions may depend on the presence of variably occlusive intraluminal thrombus superimposed on fluctuating vessel tone. Under these circumstances, physiologic lesional assessment can yield helpful information, which nonetheless must be interpreted with caution in light of the clinical context. Determination of optimal management

70 yr old Male, CFX

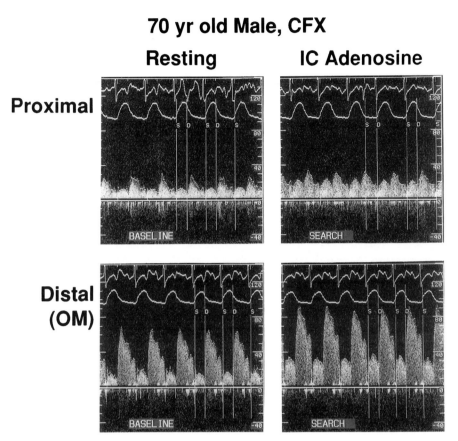

Fig. 6. Flow velocity measurements in the proximal circumflex (CFX) artery (top) and a large terminal obtuse marginal (OM) branch (bottom) at rest and hyperemia [18 µg intracoronary (IC) adenosine]. Format and abbreviations as in Figure 2.

strategies for such patients remains difficult and must await further investigation of prognosis and outcome.

ACKNOWLEDGMENTS

The authors wish to thank the J.G. Mudd Cardiac Catheterization Laboratory Team and Donna Sander for manuscript preparation.

REFERENCES

1. Ellis SG, Roubin GS, King SB III, Douglas S Jr, Weintraub WS, Thomas RG, Cox WR: Angiographic and clinical predictors of acute closure after native vessel coronary angioplasty. Circulation 77:372–379, 1988.
2. Moore JA, Kern MJ: Interventional physiology, part XII: Assessment of serial lesions in the proximal right coronary artery following intracoronary thrombolysis. Cathet Cardiovasc Diagn 33: 349–355, 1994.
3. Ganz P, Abben R, Friedman PL, Garnic JD, Barry WH, Levin DC: Usefulness of transstenotic coronary pressure gradient measurements during diagnostic catheterization. Am J Cardiol 55: 910–914, 1985.
4. Hodgson J, Reinert S, Most A, Williams D: Prediction of long-

term clinical outcome with final translesional pressure gradient during coronary angioplasty. Circulation 74:563–566, 1986.
5. Anderson H, Roubin G, Leimgruber P, Cox W, Douglas J Jr, King SB III, Gruentzig A: Measurement of transstenotic pressure gradient during percutaneous transluminal coronary angioplasty. Circulation 73:1223–1230, 1986.
6. Peterson RJ, King SB III, Fajman WA, Douglas JS Jr, Gruntzig AR, Orias DW, Jones RH: Relation of coronary artery stenosis and pressure gradient to exercise-induced ischemia before and after coronary angioplasty. J Am Coll Cardiol 10:253–260, 1987.
7. Donohue TJ, Kern MJ, Aguirre FV, Bach RG, Wolford T, Bell CA, Segal J: Assessing the hemodynamic significance of coronary artery stenoses: Analysis of translesional pressure-flow velocity relations in patients. J Am Coll Cardiol 22:449–458, 1993.
8. Moore JA, Kern MJ: Interventional physiology, part VI: Coronary flow velocity during coronary angioplasty in regions of myocardial infarction. Cathet Cardiovasc Diagn 32:187–192, 1994.
9. Ofili EO, Kern MJ, Labovitz AJ, St. Vrain JA, Segal J, Aguirre F, Castello R: Analysis of coronary blood flow velocity dynamics in angiographically normal and stenosed arteries before and after endolumen enlargement by angioplasty. J Am Coll Cardiol 21: 308–316, 1993.
10. Kern MJ, Donohue TJ, Aguirre FV, Bach RG, Caracciolo EA, Wolford T, Mechem CJ, Flynn MS, Chaitman B: Clinical outcome by differing angioplasty in patients with normal translesional pressure-flow velocity measurements. J Am Coll Cardiol 25:178–187, 1995.

Chapter 10

Translesional Pressure and Flow Responses in a Patient With a Vasoactive and Atherosclerotic Coronary Artery

Bassam Al-Joundi, MD, Morton J. Kern, MD, Richard G. Bach, MD, and Thomas J. Donohue, MD

INTRODUCTION

Coronary vasomotion superimposed on atherosclerotic lesions, a clear factor in rest angina, has also been proposed to account for variable thresholds for exercise-induced angina [1,2]. In many patients, spontaneous episodes of chest pain at rest and classical exertional angina may co-exist. Treatment for such patients may include both anti-vasospastic medications, such as nitrates and calcium channel blockers, and angioplasty or bypass of the atherosclerotic lesion if hemodynamic significance is established [3]. In the course of treatment of a young man with a vasoactive and atherosclerotic left anterior descending coronary stenosis, translesional coronary physiologic measurements were made to assess the contribution of vasomotion to the ischemic syndrome. Sympathetic stimulation with handgrip exercise and cold pressor testing, before and again after coronary balloon angioplasty and directional atherectomy, was examined. The observations in this case represent a novel demonstration of the influence of sympathetic stimuli on variability of stenosis severity and vessel resistance which can be detected by physiologic measurements.

Case Example

A 38-year-old man was admitted for chest pain with exertion which began approximately 10 days earlier. Several painful episodes also occurred at rest and during minimal exercise. Chest pain was usually spontaneously relieved within 2–3 min. The patient denied chest pain at times of much higher levels of exercise during the same period. Cardiac risk factors included smoking and positive family history. He was using no medications. An exercise treadmill test was performed during which the patient exercised for a total of 9 min, 20 sec (ACIP protocol), achieving a maximal heart rate of 151 (80% of maximal predicted heart rate). The patient developed chest pain at 5 min into exercise. At 6 min into exercise, he developed 2 mm horizontal ST segment depression in the inferolateral leads associated with ventricular bigeminy. The chest pain and electrocardiographic changes resolved spontaneously at approximately 8 min into exercise. However, the chest pain and similar ST segment depression (2–2.5 mm in the inferolateral leads) recurred at minute 9 into exercise. Exercise was terminated. The chest pain and electrocardiographic changes resolved quickly during recovery.

Two days later, coronary angiography revealed a normal circumflex coronary artery and an eccentric 80% proximal left anterior descending artery stenosis (Fig. 1). The right coronary artery demonstrated diffuse catheter-induced spasm upon engagement of the coronary ostium. Complete resolution of the right coronary artery spasm was achieved with 200 μg of intracoronary nitroglycerin and 0.4 mg sublingual nitroglycerin. Left ventricular angiography showed minimal anterolateral hypokinesis with a normal ejection fraction. After discussing the results with the patient and family, directional coronary atherectomy of the proximal left anterior descending artery stenosis was elected.

Prior to atherectomy, an evaluation of translesional hemodynamics was performed as previously described using a 0.018 inch flowire and 2.2F tracking catheter [4,5]. On passage of the guidewire beyond the stenosis, the patient complained of significant chest pain. At that point, the distal left anterior descending blood flow was minimal with an average peak velocity of <3.0 cm/sec.

38 yr old, Exercise ischemia + Spasm

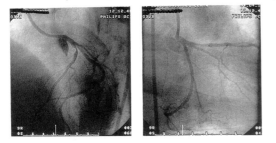

Fig. 1.   Cineangiographic frames of a proximal eccentric left anterior descending stenosis in the left anterior oblique (left) and right anterior oblique (right) projections. The plaque appears located on the medial or circumflex side of the left anterior descending artery opposite the circumflex artery without accumulation in the superior or inferior aspect (on the RAO view).

Immediate angiography showed complete occlusion of the left anterior descending artery at the site of the lesion. Intracoronary nitroglycerin (200 µg) was given with complete relief of the patient's symptoms and simultaneous improvement of the distal left anterior descending flow velocity to an average peak velocity of 12 cm/sec. A widely patent distal left anterior descending artery with brisk contrast filling (TIMI 3) was then demonstrated by angiography and the stenosis was similar to baseline in severity (80%).

Prior to the planned intervention, additional studies were performed. First translesional pressure gradients and blood flow velocity were measured during isometric handgrip exercise (Fig. 2). The baseline pressure gradient was 52 mm Hg with average peak flow velocity of 12 cm/sec. The patient exercised for 2 periods each of 2 min duration. Isometric exercise increased the mean aortic pressure by 25 mm Hg, which was associated with a mild increase in the translesional pressure gradient (60 mm Hg). With exercise, there was a 75% increase in distal left anterior descending artery average peak velocity from 12 to 20 cm/sec. No chest pain or ST segment changes occurred. Intracoronary nitroglycerin (200 µg) was given with a subsequent reduction in the baseline pressure gradient to 30 mm Hg, suggesting a vasoconstrictor tonus at the lesion was present at baseline which increased further during exercise. Subsequently, a cold pressor test was performed by putting the patient's left hand into ice slush for 90 sec, while monitoring distal left anterior descending artery flow velocity and aortic pressure (Fig. 3). Cold pressor testing increased mean aortic pressure 14 mm Hg, but without a change in the distal flow velocity (16 cm/sec).

Due to the severity and lability of the stenosis, balloon angioplasty was then elected as the initial procedure. The lesion was dilated multiple times using a 3.5 mm balloon catheter (Synergy, Mansfield Scientific, Watertown, MA) with only fair angiographic result. To better assess the results, two-dimensional intravascular ultrasound imaging of the lesion site was performed with a 3.5F Boston Scientific (Mansfield Scientific) catheter (Fig. 4). The intracoronary ultrasound catheter was advanced across the proximal left anterior descending artery. The ultrasound images (Fig. 4) showed extensive eccentric residual plaque burden present in the proximal left anterior descending artery. Based on the angiogram and two-dimensional ultrasound data, a decision was made to perform atherectomy of the proximal left anterior descending. A 7 French Atherocath was then advanced over the guidewire to the proximal left anterior descending lesion where serial atherectomy excisions were performed with a gradual increase of the atherocath balloon pressure to approximately 50–55 PSI. Two small pieces of plaque were recovered. Repeat intravascular ultrasound imaging demonstrated evidence of atherectomy cuts within the plaque area with improvement in the total luminal diameter. The post-asymmetric atherectomy angiogram revealed patency with minimal dissection at the proximal left anterior descending site, but persistent moderate stenosis. Additional balloon catheter (4.0 mm Cobra 18, Scimed Life Systems, Inc., Maple Grove, MN) dilations were performed after atherectomy.

After the final dilations, flow velocity was improved. However, within 3 min angiographic low flow was observed corresponding to flow velocity of 10 cm/sec (Fig. 5). Intracoronary verapamil (50 µg) was given with an increase in distal left anterior descending average peak flow velocity to 20 cm/sec (Fig. 5, middle). Post-procedural translesional hemodynamic assessment was then performed. After flow velocity stabilized, the isometric handgrip exercise was repeated without change in flow or gradient. The post-angioplasty resting translesional gradient was 8 mm Hg. Post-procedure angiogram revealed a residual stenosis of approximately 9% by computer caliper measurements (Fig. 6). A summary of the coronary hemodynamic data is shown in Table I. The patient did well after the procedure and has been symptom free for 4 months.

DISCUSSION
Vasomotion Complicating Fixed Coronary Artery Disease

In this young individual, coronary vasomotion was suspected on the basis of the clinical syndrome, including both rest and exertional angina. Treadmill testing gave an objective demonstration of variable angina and exercise-induced ST segment alterations with spontaneous resolution and re-induction over the course of vigorous exercise. The sensitivity of the coronary arteries to

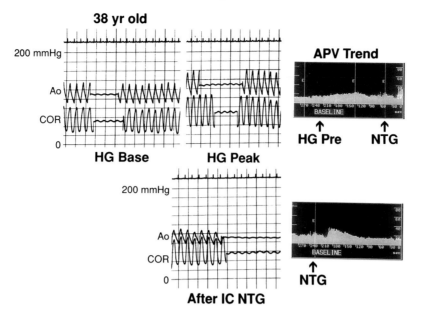

Fig. 2. Translesional pressure gradients and average flow velocity trends. Top left: Aortic (Ao) and distal left anterior descending (LAD) coronary (COR) artery pressure before handgrip (HG) isometric exercise. **Top middle:** Peak exercise response increased AO and cor pressures each by 20 mm Hg. **Top right:** 4.5 min (270 sec) continuous trend of average peak velocity (APV) during HG. Velocity scale is 0–100 cm/sec. Vertical lines (E) are event markers for onset and release of HG. **Lower middle:** Pressure gradient after intracoronary (IC) nitroglycerin (NTG). Ao = aortic pressure; COR = distal coronary artery pressure. Scale is 0–200 mm Hg. **Lower right:** Flow velocity trend shows typical hyperemic responses to NTG.

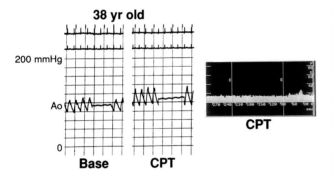

Fig. 3. Aortic (Ao) pressure and flow velocity trend during cold pressor testing (CPT). Abbreviations as in Figure 2. CPT increased mean arterial pressure 18 mm Hg without increasing average peak velocity. Format as in Figure 2.

mechanical stimulation was evident from catheter-induced vasospasm of the right coronary artery during diagnostic catheterization and, indeed, during minor guidewire stimulation on initial instrumentation of the left anterior descending coronary stenosis. Immediate resolution of the vasomotion compromising coronary blood flow in the left anterior descending artery was achieved with intracoronary nitroglycerin. The coronary vasoreactivity evident prompted alteration in the therapeutic approach by employing standard balloon angioplasty as the initial procedure. Perhaps the introduction of the atherectomy catheter would have been well toler-

ated, but the vigorous vasoconstrictor nature of the coronary artery already superimposed on a compromised lumen was felt to be an unnecessary complicating factor for this patient.

Variations of Translesional Pressure Gradients and Flow During Vasoconstriction

The influence of isometric exercise on translesional pressure and flow velocity demonstrated a response suggesting that the fixed component of the coronary artery resistance to flow was a predominant influence during this type of sympathetic stimulation. The baseline gradient of approximately 55 mm Hg was minimally increased in absolute value during peak handgrip exercise after 2 min. Aortic pressure increased from 110 to 120 mm Hg with a corresponding increase of the distal coronary pressure of 55 to 65 mm Hg. Associated with this increase in pressure gradient, coronary flow velocity increased. An increase in vasomotor tone at the lesion site or distal vessel would result in increasing flow velocity with a constant volume flow. Increased flow velocity may also reflect increased volumetric flow. Increased flow across a fixed stenosis usually increases the pressure gradient along the curvilinear pressure-flow velocity relationship. After handgrip exercise, intracoronary nitroglycerin reduced basal vasomotor tone, decreasing the baseline gradient from approximately 60 to 38 mm Hg. Intracoronary

38 yr old

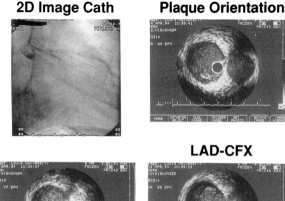

2D Image Cath   **Plaque Orientation**

LAD-CFX

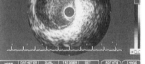

Pre Atherectomy   **Post Atherectomy**

Fig. 4. Interim and final procedural intravascular ultrasound 2-dimensional catheter images. Top left: Angiogram of imaging catheter position. Top right: Image orientation in the left main location to position the circumflex artery on the right side of the artery with plaque in the medial aspect. Bottom left: Left anterior descending lesion site after initial balloon angioplasty before atherectomy. Plaque is located on the left side of image indicated by catheter orientation to the circumflex artery. Bottom right: On 2-dimensional imaging after atherectomy, 2 cuts can be seen without major change in lumen area. Scale markers are 0.5 mm.

nitroglycerin produced a characteristic hyperemic flow response of approximately 1.6 times basal flow distal to the lesion.

Similar to isometric exercise, cold pressor testing increases systemic resistance and, in patients with coronary artery disease, coronary resistance [6–8]. In this patient, cold pressor testing increased aortic pressure from 95 to 110 mm Hg with no increase in distal flow velocity. This response is abnormal and characterizes the increased resistance of significant coronary artery lesions. Normally, cold pressor testing increases coronary blood flow in response to increased aortic pressure, resulting in unchanged or decreased coronary vascular resistance [8].

After angioplasty, repeat isometric handgrip exercise produced no increase in coronary blood flow velocity. The translesional pressure gradient, although not measured simultaneously, was <15 mm Hg. During handgrip exercise, systemic pressure increased, as occurred prior to angioplasty, but coronary flow velocity was unchanged. The attenuated flow responses may have been due to stimulation of the microcirculatory bed after an-

gioplasty/atherectomy. Cold pressor testing was not repeated following angioplasty due to the prolonged and complicated nature of the procedure.

Eccentric Plaque

Although angiographically satisfactory results were obtained using standard balloon angioplasty technique, residual intravascular plaque was evident with intravascular ultrasound, prompting a decision to proceed with atherectomy for further plaque removal. Likely due to the eccentric positioning of the plaque with a 100° arc of normal smooth muscle which had previously been characterized as highly reactive, atherectomy of the plaque was minimally successful. We speculate that the expansion of the vasoreactive segment of the artery was occurring and reduced the ability of the balloon to engage the cutter housing into the plaque at a depth great enough for sufficient plaque resection. We did not feel that a large atherectomy catheter was indicated. Due to the time constraints of the procedure, vasoreactivity testing by two-dimensional intravascular imaging was not performed.

Coronary Flow Responses to Intracoronary Verapamil

Angiographic slow flow has been associated with intravascular thrombolysis, angioplasty, directional and rotational atherectomy. The mechanism is unknown but may involve small vessel vasospasm. Low dose (50 μg) intracoronary verapamil, administered during a period of angiographically slow flow, produced only a minimal increase in hyperemia (12 to 20 cm/sec) which was delayed by about 100 sec after drug administration. During the same time intracoronary adenosine produced a 2-fold increase in coronary flow velocity. The hyperemic differences in intracoronary verapamil and adenosine during periods of slow flow have not been examined. Limited observations suggest that intracoronary verapamil may be the drug of choice for low reflow depending on the nature of the inciting incident [9].

Summary

Sympathetic stimulation produces characteristic changes in systemic and coronary hemodynamics which can be detected by pressure and flow velocity measurements in patients with coronary artery disease. In this particular patient with a highly reactive coronary vasculature in association with a fixed obstructive lesion, marked vasoreactivity produced striking differences in the resting translesional pressure gradient and flow velocity. Intracoronary nitroglycerin was immediately effective in relieving adverse vasoconstrictor tone. Studies of coronary hemodynamics during sympathetic stimulation in such patients will lead to improved understanding

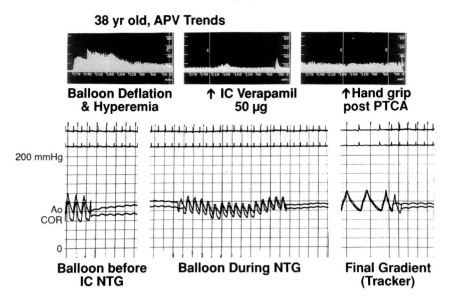

38 yr old, APV Trends

Balloon Deflation & Hyperemia   ↑ IC Verapamil 50 µg   ↑ Hand grip post PTCA

200 mmHg

Ao COR

0

Balloon before IC NTG   Balloon During NTG   Final Gradient (Tracker)

Fig. 5. Top left: Flow velocity trends after final balloon inflations. Top middle: Intracoronary verapamil 50 µg and (Top right) during isometric handgrip. Bottom: Final translesional pressure gradients with 4.0 mm deflated balloon catheter and 2.2F tracker catheter. The balloon catheter gradient was associated with vasoconstriction relieved by intracoronary nitroglycerin.

38 yr old

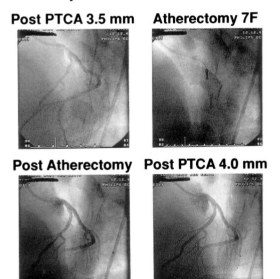

Post PTCA 3.5 mm   Atherectomy 7F

Post Atherectomy   Post PTCA 4.0 mm

Fig. 6. Top left: Cineangiograms after initial (3.5 mm) angioplasty balloon dilation. Top right: Atherectomy cutting window direct medially away from the circumflex. Bottom left: Angiograms after atherectomy. Bottom right: angiograms after final 4.0 mm balloon dilations.

TABLE I. Coronary Hemodynamic Data*

Condition	Stenosis (% diameter)	Pressure (mm Hg) MAP	Cor	▲P	Flow (cm/sec; APV)
Spasm	100	90	—	—	2.8
Nitroglycerin	80	85	—	—	12.0
Pre-PTCA					
Baseline	—	110	58	52	12.0
Handgrip	—	128	68	60	20.0
Nitroglycerin	—	90	60	30	38.0
Base	—	96	—	—	16.0
CPT	—	110	—	—	16.0
Post-PTCA/DCA					
Baseline	9	90	—	—	20.0
Handgrip	—	110	—	—	20.0
Balloon catheter	—	96	76	14	20.0
Nitroglycerin	—	96	88	8	20.0
Tracker final	—	96	88	8	20.0

*APV = average peak velocity; Cor = coronary artery pressure; CPT = cold pressor testing; DCA = directional atherectomy; MAP = mean arterial pressure; ▲P = pressure gradient.

ACKNOWLEDGMENTS

The authors thank the J.G. Mudd Cardiac Catheterization Team and Donna Sander for manuscript preparation.

REFERENCES

1. Maseri A, Severi S, DeNes M, L'Abbate A, Chierchia S, Marzilli M, Ballestra AM, Parodi O, Biagini A, Distante A: "Variant" angina: One aspect of a continuous spectrum of vasospastic myo-

of the therapeutic modalities and associated interventional techniques to treat ischemic producing vasoreactive coronary arteries.

cardial ischemia. Pathogenetic mechanisms, estimated incidence and clinical and coronary arteriographic findings in 138 patients. Am J Cardiol 42:1019–1035, 1978.

2. Waters D, Szlachcic J, Bourassa M, Scholl J, Théroux P: Exercise testing in patients with variant angina: Results, correlation with clinical and angiographic features and prognostic significance. Circulation 65:265–274, 1982.

3. Yasue H, Takizawa A, Nagao M, Nishida S, Horie M, Kubota J, Omote S, Takaoka K, Okumura K: Long-term prognosis for patients with variant angina and influential factors. Circulation 78: 1–9, 1988.

4. Donohue TJ, Kern MJ, Aguirre FV, Bach RG, Wolford T, Bell CA, Segal J: Assessing the hemodynamic significance of coronary artery stenoses: Analysis of translesional pressure-flow velocity relations in patients. J Am Coll Cardiol 22:449–458, 1993.

5. Kern MJ, Aguirre FV, Bach RG, Caracciolo EA, Donohue TJ: Translesional pressure-flow velocity assessment in patients. Cathet Cardiovasc Diagn 31:49–60, 1994.

6. Brown BG, Lee AB, Bolson EL, Dodge HT: Reflex constriction of significant coronary stenosis as a mechanism contributing to ischemic left ventricular dysfunction during isometric exercise. Circulation 70:18–24, 1984.

7. Mudge GH, Grossman W, Mills RM, Lesch M, Braunwald E: Reflex increase in coronary vascular resistance in patients with ischemic heart disease. N Engl J Med 295:1333–1337, 1976.

8. Mudge GH, Goldberg S, Gunther S, Mann T, Grossman W: Comparison of metabolic and vasoconstrictor stimuli on coronary vascular resistance in man. Circulation 59:544–550, 1979.

9. Babbitt DG, Perry JM, Forman MB: Intracoronary verapamil for reversal of refractory coronary vasospasm during percutaneous transluminal coronary angioplasty. J Am Coll Cardiol 12:1377–1381, 1988.

Part V

Rotational Atherectomy

Chapter 11

Influence of Adjunctive Balloon Angioplasty on Coronary Blood Flow After Rotational Atherectomy

Alexander F. Khoury, MD, Richard G. Bach, MD, and Morton J. Kern, MD

INTRODUCTION

Integration of coronary blood flow velocity measurements into interventional procedures has enhanced our understanding of coronary flow dynamics [1–3] and has provided new insights into coronary artery disease. Translesional flow velocity assists in the accurate and objective assessment of the severity of a coronary atherosclerotic lesion [4,5] and documents the restoration of coronary blood flow following balloon angioplasty [5]. New coronary interventional devices have recently been introduced that appear to be superior to conventional balloon angioplasty in achieving angiographic success in certain complex coronary lesions. Some calcified coronary stenoses and complex anatomic subsets, known to respond poorly to coronary angioplasty, can be successfully addressed by rotational atherectomy (Rotablator)

[6]. Although satisfactory luminal enlargement can be accomplished with the use of rotational atherectomy alone in some patients, adjunctive balloon angioplasty is necessary in most cases, to obtain a minimal residual angiographic result. The physiologic coronary responses in patients undergoing rotational atherectomy, with and without adjunctive coronary angioplasty, have not been well defined. To demonstrate the potential changes in coronary physiology induced by rotational atherectomy, serial coronary blood flow and translesional hemodynamics were measured following rotational atherectomy and again after adjunctive balloon angioplasty. The data from this case illustrate that coronary blood flow may not be normalized despite significant angiographic improvements after rotational atherectomy alone.

CASE REPORT

An 80-year-old man was admitted with unstable angina. Past history included an inferior wall myocardial infarction 8 months earlier. His post-myocardial infarction course was uncomplicated, and he was managed conservatively on medical therapy. Past medical history was also remarkable for hypertension and symptomatic bradycardia, which necessitated pacemaker implantation. A cerebrovascular accident 5 years prior to this admission was followed by right internal carotid artery endarterectomy.

The patient remained asymptomatic until 3 months earlier, when he experienced chest pain at rest unresponsive to sublingual nitroglycerin. In the emergency department, angina was controlled with intravenous nitroglycerin and morphine. He was admitted to the coronary care unit (CCU), where acute myocardial infarction was excluded. He was again discharged on medical therapy.

Two weeks prior to admission, resting chest pain recurred, which increased in frequency and intensity. Urgent cardiac catheterization was performed. Coronary angiography demonstrated total occlusion of the mid left anterior descending artery, an 80% stenosis of the first obtuse marginal, 80% stenoses of the proximal and 90% stenosis of the mid right coronary artery, and an 80% lesion at the origin of the posterior descending artery (Fig. 1). Hemodynamic assessment indicated no valvular pathology. The left ventricular ejection fraction was depressed at 30% with inferior and anterior segmental wall motion abnormalities. A myocardial radionuclide stress perfusion study was performed that showed reversible perfusion defects in the inferior and posterior distribution. In view of his overall medical condition, age, and depressed left ventricular ejection fraction, selective re-

Pre-Roto   **Pre-AP Cran**

1.75, 2.25 mm Burrs   **Post-Roto**

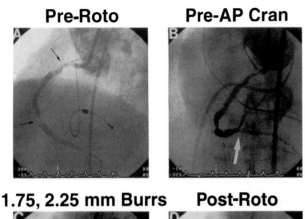

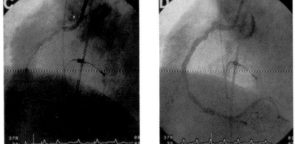

Fig. 1. **A:** Left anterior oblique projection. **B:** Anteroposterior (AP). cran, cranial projection. Right coronary artery angiography shows two sequential lesions (*arrow*) in the proximal right coronary artery and a third lesion at the takeoff of the posterior descending artery (*small white arrow*). **C:** Angiogram showing Rotablator burr during procedure. **D:** Angiographic results following rotational atherectomy.

vascularization of the highly calcified right coronary artery appeared to be a satisfactory initial approach to relieve unstable angina.

Physical examination on admission revealed an elderly white male. Blood pressure was 105/70 mm Hg. Pulse was 80/min and regular. Respiratory rate was 16/min and unlabored. The carotid artery examination was normal. There was no jugular venous distension. Chest examination was remarkable for a grade II/VI holosystolic murmur at the apex with normal heart sounds. The remainder of the examination was unremarkable.

Because of the highly calcified right coronary artery, rotational atherectomy was elected. To provide hemodynamic support and improve coronary perfusion, an intra-aortic balloon pump was inserted prior to the initiation of the procedure. To assess the influence of rotational ablation on coronary physiology, coronary blood flow velocity was measured with a 0.018-inch Doppler guidewire. The method and validation of the Doppler coronary flow measurements (FloWire, Cardiometrics, Inc., Mountain View, CA) have been previ-

ously reported [7]. Baseline and hyperemic (intracoronary adenosine, 12 μg) flow velocity were obtained proximal to the mid right coronary artery stenosis and distally within the posterior descending coronary artery (Fig. 2). Before rotational atherectomy, average peak velocities in the proximal and distal segments were 17 and 12 cm/sec, respectively with abnormal diastolic-to-systolic velocity ratios (DSVR) in both the proximal and distal segments (1.0 and 1.3, respectively). Coronary flow reserve was also impaired in both the proximal and distal regions (1.6 and 1.2, respectively). A translesional pressure gradient measured across the distal stenosis [Tracker-18 (2.7F) catheter] was 70 mmHg (Fig. 3). On catheter pullback to the proximal right coronary artery lesion, the gradient decreased to 12 mm Hg, with no intrinsic pressure gradient in the guide catheter.

The flow wire was exchanged for a 0.009-inch rotablator guidewire, positioned in the distal posterior descending artery. Rotational atherectomy using 1.75-mm and 2.25-mm burrs enlarged the ostial and mid right lesions. The distal posterior descending coronary artery lesion was treated with a 1.75-mm burr only. The patient tolerated rotational atherectomy without problems and with angiographic TIMI grade III flow. The 0.009-inch rotablator wire was exchanged for the Doppler guidewire, and flow velocity data were again obtained prior to adjunctive balloon angioplasty. Both proximal and, more importantly, distal blood flow velocity was slightly increased compared to the pre-rotablator values (Table I). Distal average peak velocity increased from 12 cm/sec to 22 cm/sec, with no change in the diastolic-to-systolic velocity ratio. Coronary flow reserve was mildly increased (1.5) in the distal segment. The alterations in coronary flow occurred with mean arterial blood pressure and heart rate comparable to pre-rotablator conditions.

Adjunctive balloon angioplasty was then performed with a 3.5-mm balloon catheter and then a 4.0-mm balloon catheter (Synergy Catheters, Mansfield, Inc., Boston, MA). Flow velocity data were again obtained (Fig. 4). Average peak velocity (27 cm/sec) and coronary flow reserve (2.0) were significantly increased with a diastolic-to-systolic velocity ratio of 1.5. The final pressure gradient across the most distal lesion was 30 mm Hg; the gradient across the proximal lesion was zero (Fig. 3, bottom right). At the end of the procedure, quantitative coronary angiography identified a 20% residual narrowing in the proximal right coronary artery, a 20% residual lesion in the mid right coronary artery, and a 5% residual lesion in the posterior descending artery (Fig. 5). The intra-aortic balloon pump was maintained for 24 hr with intravenous heparin. The post-procedure course was uncomplicated and he was discharged. At follow-up, he was free of exertional chest pain and fully active on medical therapy.

Pre-Roto   **CFR**

Proximal

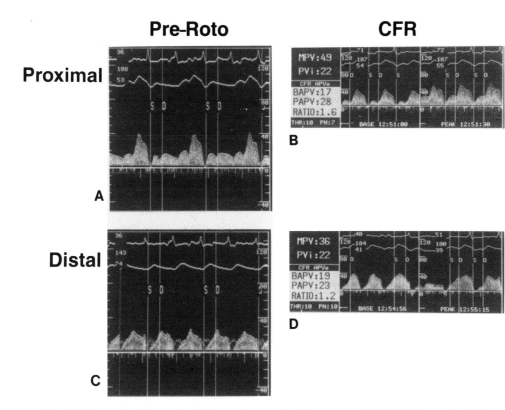

A

B

Distal

C

D

Fig. 2. Coronary Doppler flow velocity spectra before rotational ablation. Baseline proximal (A) and distal flow velocity (C), and coronary flow reserve (B, D). Proximal velocity spectra demonstrate effect of 2:1 intra-aortic balloon pumping. Average peak velocity (APV) is 18 cm/sec. Intra-aortic balloon pumping increased maximal velocity to 40 cm/sec. Distal average peak velocity was recorded with intra-aortic balloon pump off. Average peak velocity was 12–19 cm/sec. B: Proximal coronary flow reserve (ratio) was 1.6. D: Distal coronary flow reserve was 1.2. BAPV, baseline average peak velocity; PAPV, peak hyperemic average peak velocity. Velocity scale is 0–160 cm/sec. S and D demarcate systolic and diastolic periods.

DISCUSSION

This case illustrates the effects rotational atherectomy and adjunctive angioplasty on coronary flow velocity indices after treating hemodynamically significant coronary lesions. Translesional hemodynamic (flow/pressure) assessment prior to revascularization unequivocally established the severity of each of the sequential lesions described. The decrease in average peak velocity (<20 cm/sec) distal to the lesions was associated with reduced diastolic-to-systolic velocity ratio and coronary flow reserve. The severe translesional pressure gradient across the two most distal lesions was >30 mm Hg with a proximal-to-distal flow velocity ratio of >1.7. Following rotational atherectomy alone, coronary flow improved, with both the average peak velocity (12 cm/sec to 22 cm/sec) and diastolic-to-systolic velocity ratio (1.4) increasing. Coronary flow reserve increased only slightly (1.5).

Changes in coronary flow after rotablator alone have not been described. Prior studies demonstrate that intra-aortic balloon pumping does not significantly improve flow distal to critical stenoses [8]. Following successful

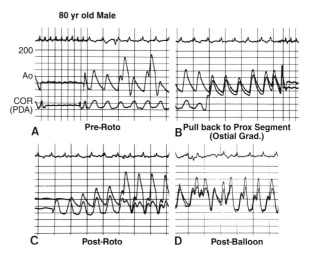

Fig. 3. A, B: Translesional pressure gradient before rotational atherectomy (pre-Roto). Following rotational atherectomy (C) and after adjunctive balloon angioplasty (D), the gradient is reduced. The effect of intra-aortic balloon pumping on aortic and distal coronary artery pressure can be appreciated. Ao, aortic pressure; Cor, distal coronary artery pressure, 0–200 mmHg scale; PDA, posterior descending artery.

TABLE I. Translesional Hemodynamics After Rotational Atherectomy and Adjunctive Balloon Angioplasty

	Average peak velocity (cm/sec)		Diastolic/systolic velocity ratio (units)		Coronary flow reserve (units)		Translesional pressure gradient (mmHg)	
	Proximal	Distal	Proximal	Distal	Proximal	Distal	IABP Off	IABP On
Pre-rotablator	17	12	1.0	1.3	1.6	1.2	70	100
Post-rotablator	18	22	1.0	1.4	1.9	1.5	24	40
Post-PTCA	—	27	—	1.5	—	2.0	24	5

Abbreviations: IABP, intra-aortic balloon pump; PTCA, percutaneous transluminal coronary angioplasty.

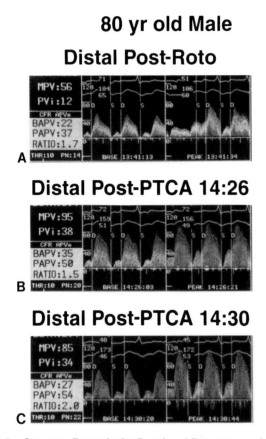

Fig. 4. Coronary flow velocity (base) and flow reserves (ratio) following rotational (roto) atherectomy (A) and after balloon angioplasty over time (B) and 4 min later (C). Format and appreciation as in Figure 2. Coronary flow reserve ratio increased from 1.7, 1.5, to 2.0. However, peak hyperemic velocity remained 50–54 cm/sec.

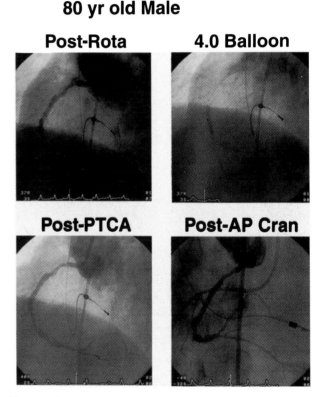

Fig. 5. Right coronary artery angiography following rotational atherectomy (Roto) and balloon angioplasty (PTCA). AP, anteroposterior projection; cran, cranial projection.

coronary angioplasty of severe coronary obstructions, intra-aortic balloon pumping markedly augments both proximal and distal coronary blood flow velocity [8]. In this patient, rotational atherectomy alone enlarged the lumen to permit enhanced diastolic coronary flow, which was further augmented during intra-aortic balloon pumping (Fig. 4). Intra-aortic balloon pump diastolic pressure augmentation was further and substantially increased by the larger lumen following coronary angioplasty (Fig. 3).

Interestingly, after rotational atherectomy, although distal coronary pressure and flow signals displayed sig-

nificant intra-aortic balloon pumping flow velocity augmentation compared to the tracings before rotational atherectomy, coronary flow reserve was unaffected by intra-aortic balloon pumping.

Preliminary studies have compared the post-procedural degree of change of distal vessel velocity indices after atherectomy, angioplasty, or balloon expandable coronary stents [9–11]. Younis et al. [9] found no difference in the increase in post-procedural flow velocity when comparing stent, atherectomy, and angioplasty procedures with similar angiographic results. By contrast, the data reported by Deychak et al. [10] demonstrated that flow velocity did not improve following routine coronary atherectomy, with the magnitude of the flow increase remaining below levels seen with angioplasty. The mechanism of this response is unknown. In most studies, distal flow parameters, except for coronary vasodilatory reserve, tend to increase to values found in angiographically normal vessels, irrespective of the intervention used. However, the mechanism of rotational atherectomy differs in that the production of minute (<4 μm) plaque debris may compromise the distal microvascular circulation. It is plausible that distal flow parameters would not necessarily normalize after rotational atherectomy, as would be expected to occur after conventional balloon angioplasty or directional atherectomy, where distal embolization of microparticulate debris is rarely appreciated as a complicating factor. A preliminary report by Kumar et al. [12] indicates that rotablator plus adjunctive balloon angioplasty does not normalize post-stenotic coronary vasodilatory reserve.

In this case, rotational coronary atherectomy marginally improved diastolic-to-systolic velocity ratios from 1.3 to 1.4; balloon angioplasty appeared to confer only slight additional benefit, with a final diastolic-to-systolic velocity ratio of 1.5, suggesting that although lumen enlargement could transmit flow (as evidenced by intraaortic balloon pump responses), the post-rotablator result remained suboptimal for flow normalization. The increase in phasic pattern after angioplasty suggested conduit enlargement without important myocardial contractile loss.

While normal coronary flow velocities may be restored following successful revascularization, vasoregulatory (compensatory) mechanism as assessed by flow velocity responses to intracoronary adenosine can remain severely impaired. The time course of this flow reserve normalization has been the subject of a number of studies assessing microcirculatory vasoregulatory function following angioplasty [13,14]. Marked improvements after adjunctive balloon angioplasty in this patient occurred within <5 min, to a value of 2.0.

This case represents one of the first explorations into the coronary physiology of rotational atherectomy with adjunctive balloon angioplasty. Further data should establish the impact of rotational atherectomy on coronary flow dynamics and coronary flow reserve as compared with other percutaneous modes of revascularization producing similar degrees of angiographic improvement. These data may assist in determining the physiologic mechanisms responsible for various clinical outcomes.

ACKNOWLEDGMENTS

The authors thank the J.G. Mudd Cardiac Catheterization Laboratory Team and Donna Sander for manuscript preparation.

REFERENCES

1. Straur B: The significance of coronary reserve in clinical heart disease. J Am Coll Cardiol 15:775–783, 1990.
2. Demer L, Gould KL, Kirkeeide RL: Assessing stenosis severity: Coronary flow reserve, collateral function, quantitative coronary arteriography, positron imaging, and digital subtraction angiography: A review and analysis. Prog Cardiovasc Dis 30:307–322, 1988.
3. Kern MJ, Donohue TJ, Bach RG, Aguirre FV, Caracciolo EA, Ofili EO: Quantitating coronary collateral flow velocity in patients during coronary angioplasty using a Doppler guidewire. Am J Cardiol 71(14):34D–40D, 1993.
4. Ofili EO, Labovitz AJ, Kern MJ: Coronary flow velocity dynamics in normal and diseased arteries. Am J Cardiol 71(14):3D–9D, 1993.
5. Ofili EO, Kern MJ, Labovitz AJ, St. Vrain JA, Segal J, Aguirre F, Castello R: Analysis of coronary blood flow velocity dynamics in angiographically normal and stenosed arteries before and after endolumen enlargement by angioplasty. J Am Coll Cardiol 21:308–316, 1993.
6. Warth DC, Leon MB, O'Neill W, Zacca N, Polissar NL, Buchbinder M: Rotational atherectomy multicenter registry: Acute results, complications and 6-month angiographic follow-up in 709 patients. J Am Coll Cardiol 24:641–648, 1994.
7. Doucette JW, Corl PD, Payne HM, Flynn AE, Goto M, Nassi M, Segal J: Validation of a Doppler guidewire for intravascular measurement of coronary flow velocity. Circulation 85:1879–1911, 1992.
8. Kern MJ, Aguirre F, Bach R, Donohue T, Siegel R, Segal J: Augmentation of coronary blood flow by intra-aortic balloon pumping in patients after coronary angioplasty. Circulation 87:500–511, 1993.
9. Younis L, Kern MJ, Bach R, Donohue T, Aguirre FV, Mechem C, Cauley M, Stonner T: Post-procedural normalization of coronary flow dynamics following successful atherectomy, PTCA and stenting: Analysis of intracoronary spectral Doppler. J Am Coll Cardiol 21:79A, 1993 (abst).
10. Deychak YA, Thompson MA, Rohrbeck SC, et al: A Doppler guidewire used to assess coronary flow during directional coronary atherectomy. Circulation 86:I-122, 1992 (abst).
11. Kern MJ, Bach RG, Donohue TJ, Caracciolo EA, Aguirre FV, Mechem C, Cauley M, Abbott L: Clinical utility of continuous coronary flow velocity monitoring during interventional studies. Cathet Cardiovasc Diagn 29:81, 1993.
12. Kumar K, Dorros G, Jain A, Dufek CA, Mathiak LM: Coronary flow measurements following rotational ablation (atherectomy). Cathet Cardiovasc Diagn 32(1):97 (P43), 1994 (abst).
13. Eichhorn EJ, Grayburn PA, Willard JE, et al: Spontaneous alterations in coronary blood flow velocity before and after coronary angioplasty in patients with severe angina. J Am Coll Cardiol 17:43–52, 1991.
14. Kern MJ, Donohue T, Bach R, Aguirre F, Bell C: Monitoring cyclical coronary blood flow alterations following coronary angioplasty for stent restenosis using a Doppler guidewire. Am Heart J 125:1159–1160, 1993.

Part VI

Stents

Chapter 12

Alterations of Coronary Flow Velocity Distal to Coronary Dissections Before and After Intracoronary Stent Placement

Morton J. Kern, MD, Frank V. Aguirre, MD, Richard G. Bach, MD,
Eugene A. Caracciolo, MD, Thomas J. Donohue, MD, Michael S. Flynn, MD,
and Joseph A. Moore, MD

INTRODUCTION

Translesional flow velocity can identify hemodynamically significant stenoses [1–3]. In addition to loss of the absolute distal translesional flow velocity and distal coronary hyperemic response to maximal intracoronary vasodilators, the predominant diastolic-to-systolic phasic flow pattern is usually severely impaired [3, 4]. The diastolic-to-systolic velocity ratio (DSVR) is related not only to epicardial coronary obstruction but also be abnormal myocardial contractility and ischemic dysfunction [5]. Furthermore, the new appearance of an abnormal from previously normal DSVR pattern should indicate an important flow altering event which may not be immediately apparent based on clinical or angiographic findings. In this Interventional Physiology review, we describe two patients undergoing coronary angioplasty which was complicated by coronary dissection. Alterations of the flow velocity patterns could be readily identified suggesting significantly impaired coronary lumina and flow. Restoration of the angiographic appearance and normalization of the distal flow velocity pattern were achieved after coronary stent placement. Recognition of abnormal distal coronary flow may assist in decision making for similar interventional procedures.

CASE 1: RIGHT CORONARY ARTERY DISSECTION

A 59-year old woman with angina pectoris and positive exercise thallium-201 scintigraphy had coronary arteriography which showed a severe, irregular, 8 mm long, 95% stenosis in the proximal right coronary artery (Fig 1, top panels). Angiographic collateral opacification during left coronary arteriography was not seen. Elective angioplasty was performed in a routine fashion from the right femoral artery using a standard Judkins 8F guiding catheter (0.084 in. Judkins 4 cm right, Cordis Corp., Miami, FL) through an 8F femoral arterial sheath. The diameter of the vessel was estimated to be 3.0 mm without significant tortuosity or excessive calcification. A 3.0 mm minimally compliant 0.018 in. guidewire-compatible balloon catheter (Olympix, Cordis Corp.) was selected. A 0.018 in. medium soft Doppler-tipped angioplasty FloWire (Cardiometrics, Inc., Mountain View, CA) was used as the primary crossing wire. The validation and method of use of the flowire have been described previously [1–3].

Coronary flow velocity was measured approximately 1 cm proximal and 3 cm distal to the lesion (Fig. 1, bottom panels). In this severely stenosed right coronary artery, the flow velocity demonstrates several findings of impaired flow. First, in the proximal location the flow pattern is systolic predominant with a DSVR of 0.7 (normal > 1.2 in proximal right coronary artery and > 1.5 in left coronary artery). After crossing the stenosis, distal flow velocity is diminished with marked blunting of the phasic pattern. The mean velocity decreased from 20 to

J.M., RCA, Positive Thallium

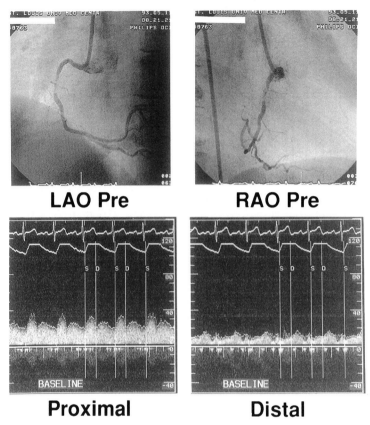

LAO Pre   **RAO Pre**

Proximal   **Distal**

Fig. 1. Top: Cineangiograms in the left and right anterior oblique (LAO, RAO) projections showing 95% proximal stenosis in the right coronary artery (RCA) (arrow). Locations of proximal and distal flow velocity measurements is shown by large open arrows. Pre = before angioplasty. Bottom: Proximal and distal flow velocity spectra show abnormal phasic pattern and diminished distal mean velocity.

10 cm/sec. There was no hyperemic response to intracoronary adenosine (6–8 μg). A translesional proximal/distal flow velocity integral ratio > 1.7 has been associated with translesional pressure gradients > 30 mm Hg in branching systems [3]. In non-branched vessels, such as right coronary artery with minimal proximal branching (as shown here), or saphenous vein or internal mammary artery grafts, a proximal/distal ratio often cannot be used. In this case, distal flow is diminished (proximal/distal ≈ 2.0) relative to proximal flow with only a trivial right ventricular branch interposed. A significant lesion was also characterized by loss of phasic pattern and impaired coronary flow reserve [1–3].

The guidewire was advanced to a posterolateral branch before positioning the balloon across the lesion. During balloon occlusion (Fig. 2, botton left), distal flow velocity revealed both antegrade and retrograde flow velocities consistent with collateral flow recruitment. Flow velocity reversal from collateral branch input is identified

by a negative spectral flow velocity below the zero baseline [6,7], especially evident during antegrade coronary flow cessation. The pattern of collateral flow was predominantly monophasic, most likely to result from intramyocardial collateral channels, such as could be expected during acute recruitment compared to angiographically visible mature epicardial collateral routes. Figure 3 shows a monophasic unidirectional collateral flow. The simultaneous antegrade and retrograde velocity during occlusion most likely indicates the collateral input source is upstream from the tip of the flowire with the majority of collateral flow occurring during systole. A detailed discussion of collateral flow velocity will be available in future Interventional Physiology presentations. As expected in patients with collateral circulation, coronary occlusion was well tolerated with minimal electrocardiographic or hemodynamic consequences. The immediate post-angioplasty result (Fig. 2, top panel) appeared highly satisfactory in the left anterior oblique view with

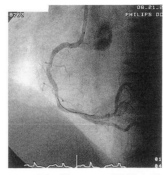

After Balloon Dilation

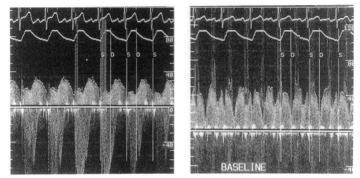

Post. Lat. Collaterals
During Occlusion   **Post PTCA**
Distal

Fig. 2. Top: Left anterior oblique projection immediately after angioplasty without evidence of dissection. Bottom left: Flow velocity during balloon occlusion shows systolic collateral flow reversal with persistent antegrade flow in the posterolateral (Post. Lat.) branch. Wire is distal to collateral input source. Bottom right: Flow velocity after angioplasty with improvement in mean velocity and phasic pattern.

a striking improvement in coronary flow velocity. The average velocity increased from 10 to 30 cm/sec with near normalization of the phasic flow velocity pattern (DSVR = 1.1; Fig. 2, bottom right panel). However, an angiogram in the right anterior oblique view a few minutes after dilation revealed a significant spiral dissection (Fig. 4, top left panel). Because of satisfactory post-percutaneous transluminal coronary angioplasty (PTCA) flow despite a dissection, a translesional pressure gradient was measured with a 2.2F tracking catheter. The gradient was 5 mm Hg. Distal flow velocity was continuously monitored and within 6 min an abnormal phasic flow velocity pattern emerged with a DSVR of 0.7 with a systolic predominant flow pattern (Fig. 4, bottom left panel). Mean velocity had also fallen to 18 cm/sec. Because of the large dissection with evidence of impaired flow, a 3.0 mm balloon expandable stent (Cook, Inc., Bloomington, Indiana) was inserted over the flowire through the 0.084 in. guide catheter. The angiographic result was excellent (Fig. 4, top middle and right panels) with a marked increase in distal flow and improvement

in the DSVR to 1.0 (Fig. 4, bottom middle panel). On withdrawal of the flowire to the proximal location, mean flow velocity is similar to distal flow > 45 cm/sec (twice that of flow velocity before angioplasty), but has a persistently systolic predominant flow pattern (DSVR = 0.9). This final DSVR is improved relative to that before angioplasty. This pattern can occasionally be seen in some non-diseased proximal regions of large right coronary arteries. The precise mechanism of the systolic predominant right coronary arter DSVR is incompletely understood.

CASE 2: SERIAL DISSECTIONS IN A LEFT ANTERIOR DESCENDING ARTERY

A 57-year-old man with insulin-dependent diabetes mellitus, hypertension, and renal insufficiency developed unstable angina prior to planned renal transplantation [8]. Despite optimal medical therapy, anginal chest pain recurred at rest associated with anterior ST depres-

Collateral Flow Reversal During Balloon Occlusion

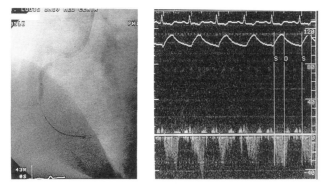

Fig. 3. Typical monophasic inverted flow velocity signal (right) during balloon occlusion (left). Note flow is predominantly occurring during the systolic period.

sion. Coronary arteriography demonstrated multiple severe left anterior descending coronary artery narrowings (Fig. 5, top panel). The left circumflex and right coro-

nary arteries had mild, non-critical (<50%) diameter narrowings.

Coronary angioplasty was performed with a 0.018 in. Doppler flowire (Cardiometrics, Inc.) and a 2.5 mm angioplasty balloon (Olympix, Cordis Corp.) through a routine femoral arterial approach. Sequential balloon inflations were performed for lesions A, B, and C (Fig. 5, top panel). Coronary flow velocity (Fig. 5, bottom left) obtained proximal to the left anterior descending lesion A was normal in phasic pattern (DSVR = 1.9) and mean velocity (38 cm/sec). The flowire was then advanced beyond the lesion C where coronary flow velocity was reduced to 18 cm/sec (mean velocity) with an abnormal DSVR of 1.2, with a diastolic predominant pattern (Fig. 5, bottom right). The proximal-to-distal flow velocity ratio of 2.1 suggested a transarterial pressure gradient >30 mm Hg. After the first series of balloon inflations for the three lesions, two areas of coronary dissection could be seen at locations B and C (Fig. 6, top left panel, labeled D). The angiographic flow appeared adequate without ischemic electrocardiogram abnormalities or symptoms. However, distal coronary flow velocity had a

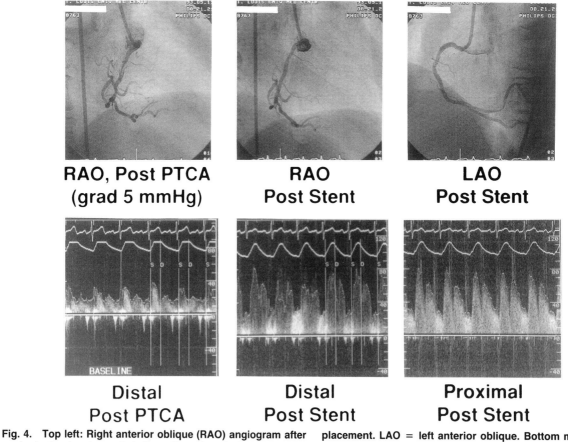

RAO, Post PTCA (grad 5 mmHg)	RAO Post Stent	LAO Post Stent
Distal Post PTCA	Distal Post Stent	Proximal Post Stent

Fig. 4. Top left: Right anterior oblique (RAO) angiogram after angioplasty showing spiral dissection. Translesional gradient (grad) was 5 mm Hg. Bottom left: Flow velocity 6 min after angiogram above showing abnormal systolic predominant flow velocity pattern. Top middle, right: Angiograms after stent placement. LAO = left anterior oblique. Bottom middle, right: Flow velocity after stent placement shows marked improvement in mean velocity (45 cm/sec) and DSVR. Proximal DSVR of 0.9 is still abnormal despite markedly improved flow.

57 yr old Male, LAD, DM, Multiple Lesions

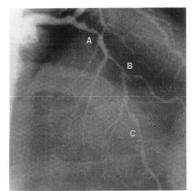

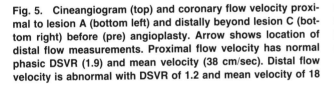

Pre PTCA

Fig. 5. Cineangiogram (top) and coronary flow velocity proximal to lesion A (bottom left) and distally beyond lesion C (bottom right) before (pre) angioplasty. Arrow shows location of distal flow measurements. Proximal flow velocity has normal phasic DSVR (1.9) and mean velocity (38 cm/sec). Distal flow velocity is abnormal with DSVR of 1.2 and mean velocity of 18 cm/sec. Velocity scale is 0–200 cm/sec. Electrocardiogram and arterial pressure are displayed at top of flow scale. Vertical lines mark systolic (S) and diastolic (D) flow periods. (Modified with permission from the *American Heart Journal* 127:436–438, 1994.)

new and abnormal systolic predominant flow pattern (DSVR = 0.6) with an unchanged mean flow velocity (22 cm/sec) (Fig. 6, bottom left panel). Because of the unsatisfactory angiographic and flow velocity findings, prolonged (5 min) balloon inflations were performed. A reperfusion balloon catheter could not negotiate the tortuous and dissected segments beyond lesion B. After prolonged balloon inflations, mild angiographic improvement (Fig. 6, top middle panel) was associated with only minimally improved distal flow velocity. The distal mean flow velocity was 16 cm/sec with a DSVR of 1.1 (Fig. 6, bottom middle panel). Because of the extensive dissection in both distal and mid left anterior descending angioplasty sites with impaired coronary flow velocity, 2 serial 2.5 × 20 mm stents (Cook, Inc.) were inserted into the dissected portions of the artery at locations B and C. Angiographic results were improved with residual evidence of dissection at lesion B. Part of the mid vessel dissection at location B remained angiographically visible despite stent placement covering

nearly all of the dissection length (Fig. 6, top right). Distal flow velocity normalized with a mean velocity of 39 cm/sec and DSVR of 2.2 (Fig. 6, bottom right). With restoration of normal distal flow, further dilations and stent placements were deemed unnecessary. Despite intravenous heparin for 48 hr with adequate anticoagulation, the patient developed angina associated with 0.5–1 mm anterior ST segment elevations on electrocardiogram and was sent for urgent bypass surgery. The patient did well post-operatively.

DISCUSSION

Decisions regarding the results of coronary interventions can be difficult at times due to the well-known limitations of angiography [9,10]. Using continuously measured coronary flow velocity, the physiologic significance of various post-procedural angiographic findings such as haziness, dissections, or intermediately severe stenoses can be assessed [1–3].

These cases demonstrate that abnormal phasic patterns

57 yr old Male, LAD, DM, Multiple Lesions

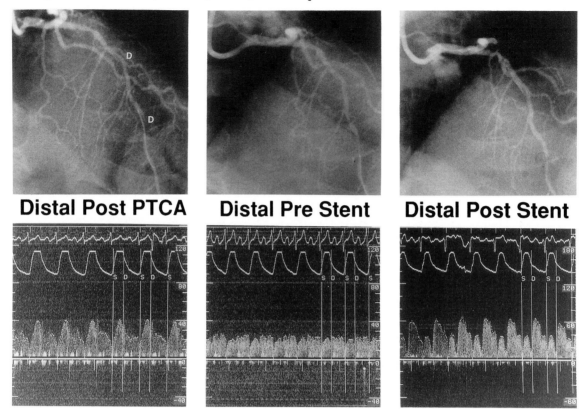

Fig. 6. Cineangiograms (top) and corresponding flow velocity data (bottom left) after coronary angioplasty (PTCA), before stent placement at dissected (D) regions (bottom middle), and after two serial stent implantations (bottom right). Distal flow velocity after serial balloon inflations showed abnormal systolic precominant flow pattern (DSVR = 0.6, bottom left). Prolonged balloon dilations improved the DSVR, but did not normalize phasic flow (bottom middle). After stent placement, distal flow velocity is normal in phasic pattern (DSVR = 2.2) and is equivalent to proximal pre-procedural values (40 cm/sec, bottom right). Velocity scale is 0–200 cm/sec for pre-stent angioplasty panels and 0–300 cm/sec for post-stent velocity scale.

of coronary flow beyond significant lesions can be restored with angioplasty and then may revert to an abnormal pattern when flow-limiting dissections compromise the lumina. Based on angiography alone, a decision against a stent in the first case may have been made based on the left anterior oblique angiogram and low translesional gradient. Flow monitoring demonstrated abnormal flow in the absence of clinical or new angiographic findings. Similarly, in case 2, the dissections were associated with marginal but acceptable angiographic results which could have been managed with observation and prolonged heparin therapy. The abnormal flow pattern was further physiologic evidence of limited flow which was normalized after serial stent placement.

Systolic Predominant Flow

Abnormal phasic flow velocity patterns were reported by Segal et al. [1] distal to severe lesions. Normalization of DSVR was associated with angiographic improvement [1,2]. Similar data were reported by Ofili et al. [2] in which at least 30% of patients undergoing angioplasty had abnormal distal DSVR. The precise mechanism by which a systolic predominant flow pattern occurs is unknown but several investigators [4,5] postulate abnormal flow due to arterial luminal narrowing, myocardial contractility, microvascular abnormalities, or absence of left ventricular myocardial supply. The low DSVR is usually due to an abnormally low diastolic flow velocity integral and not secondary to an elevated systolic flow velocity integral. Normalization of the DSVR is usually accomplished by an increase in the diastolic component of flow. The normal proximal right coronary artery has a lower DSVR than the left coronary artery [4], which may reflect the lower compressive effects of contraction of right compared to left ventricular myocardium.

Severe dissections with adequate angiographic flow may be associated with a markedly abnormal systolic predominant flow pattern. Further reparative dilations aimed at improving the angiographic appearance may be performed with only minor improvement in distal flow velocity as shown. Complete normalization of distal flow velocity was achieved with stent placement both singly in the right coronary artery and serially in the left anterior descending artery. It should be recognized that immediate post-stent flow may not predict impending abrupt vessel closure which can occur despite restoration of a normal diastolic predominant pattern. It has also been acknowledged that small stents (<2.5 mm) and diffuse arterial disease are significant risk factors for post-intervention arterial compromise or closure [9,10], which likely played a significant role in case 2. Several studies indicate that arteries receiving stents of 2.5 mm diameter or smaller have higher subacute rates of thrombosis than vessels with stents >3.0 mm, despite equivalent angiographic results and identical vigorous anticoagulation regimens [9,10]. Normal flow velocity after stent placement was seen with the persistence of an angiographic dissection.

Because of the difficulty in recrossing multiple lesions after balloon dilations, differential flow velocity between serial lesions was not assessed. Using distal flow, the effects of the serial dilations of the more proximal lesions could be assessed. However, in the particular case example, flow did not improve until all lesions were dilated. It was interesting to note that placement of the initial distal stent at location C did not completely normalize flow. Only after the more proximal stent implantation was completed did flow velocity normalize.

Preliminary experience with flow velocity monitoring during coronary interventions has identified several patterns of unstable or unsatisfactory flow velocity which include cyclical flow variations on thombus formation [11,12], continuous decline of mean velocity trend of impending vessel occlusion [13], abrupt flow cessation due to spasm or vasovagal hypotension [14], and transiently accelerated flow velocity of coronary spasm (and reversal of both velocity and artery spasm after nitroglycerin) [15]. Abnormal systolic predominant coronary phasic flow velocity patterns can be reversed after angioplasty and, as currently demonstrated, normalized after stent placement. Use of distal flow velocity and physiologic responses should facilitate decision making during coronary interventions when angiographic results remain in question.

ACKNOWLEDGMENTS

The authors thank the J.G. Mudd Cardiac Catheterization Laboratory team, Trina Stonner, RN, MSN, Marilyn Cauley, Carol Mechem, RN, and Lisa Abbott and Donna Sander for manuscript preparation.

REFERENCES

1. Segal J, Kern MJ, Scott NA, King SB III, Doucette JW, Heuser RR, Ofili E, Siegel R: Alterations of phasic coronary artery flow velocity in man during percutaneous coronary angioplasty. J Am Coll Cardiol 20:276–286, 1992.
2. Ofili EO, Kern MJ, Labovitz AJ, St Vrain JA, Segal J, Aguirre F, Castello R: Analysis of coronary blood flow velocity dynamics in angiographically normal and stenosed arteries before and after endoluminal enlargement by angioplasty. J Am Coll Cardiol 21: 308–316, 1993.
3. Donohue TJ, Kern MJ, Aguirre FV, Bach RG, Wolford T, Bell CA, Segal J: Assessing the hemodynamic significance of coronary artery stenoses: Analysis of translesional pressure-flow velocity relationships in patients. J Am Coll Cardiol 22:449–458, 1993.
4. Spaan JAAE, Breuls NPW, Laird JD: Diastolic-systolic coronary flow differences are caused by intramyocardial pump action in the anesthetized dog. Circ Res 49:584–593, 1981.
5. Goto M, Flynn AE, Doucette JW, Kimura A, Hiramatsu O, Yamamoto T, Ogasawara Y, Tsujioka K, Hoffman JIE, Kajiya F: Effect of intracoronary nitroglycerin administration on phasic pattern and transmural distribution of flow during coronary artery stenosis. Circulation 85:2296–2304, 1992.
6. Kern MJ, Donohue TJ, Bach RG, Aguirre FV, Caracciolo EA, Ofili EO: Quantitating coronary collateral flow velocity in patients during coronary angioplasty using a Doppler guidewire. Am J Cardiol 71(14):34D–40D, 1993.
7. Ofili E, Kern MJ, Tatineni S, Deligonul U, Aguirre F, Serota H, Labovitz AJ: Detection of coronary collateral flow by a Doppler-tipped guidewire during coronary angioplasty. Am Heart J 122: 221–225, 1991.
8. Kern MJ, Aguirre FV, Bach RG, Donohue TJ, Caracciolo EA: Restoration of normal phasic flow velocity after multiple coronary artery stent placement. Am Heart J 127:436–438, 1994.
9. Roubin GS, Cannon AD, Agrawal SK, Macander PJ, Dean LS, Baxley WA, Breland J: Intracoronary stenting for acute and threatened closure complicating percutaneous transluminal coronary angioplasty. Circulation 85:916–927, 1992.
10. Schatz RA, Baim DS, Leon M, Ellis SG, Goldberg S, Hirshfeld JW, Cleman MW, Cabin HS, Walker C, Stagg J, Buchbinder M, Teirstein PS, Topol E, Savage M, Perez JA, Curry RC, Whitworth H, Sousa EJ, Tio F, Almagor Y, Ponder R, Penn IM, Leonard B, Levine SL, Fish RD, Palmaz JC: Clinical experience with the Palmaz-Schatz coronary stent. Circulation 83:148–161, 1991.
11. Eichhorn EJ, Grayburn PA, Willard JE, et al.: Spontaneous alterations in coronary blood flow velocity before and after coronary angioplasty in patients with severe angina. J Am Coll Cardiol 17:43–52, 1991.
12. Anderson HV, Kirkeeide RL, Stuart Y, Smalling RW, Heibig J, Willerson JT: Coronary artery flow monitoring following coronary interventions. Am J Cardiol 71(14):62D–69D, 1993.
13. Kern MJ, Aguirre FV, Donohue TJ, Bach RG, Caracciolo EA, Flynn MS: Coronary flow velocity monitoring after angioplasty associated with abrupt reocclusion. Am Heart J, 1993.
14. Kern MJ, Bach RG, Donohue TJ, Caracciolo EA, Aguirre FV, Mechem C, Cauley M, Abbott L: Clinical utility of continuous coronary flow velocity monitoring during interventional studies. Cathet Cardiovasc Diagn 29:81, 1993 (Abstract).
15. Donohue T, Kern MJ, Wolford T, Bach R, Aguirre F, Miller L: The effects of epicardial coronary spasm on intracoronary flow velocity and pressure gradient in a patient after cardiac transplantation. Am Heart J 124:1645–1648, 1992.

Part VII

Collateral Blood Flow

Chapter 13

Collateral Flow Velocity Alterations in the Supply and Receiving Coronary Arteries During Angioplasty for Total Coronary Occlusion

Morton J. Kern, MD, Jan J. Piek, MD., Frank V. Aguirre, MD, Richard G. Bach, MD, Eugene A. Caracciolo, MD, and Thomas J. Donohue, MD

INTRODUCTION

The study of collateral flow in patients with coronary artery disease has been confined principally to a semi-quantitative angiographic methodology based on an arbitrary visual grading system of the degree of collateral vessel opacification. The correlation between the degree of opacification and collateral coronary flow in animal models is fair, but poorly quantitated in man due to limitations of the available technology to measure collateral flow [1, 2]. Due to methodologic problems of establishing animal models of coronary artery disease with collaterally supplied regions, precise quantitation within the animal experimental arena has had limited usefulness in extrapolating findings to patients. With the recent development of the Doppler-tipped angioplasty guidewire (Cardiometrics, Inc., Mountain View, CA.), collateral flow velocity can be detected acutely during coronary balloon occlusion. Collateral flow velocity is quantitated as persistent retrograde or antegrade flow velocity signals during artery occulsion. The direction of flow approaching the Doppler guidewire tip as it resides within the distal portion of the collaterally supplied vessel will the distal portion of the collaterally supplied vessel will be determined by the input supply location [3]. Flow beyond chronically occluded artery segments supplied by collat-

eral vessels can be studied after crossing the obstruction with the Doppler flowire.

Analysis of spectral flow velocity changes in the contralateral artery during coronary angioplasty has been recently described as a new method for assessing collateral flow [4]. This method of examination of flow velocity in the contralateral supply artery during angioplasty demonstrated that collateral flow resistance of the receiving vascular bed was significantly reduced when angiographic collateral vessels were present during coronary occlusion. The contribution of collateral supply during coronary balloon occlusion was evidenced by a significant increase in flow velocity in the contralateral artery due to reduced resistance in the collateral vascular bed. Using 2 flow velocity guidewires, one in the collateral supply artery and the other in the distal part of the receiving artery, the simultaneous alterations in collateral flow and resistance can be examined. This simultaneous method provides the ability to study the important contribution and physiologic responses of collateral flow in patients. In this discussion of interventional physiology, 2 patients will be presented describing transient alterations in both contralateral and ipsilateral coronary blood flow related to collateral flow during coronary angioplasty. These novel observations will demonstrate dynamic alterations in coronary flow as perfusion pressure is improved with epicardial luminal enlargement.

33 yr old Male, Ant NQMI, LAD 100%

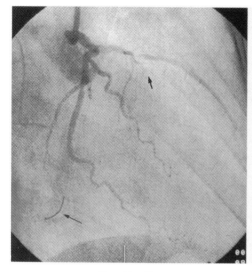
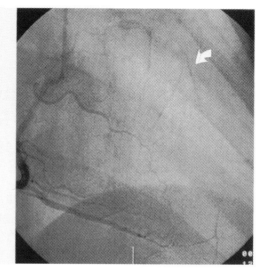

LCA

RCA
Collaterals

Fig. 1.   Left: Frames from cineangiogram of a 33-year-old man with a non-Q wave myocardial infarction. Left coronary artery (LCA) angiography revealed total occlusion of the left anterior descending (LAD, arrow) and no collateral filling of the right coronary artery. A Doppler flowire is positioned in the non-opacified right coronary artery (RCA) in this view (arrow). Right: Right coronary angiography in the right anterior oblique projection showing a late frame of right coronary filling with opacification of the left anterior descending collateral bed (white arrow).

Collateral Flow in Total Left Anterior Descending Artery With Right-to-Left Septal Collaterals

A 33-year-old man had a non-Q wave anterior myocardial infarction with mild post-infarction anginal pain. Thallium scintigraphy revealed a reversible anterior perfusion defect. Coronary arteriography showed totally occluded left anterior descending vessel at the proximal portion immediately after the first septal perforator with Rentrop grade II collateral filling from the right coronary artery (Fig. 1). Coronary angioplasty was planned with assessment of collateral function using a 2-flow velocity guidewire technique. A 0.018 in. Doppler flow velocity guidewire was positioned distal to the total occlusion in the left anterior descending artery prior to angioplasty through the right femoral artery, cannulated with an 8F sheath. Placement of a second coronary flow velocity guidewire in the posterior descending branch of the right coronary artery through a 5F right Judkins catheter positioned through the left femoral artery was performed without difficulty. The method of use of Doppler-tipped angioplasty has been described elsewhere [3]. Angioplasty was performed using a JL4 large lumen guiding catheter positioned in the ostium of the left coronary artery. Prior to angioplasty, the left anterior descending artery occlusion was easily traversed with the 0.018 in. Doppler flowire. Simultaneous flow velocity signals for the left anterior descending and posterior descending coronary arteries are shown on Figure 2.

Flow velocity data obtained in the proximal left anterior descending artery before crossing the total occlusion had a normal phase diastolic/systolic flow velocity ratio (>2.0) with a mean flow velocity of 31 cm/sec (Fig. 2A, top left). After crossing the left anterior descending artery occlusion, distal flow velocity fell to < 10 cm/sec. The flow velocity was predominantly antegrade since the tip of the flowire was distal to the septal artery collateral input location. Coronary occlusion with the balloon catheter caused a shift in collateral flow velocity input (Fig. 2A, top right) as evidenced by increased antegrade and retrograde signals. After successful angioplasty (Fig. 2A, middle left), distal left anterior descending flow velocity was entirely antegrade with an improved but mildly abnormal diastolic/systolic flow velocity ratio (1.4). The mean flow velocity increased from 10 to 27 cm/sec (Fig. 2A, middle left). After 12 min of observation, left anterior descending flow velocity improved further with a diastolic/systolic flow velocity ratio of >2.0 and mean flow velocity of 43 cm/sec (Fig. 2A, middle right).

Simultaneous continuous flow velocity trends of the average peak velocity during left anterior descending balloon occlusion and deflation and during administration of intracoronary adenosine to produce coronary hyperemia are shown in Figure 2B. The trend of average peak flow velocity in the left anterior descending (Fig. 2B, top left) can be seen to decrease from 30 to < 10 cm/sec on crossing the obstruction. Posterior descending artery flow is stable at 20 cm/sec (Fig. 2B, bottom left). There is no increase in posterior descending artery flow during left anterior descending balloon inflation. The velocity trend in the left anterior descending artery registers zero (during retrograde flow), but on balloon deflation produces a striking increase in antegrade flow. Simultaneous posterior descending artery flow decreases 10–15% for 60 sec (Fig. 2B, lower left panel, balloon down arrow). A second balloon inflation produced a similar but lesser magnitude flow response in both the left anterior descending and posterior descending arteries with a gradual reduction (5–10%) in posterior descending artery flow velocity, while left anterior descending flow stabilized to a higher level in the 10–15 min period after angioplasty.

To assess collateral responses to coronary vasodilators, intracoronary adenosine was given in the right coronary artery supplying the anterior wall infarct zone. Intracoronary adenosine (12 μg) produced no hyperemia and had no effect on left anterior descending artery flow and a minimal effect on posterior descending artery with a blunting of the previously observed flow decrease on release of left anterior descending balloon occlusion (Fig. 2B, Adeno [RCA], Ad [LAD] arrows). Intracoronary adenosine had no effect on right coronary artery distal flow when given in the left anterior descending after angioplasty. It is interesting to note the lack of adenosine hyperemia in both left anterior descending and right coronary artery regions in the post-infarction periods.

Final coronary angiography (Fig. 3) indicated a patent left anterior descending artery with no evidence of right-to-left collateral flow in this patient.

Collateral Flow in Total Right Coronary Artery Occlusion With Left-to-Right Septal Collaterals

A 68-year-old woman was referred for coronary angioplasty because of anginal pain, functional class 3 according to the classification of the Canadian Cardiovascular Society. The patient did not have a history of a previous myocardial infarction. An exercise electrocardiogram revealed ST segment depression of >0.1 mV in leads II, III, and aVF.

Coronary angiography demonstrated a total occlusion at the middle segment of the right coronary artery with Rentrop grade III collateral filling from the normal left coronary artery (Fig. 4). Angioplasty was performed using an 8F JR4 guiding catheter positioned in the ostium of the right coronary artery. The right coronary artery occlusion was traversed with a 0.014 in. high torque floppy wire and was exchanged for a 0.014 in. Doppler flow velocity guidewire prior to angioplasty. The distal right coronary artery flow velocity during balloon occlusion was predominantly antegrade since the tip of the guidewire was distal to the septal artery collateral input location. The mean flow velocity was 6 cm/sec, the maximal diastolic flow velocity was 14 cm/sec. To assess collateral hyperemia, 0.2 mg nitroglycerin was administered in the left coronary artery during balloon coronary occlusion. Mean collateral flow velocity increased from 6 to 11 cm/sec and maximal diastolic flow velocity increased from 14 to 20 cm/sec (Fig. 5). After administration of 12.5 mg papaverine in the left coronary artery during a subsequent balloon coronary occlusion, mean flow velocity increased from 7 to 10 cm/sec and maximal diastolic flow velocity increased from 13 to 16 cm/sec (Fig. 6). Coronary wedge pressure was measured through the fluid-filled lumen during subsequent balloon inflations after withdrawal of the guidewire. The administration of nitroglycerin and papaverine was repeated during successive balloon inflations for assessment of its effect on the coronary wedge pressure. The coronary wedge pressure/aortic pressure ratio increased from 0.40 to 0.50 after the administration of nitroglycerin and remained unchanged after the administration of papaverine. After successful angioplasty, distal right coronary artery flow velocity was entirely antegrade with a mean flow velocity of 16 cm/sec and normal distal phasic velocity pattern with a diastolic/systolic velocity ratio of 1.9.

DISCUSSION

These cases illustrate unique properties of collateral flow as measured by changes in the supply and receiving vascular beds. No similar observations have been available in experimental animal models and these findings will require confirmation with larger and more controlled studies. The dynamics of the collateral circulation in chronic coronary occlusion have been evaluated predominantly by thallium-201 scintigraphy [5–7]. These investigators focused attention on the interpretation of perfusion defects in the assessment of the functional capacity of the collateral circulation during exercise. The unique properties of the Doppler flow velocity guidewire system enable the assessment of coronary flow beyond coronary narrowings. In contrast to perfusion scintigraphy, this new investigational tool facilitates the study of the hemo-

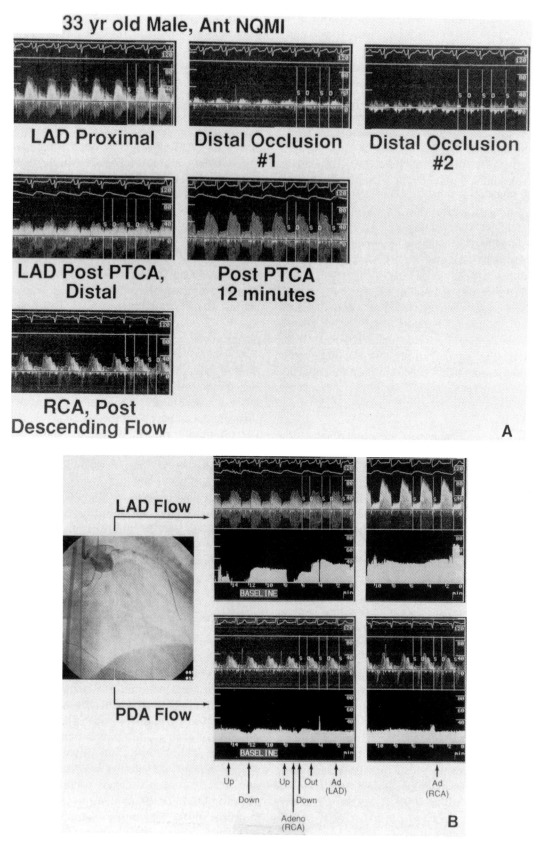

Fig. 2.

dynamics of the collateral circulation in a more direct way.

One of the major issues regarding changes in supply and receiving vessels is the question about whether the observed alterations truly reflect collateral flow or are related to other features of the coronary circulation in which a change in flow velocity occurs during transient ischemia. It is important to consider that brief coronary occlusion may be associated with alterations in arterial pressure, heart rate, or myocardial preload and thus induce coronary flow increases to compensate for the changes in myocardial demand. However, during the transient coronary occlusion of 60–120 sec, these findings occur rapidly, but are generally stable so that changes in flow velocity should reflect the reduction of collateral flow resistance or the stimulation of flow due to balloon coronary artery occlusion. Simultaneous assessment of both contralateral supply flow and recipient collateral flow help to delineate changes in flow due to changes in collateral resistance vs. myocardial demand factors.

The magnitude of volume flow changes in coronary

collateral circulation depend on the alterations in flow velocity and cross-sectional area of the supply and receiving artery. These arteries were not simultaneously imaged for vessel area analysis, but it is unlikely that the cross-sectional area would significantly be increased by transient balloon occlusion. The vasomotor properties and diameter changes of the distal bed during angioplasty have yet to be systematically studied.

There may be several conclusions that can be drawn from observations of the collateral flow responses in the contralateral supply artery. First, it is noteworthy that contralateral collateral flow velocity was diminished simultaneous with restoration of antegrade left anterior descending artery flow. The increased pressure and antegrade flow in the left anterior descending artery would close the septal collateral circuits or reduce flow through the collateral bed. This increased resistance was suggested by the transient decrease in the posterior descending artery supply region.

Based upon both experimental and clinical observations [4,8], the 10–15% sudden decrease of contralateral coronary flow after balloon deflation likely reflects the contribution of collateral flow. Right coronary artery flow velocity was re-established after the first left anterior descending coronary occlusion. After the second left anterior descending coronary occlusion, a transient but lesser reduction in collateral supply could again be demonstrated for the right coronary artery supply response. As coronary flow stabilized, the left anterior descending coronary flow gradually increased while the right remained constant. Flow velocity was unaffected by adenosine given either in the left or right coronary artery. The impaired vasodilatory responses of the 2 beds may be due to the setting of acute myocardial ischemia and re-establishment of supply. Nevertheless, a reduced response in 2 vascular beds requires careful interpretation as it may also be related to technical failure.

The observations in the second patient are a clear example of pharmacologic modulation of collateral flow in chronic coronary occlusion. The administration of nitroglycerin as well as papaverine in the contralateral artery resulted in a significant increase of flow in the ipsilateral artery. The magnitude of volume flow changes in the coronary collateral circulation depends on the alterations in flow velocity and cross-sectional area of the artery. The ipsilateral artery was not simultaneously visualized during the flow velocity assessment. Consequently, the direct effect of the administration of the vasodilators on the cross-sectional area remains unknown. The coronary wedge/aortic pressure ratio increased after the administration of nitroglycerin, indicating that pressure changes may also have affected the cross-sectional area. In contrast to the situation in acute coronary occlusion, a chronic coronary occlusion constitutes a ''stable'' condition fa-

---

Fig. 2. **A:** Phasic patterns of flow velocity for the left anterior descending (LAD) and right coronary artery (RCA) during the various balloon inflations to indicate the phasic patterns. Top panel, left: proximal left anterior descending shows normal phasic pattern. Middle panel, top: during balloon occlusion, there is a minimal collateral flow reversal with persistent antegrade signal of collateral flow. Right panel, top: during subsequent occlusion, both antegrade and retrograde collateral flow velocity can be detected. A small change in wire position relative to the collateral input source may also produce this pattern. Middle panel, left: following coronary angioplasty, left anterior descending coronary flow is markedly increased with a normal pattern and continues to increase over the following 12 min (middle panel, right). Bottom panel: Right coronary artery flow was normal in its phasic pattern in the posterior descending artery. The scale is 0–200 cm/sec. S and D = systolic and diastolic time periods based on the electrocardiogram algorithm. **B:** Trend of average peak flow velocity spectra in patient 1 with flow velocity guidewires placed in both the left anterior descending (LAD) and posterior descending coronary arteries (PDA) (angiogram). Trend panels demonstrate flow trend during balloon occlusions (up arrows), deflations (down arrows), and intracoronary adenosine (Adeno, Ad; arrows). Top trend panels represent left anterior descending flow velocity with simultaneous posterior descending artery flow on the lower panels. RCA = right coronary artery. The trend of average peak flow velocity is shown over a 15 min time base on a 0–100 cm/sec scale. The trend panels are split into phasic display on top and trend flow on lower panel. Note that with balloon deflation, flow increases in the left anterior descending coronary artery and decreases in the contralateral posterior descending vessel. This decrease in flow is then returned to baseline and stabilized. With a second balloon deflation, again, a smaller drop in right coronary artery flow was observed. Adenosine had minimal effect on either coronary vascular bed.

33 yr old Male, Post LAD PTCA

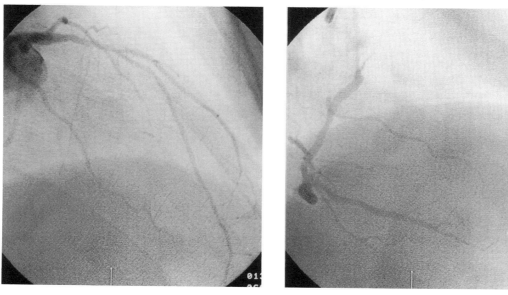

LCA   **RCA**

Fig. 3.   Coronary angiography after left anterior descending coronary angioplasty indicated a patent left anterior descending artery with disappearance of the right-to-left collateral vessels in this patient.

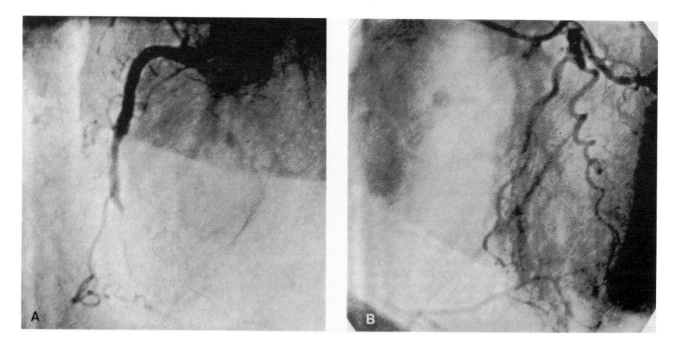

Fig. 4.   (A) Contrast injection of the right coronary artery demonstrating a total coronary occlusion at the middle segment and (B) complete opacification of the distal part after contrast injection of the left coronary artery (grade III according to Rentrop's classification).

RCA distal

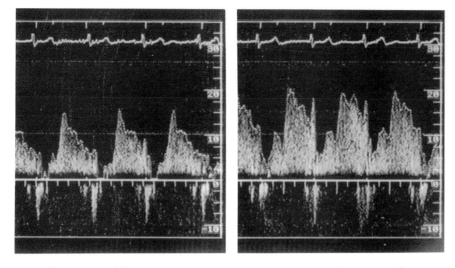

baseline   nitroglycerin

Fig. 5. Coronary flow velocity in the distal part of the right coronary artery during balloon inflation and the response after administration of 0.2 mg nitroglycerin in the left coronary artery. Velocity scale is 0–40 cm/sec.

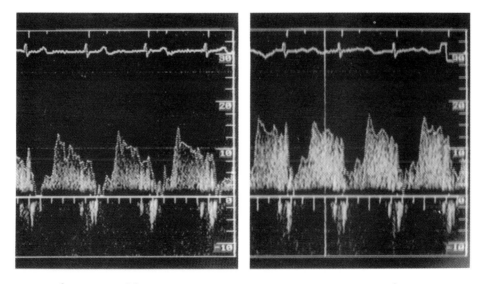

baseline   papaverine

Fig. 6. Coronary flow velocity in the distal part of the right coronary artery during balloon inflation and response after administration of 12.5 mg papaverine in the left coronary artery. Velocity scale is 0–40 cm/sec.

cilitating evaluation of the pharmacological responsiveness of the collateral circulation. Assessment of collateral flow by scintigraphic means has exhibited improvement of flow in the collateral-dependent vascular areas after administration of nitrates [9]. However, this improvement of myocardial perfusion may be the result of altered myocardial loading conditions and does not necessarily reflect enhanced collateral flow. The observation in the presented patient coincides with the scintigraphic results demonstrating enhanced collateral flow after administration of vasodilators. Obviously, the reproducibility of this observation needs to be established in larger patient cohorts. The factors influencing the magnitude of the pharmacological responsiveness of the collateral circulation in chronic coronary occlusion are at present unknown.

Summary

The unique observations of contralateral and ipsilateral coronary artery collateral supply before and after angioplasty suggest highly responsive conduits to hemodynamic conditions. The study of collateral supply system is not only significant for our current understanding of the dynamic behavior of the collateral circulation, but may also have important clinical implications for the treatment of patients with a chronic coronary occlusion.

ACKNOWLEDGMENTS

The authors thank the J.G. Mudd Cardiac Catheterization Laboratory Team and Donna Sander for manuscript preparation.

REFERENCES

1. Schaper W, Flameng W, Winkler B, et al.: Quantification of collateral resistance in acute and chronic experimental coronary occlusion in the dog. Circ Res 39:371–377, 1976.

2. Rentrop KP, Cohen M, Blanke H, Phillips RA: Changes in collateral channel filling immediately after controlled coronary artery occlusion by an angioplasty balloon in human subjects. J Am Coll Cardiol 5:587–592, 1985.

3. Kern MJ, Donohue TJ, Bach RG, Aguirre FV, Caracciolo EA, Ofili EO: Quantitating coronary collateral flow velocity in patients during coronary angioplasty using a Doppler guidewire. Am J Cardiol 71(14):34D–40D, 1993.

4. Piek JJ, Koolen JJ, Metting van Rijn AC, Bot H, Hoedemaker G, David GK, Dunning AJ, Spaan JAE, Visser CA: Spectral analysis of flow velocity in the contralateral artery during coronary angioplasty: A new method for assessing collateral flow. J Am Coll Cardiol 21:1574–1582, 1993.

5. Rigo P, Becker LC, Griffiths LSC, Alderson PO, Bailey IK, Pitt B, Burrow RD, Wagner HN: Influence of coronary collateral vessels on the results of thallium-201 myocardial stress imaging. Am J Cardiol 44:452–458, 1979.

6. Wainwright RJ, Maisey MN, Edwards AC, Sowton E: Functional significance of coronary collateral circulation during dynamic exercise evaluated by thallium-201 myocardial scintigraphy. Br Heart J 43:47–55, 1980.

7. Tubau JF, Chaitman BR, Bourassa MG, Lesperance J, Dupras G: Importance of coronary collateral circulation in interpreting exercise test results. Am J Cardiol 47:27–32, 1981.

8. Fujita M, McKown DP, McKown MD, Franklin D: Electrocardiographic evaluation of collateral development in conscious dogs. J Electrocardiol 21:55–64, 1988.

9. Aoki M, Sakai K, Koyanagi S, Takeshita A, Nakamura M: Effect of nitroglycerin on coronary collateral function during exercise evaluated by quantitative analysis of thallium-201 single photon emission computed tomography. Am Heart J 121:1361–1366, 1991.

Chapter 14

Patterns of Phasic Coronary Collateral Flow Velocity in Patients

Richard G. Bach, MD, Morton J. Kern, MD, Thomas J. Donohue, MD, Thomas Wolford, MD, Joseph A. Moore, MD, and Michael S. Flynn, MD

INTRODUCTION

In most mammalian hearts, small vascular channels called collaterals link large coronary arteries one to another [1]. The functional significance of coronary collateral flow has been extensively documented, as collateral flow has been extensively documented, as collaterals can provide perfusion to regions of myocardium which cannot receive adequate antegrade flow. Thus, collateral flow, potentially preserves myocardial viability and function. In some patients with severe coronary obstructions but adequate collaterals, a symptom-free existence under many conditions remains possible [2]. Ischemia, among other factors appears to be a major stimulus for the development of coronary collaterals in a vascular network, modifying the effects of occlusive coronary atherosclerotic disease [3].

In humans, the serial assessment of collateral development and function has been hindered due to limited semi-quantitative angiographic techniques for studying collateral flow. Nevertheless, the angiographic quality of collateral flow has been correlated with functional significance, the presence or absence of ischemia, and tolerance to coronary balloon occlusion in some patients [4]. With the recent development of intravascular flow velocity monitoring using a Doppler guidewire before and during coronary angioplasty, patterns of coronary collateral flow velocity have emerged [5].

This Interventional Physiology discussion describes several patterns of coronary flow velocity in preparation for future studies of quantitative correlations with functional outcomes. The use of flow velocity measurements identifying coronary collateral flow velocity during interventional procedures may permit prolonged balloon inflations and/or tolerance to ischemia which would not otherwise be appreciated by the operator.

METHOD OF MEASURING IPSILATERAL CORONARY COLLATERAL FLOW VELOCITY

Figure 1 diagrams the methods of measuring ipsilateral coronary collateral flow velocity during coronary balloon angioplasty. During balloon occlusion of a left anterior descending artery supplied by collaterals, antegrade or retrograde flow can appear in the distal vessel beyond the occlusion. If septal communications carry most of the collateral flow and enter the distal vessel proximal to the Doppler wire, antegrade flow across the wire tip will be detected as a spectral signal above the zero line. The quantitative assessment of the collateral flow can be obtained from the flow velocity spectral tracings and diameter of the vessel under study [6]. On the other hand, if collateral flow appears from the epicardial route through the apical segment and travels up the occluded left anterior descending, a retrograde coronary flow signal will be evident as a spectral signal below the zero line and can likewise be quantitated. On cannulation of a contralateral (right coronary) artery in this model, changes in flow velocity in the supply artery reflect recruitment of collateral flow supplied to the collateralized contralateral bed [7]. Intracoronary injection of adenosine or nitroglycerin into the right coronary artery can be used to study the pharmacologic influence of vasodilators on left anterior descending collateral flow. Serial studies using both flow velocity and balloon occlusion pressure during contralateral pharmacologic administration can provide information regarding pressure and flow changes in the distal segment. These studies may aid in appreciating the complex components of collateral blood flow in relation to coronary physiology for such patients. Unfortunately, simultaneous flow and pressure measurements in the distal segment are rarely available.

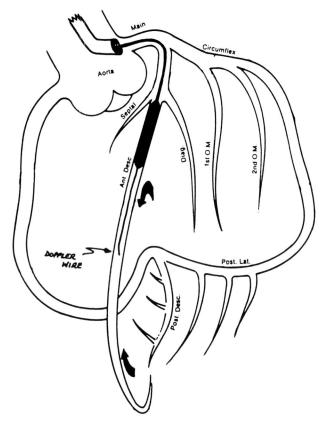

Fig. 1. Method of measurement of ipsilateral collateral flow velocity. Diagram of a left anterior descending coronary artery occlusion with balloon angioplasty catheter over distally located Doppler guidewire. The direction of flow to or away from the tip of the flowire will be evident on the velocity spectral.

CASE REPORTS

Case 1: Bidirectional Coronary Collateral Flow During Coronary Angioplasty

A 75-year-old hypertensive man had class III angina despite treatment with aspirin and metoprolol. Physical examination was unremarkable. A routine exercise radionuclide perfusion study was found to be markedly abnormal. Exercise was terminated after 9 min secondary to substernal pain typical of angina pectoris. Electrocardiography (ECG) was positive for prominent ST segment changes in the anterior and inferior leads. The myocardial perfusion study showed large anteroapical and anteroseptal reversible defects consistent with myocardial ischemia.

Coronary angiography showed a totally occluded mid left anterior descending artery and severe stenosis in the mid right coronary artery. Figure 2 demonstrates the total occlusion of the left anterior descending artery, which filled distally from septal collateral flow as evidenced by contrast injection into the right coronary artery (Fig. 3). Subsequent angioplasty was performed with a 0.018-inch Doppler-tipped flowire. The left anterior descending flow signal proximal to the occlusion demonstrated a normal phasic pattern with an average peak velocity of approximately 22 cm/sec. Intracoronary adenosine was administered and hyperemia increased flow velocity to approximately 56 cm/sec for a coronary reserve (hyperemic/basal flow) of 2.4. After traversing the left anterior descending coronary artery occlusion with the flowire

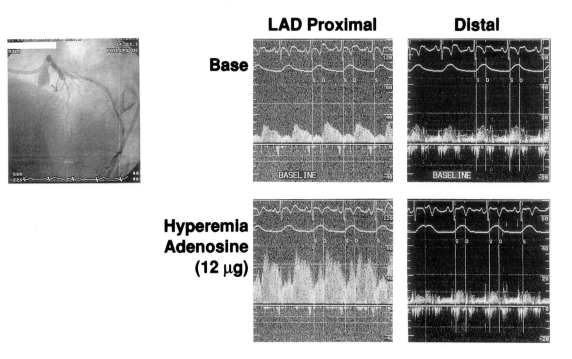

Fig. 2. Top: Left anterior oblique cineangiogram demonstrating occlusion of the left anterior descending artery (*arrow*). Bottom: Proximal and distal flow velocity at baseline and during hyperemia induced with intracoronary adenosine. Velocity scale for the proximal spectra is 0–200 cm/sec and 0–80 cm/sec for distal data.

prior to balloon inflation, distal coronary flow velocity, representing collateral supply, demonstrated an abnormal phasic pattern with bidirectional coronary flow (Fig. 2, bottom). Before angioplasty, collateral coronary flow velocity predominantly occurred in systole and was unaffected by adenosine injected directly into the left coronary artery. With the left anterior descending coronary flow velocity guidewire in place and the angioplasty balloon inflated (Fig. 3A,B), contralateral contrast injection of the right coronary artery demonstrated septal and apical collateral supply. During balloon occlusion (Fig. 3C,D), coronary collateral flow velocity was markedly augmented through septal channels producing a large antegrade systolic-predominant coronary flow velocity signal with an average peak velocity of approximately 30 cm/sec, demonstrating striking recruitable collateral flow during balloon occlusion. To assess collateral vessel vasodilator function, adenosine (12 μg) was injected into the right coronary artery, while balloon occlusion was maintained in the left anterior descending artery. Collateral flow velocity actually diminished (20 cm/sec). Intracoronary nitroglycerin (200 μg) further reduced the absolute magnitude of coronary flow velocity (14 cm/sec), associated with a decrease in arterial perfusion pressure to the collateral zone. Note peak systolic velocity decreased from 60 cm/sec to 50 cm/sec to 28 cm/sec during these pharmacologic interventions, respectively. After successful coronary angioplasty with a 2.5-mm balloon, distal coronary flow was now entirely antegrade and normal in its phasic pattern (Fig. 4B,C). Adenosine now increased distal coronary flow velocity from 40 cm/sec to approximately 75 cm/sec (CVR = 1.9).

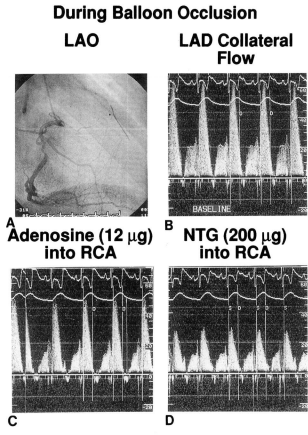

Fig. 3.   A: Angiogram of the right coronary artery showing septal collateral filling of the left anterior descending artery with a flowire positioned through the left anterior descending balloon catheter during occlusion. B–D: Flow velocity spectra during balloon occlusion. Velocity scale is 0–80 cm/sec. S and D indicate onset of systole and diastole.

Post LAD PTCA

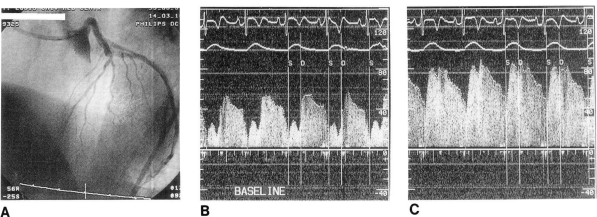

Fig. 4.   A: Angiogram after left anterior descending artery after angioplasty. B,C: Flow velocity spectra in the distal region after angioplasty. Velocity scale is 0–200 cm/sec. S and D indicate onset of systole and diastole.

RCA Pre-PTCA

Proximal   **Distal**

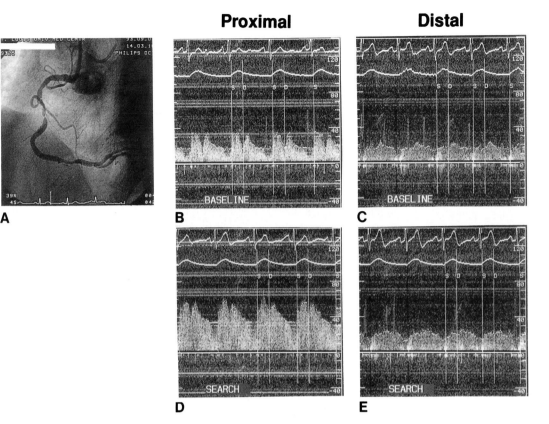

Fig. 5. A: Angiogram of right coronary artery showing severe mid vessel stenosis. **B,C:** Flow velocity spectra in the proximal and distal regions at baseline and **(D,E)** after intracoronary adenosine (8 μg). Velocity scale is 0–200 cm/sec.

After satisfactory dilation of the left anterior descending artery, angioplasty of the right coronary artery was then performed. The right coronary artery, in the left anterior oblique projection (Fig. 5), had a severe mid vessel stenosis. Proximal right coronary flow velocity showed an equiphasic systolic and diastolic flow pattern, not unusual for this location. The average peak velocity was approximately 18 cm/sec. Intracoronary adenosine (Fig. 5D,E) produced ≥2× basal proximal flow velocity. On crossing the lesion, distal coronary flow velocity was diminished and its phasic pattern impaired. There was no evidence of distal hyperemia after intracoronary adenosine (Fig. 5E). Right coronary artery angioplasty was then successfully performed with improvement of the stenosis from 90% to approximately 25% by visual estimation (Fig. 6). The distal right coronary artery flow velocity pattern during balloon occlusion demonstrated retrograde collateral flow with an inverted spectral signal of flow velocity (Fig. 6B), originating now from the left circulation through septal channels contributing reversed flow to the distal right coronary artery (confirmed an-

giographically, not shown). The phasic pattern of this collateral flow velocity was again systolic-predominant (preceded by a short systolic contraction artifact). Following angioplasty, antegrade distal coronary flow increased dramatically to a mean velocity of 21 cm/sec, and hyperemia could now be detected after administration of adenosine (Fig. 6C,D).

This case demonstrated functionally bidirectional coronary collaterals with prominent demonstrable collateral flow velocity via septal channels recruited from the right coronary artery during mid left anterior descending artery balloon occlusion, and then from the left anterior descending artery during mid right coronary artery balloon occlusion.

Case 2: Normal Antegrade Coronary Flow Velocity Pattern Due to Grade III Epicardial Angiographic Collateral Flow

A 49-year-old man with diabetes mellitus, hypertension, coronary artery disease, and renal transplant secondary to polycystic kidney disease, complained of 2

Post RCA PTCA

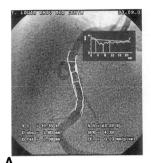

A

Distal RCA During Occlusion

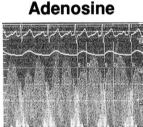

B

Post PTCA Base

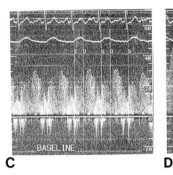

C

Post PTCA Adenosine

D

Fig. 6. A: Angiogram of the right coronary artery after angioplasty. B–D: Flow velocity during balloon occlusion, post-angioplasty, and post-angioplasty hyperemia. Velocity scale is 0–80 cm/sec. S and D indicate onset of systole and diastole.

LAD R→L Collaterals

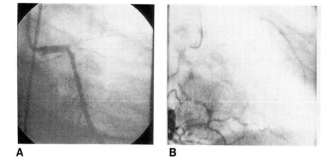

A   **B**

Fig. 7. A: Angiogram of the left coronary artery with totally occluded proximal left anterior descending artery. Flowire is across the occlusion, and its tip resides in the mid vessel. B: Contrast opacification of the right coronary artery fills the distal left anterior descending through septal collaterals.

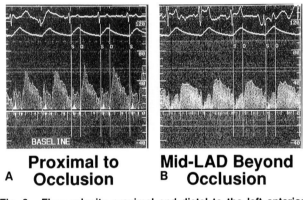

Proximal to Occlusion

A

Mid-LAD Beyond Occlusion

B

Fig. 8. Flow velocity proximal and distal to the left anterior descending occlusion was obtained with the flowire in position indicated in Figure 7. Note normal antegrade phasic collateral left anterior descending pattern distal to the left anterior descending occlusion. Velocity scale is 0–160 cm/sec. S and D indicate onset of systole and diastole.

years of stable angina relieved by rest and nitroglycerin. A recent increase in substernal pain associated with shortness of breath and diaphoresis prompted admission to the coronary care unit and treatment with intravenous nitrates and heparin. Substernal pain persisted despite intravenous nitroglycerin. The patient was taking aspirin, nifedipine, labetalol, prednisone, cyclosporine, NPH insulin, and nitropaste. Physical examination was remarkable for an S_4 gallop and normal pulses. The ECG demonstrated left ventricular hypertrophy with strain without evidence of myocardial infarction.

Cardiac catheterization was performed which revealed 100% occlusion of the proximal left anterior descending artery with evidence of calcification (Fig. 7). There was angiographic grade III (complete epicardial filling) left-to-left and right-to-left collateral filling of the distal left anterior descending artery (Fig. 7). Left ventricular ejection fraction was 65%. There was, however, severe hypokinesis of the anterolateral and apical segments. Because of the persistent angina despite the collaterally-supplied left anterior descending artery, angioplasty was performed. A 0.018-inch Doppler-tipped guidewire was

used to cross the total occlusion. Flow velocity data were measured proximal and distal to the total occlusion as shown in Figure 7. Proximal flow velocity demonstrated a normal phasic pattern with a mean velocity of approximately 31 cm/sec (Fig. 8). Of interest, distal to the total occlusion, antegrade flow, (documented as collateral flow by contrast injection showing the flowire tip distal to the total occlusion in a segment opacified solely via septal channels from the right coronary artery), demonstrated a normal diastolic-predominant antegrade flow velocity pattern with an average peak velocity of approximately 24 cm/sec. It is remarkable that this collateral flow has a normal phasic pattern and velocity. After the flowire was advanced distally, during mid left anterior descending balloon occlusion, collateral flow was altered (Fig. 9). The phasic flow velocity diminished,

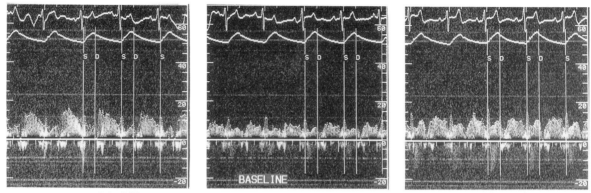

Distal LAD   **Balloon Up**   **Balloon Up + Adenosine**

Fig. 9.   Distal coronary flow velocity spectra before and during balloon occlusion, and during occlusion with contralateral administration of intracoronary adenosine (8 μg). Velocity scale is 0–80 cm/sec.

likely due to partial occlusion of the septal collateral feeding artery by the angioplasty balloon. During balloon occlusion, the administration of intracoronary adenosine in the contralateral (right) coronary artery moderately augmented collateral coronary flow (Fig. 9). Following coronary angioplasty with relief of the obstruction, distal flow achieved a normal pattern similar to that of the proximal flow velocity prior to angioplasty both in phasic pattern and velocity magnitude (Fig. 10).

Collateral flow in this patient was unique in that the grade III angiographic collaterals were correlated with a flow velocity of normal magnitude with a normal phasic pattern. Despite the normal pattern and magnitude of flow velocity as assessed by the flowire, this patient has hypokinesis of the anterolateral segment. Similarly, in a small series of patients so studied [6], the magnitude of collateral flow velocity did not correlate significantly with the degree of segmental wall motion abnormality by contrast ventriculography. It is also interesting that during balloon occlusion, the distal collateral flow pattern became abnormal, likely due in part to some limitation of antegrade collateral flow input. Comparing this patient's collateral flow velocity spectra (Fig. 9) to that seen in Case 1, it can be appreciated that phasic patterns and magnitudes of collateral flow velocity spectra can vary widely between patients.

Case 3: Retrograde Collateral Flow With an Inverted Normal Phasic Pattern

Collateral flow velocity in an artery during balloon occlusion can appear to have a normal antegrade flow pattern, as previously demonstrated. An inverted signal indicates collateral flow is coming toward the tip of the flow velocity guidewire. Collateral flow velocity spectra in some vessels may be inverted but is otherwise entirely

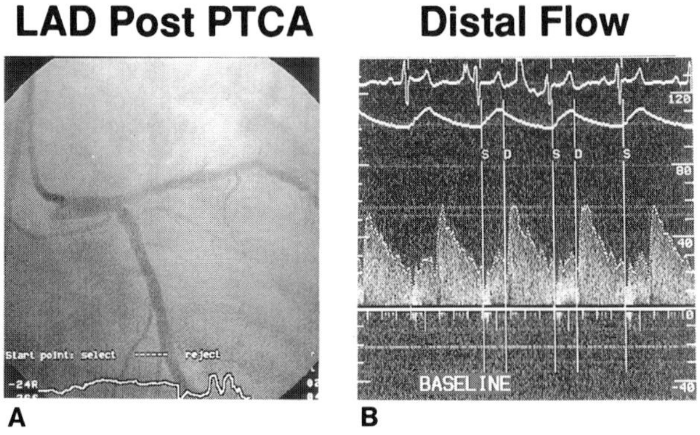

LAD Post PTCA   Distal Flow

A   **B**

Fig. 10.   A: Angiogram after left anterior descending artery after angioplasty. B: Distal coronary flow velocity after angioplasty has similar magnitude and phasic pattern compared to left anterior descending flow proximal to the occlusion shown in Figure 8. Velocity scale is 0–160 cm/sec.

normal in phasic pattern. As shown in Figure 11, during left anterior descending artery balloon occlusion in a patient with large right-to-left grade III epicardial collateral supply from the right coronary artery, the collateral flow velocity signal is inverted with an average peak velocity of (−)28 cm/sec and normal phasic (diastolic-predominant) components. The collateral epicardial supply to this vessel provided nearly identical flow parameters when compared to that obtained in antegrade fashion demonstrated in Case 2. Intravenous adenosine (in a dose sufficient to produce coronary hyperemia equivalent to the intracoronary route) augmented collateral coronary flow velocity (Fig. 11B). During repeated balloon occlusions, there was further recruitment of collateral flow above baseline values. These findings have been duplicated in a preliminary series of 12 patients in whom the

Collateral Flow-LAD (R→L)

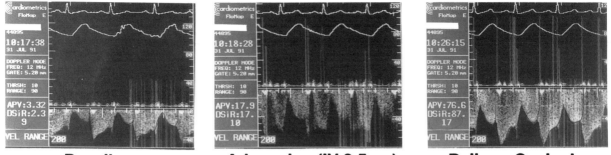

Baseline   **Adenosine (IV 2.5mg)**   **Balloon Occlusion**

Fig. 11. Collateral flow velocity in a patient with left anterior descending occlusion with right-to-left large epicardial collaterals. Baseline retrograde flow velocity with normal and phasic pattern. Intravenous adenosine given in the right atrium produced minimal augmentation of collateral flow velocity. However, repeated balloon occlusion produced a marked increase in the coronary collateral flow velocity magnitude with persistence of the normal phasic pattern. Flow velocity is on a 0–200-cm/sec velocity scale.

hyperemic stimuli of adenosine and nitroglycerin given into contralateral (collateral supply) arteries were compared to hyperemia by repeated balloon occlusions [8] (Fig. 12). The relationship of perfusion pressure to collateral flow appears to be important for both pharmacologically and mechanically induced responses. Nitroglycerin appears frequently to produce a pressure-dependent reduction in collateral flow (Fig. 13). In the current study, the left anterior descending collateral supply to the distal right coronary artery was angiographically evident. Distal coronary flow with the Doppler guidewire demonstrated biphasic flow which increased during intracoronary adenosine. However, intracoronary nitroglycerin (200 μg) decreased collateral coronary flow velocity. Both perfusion pressure and distal coronary occlusion (collateral) pressure responded differently in response to adenosine and nitroglycerin. Adenosine reduced distal perfusion pressure with no effect on aortic pressure, whereas nitroglycerin reduced both distal pressure and aortic pressure, likely diminishing coronary collateral flow on a hemodynamic basis.

DISCUSSION

The development of coronary collateral channels in animals has been extensively studied by Schaper and colleagues [1,2], who noted the transformation of small vessels in response to myocardial ischemia to mature collateral channels. Investigators have described phases of initial transformation due to perivascular inflammation and a subacute period of vascular growth facilitated by mitotic division of endothelial, smooth muscle, and fibroblastic cells in the vessel wall. Protein synthesis in

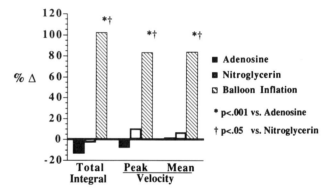

Fig. 12. Percentage change for total flow velocity integral, peak and mean velocity in response to adenosine, nitroglycerin, and repeated balloon inflations. Repeated balloon inflations had largest percent increase in coronary collateral flow velocity in 12 patients.

vascular smooth muscle cells begins immediately after the onset of ischemia [2] and, in animal models, initial collateral development can be demonstrated approximately 24 hr from the onset of ischemia.

Collateral channels have been differentiated microscopically from normal coronary arteries of similar size mainly by small defects in the internal elastic lamina, potentially responsible for the typical high tortuosity of such collateral channels. Compared to conduit coronary arteries, innervation of collateral vessel is reduced and subintimal proliferation of smooth muscle occasionally causes obliteration of the vascular lumen. In animal models, the functional capacity of collateral channels appears nearly maximal at 4 weeks following coronary occlusion.

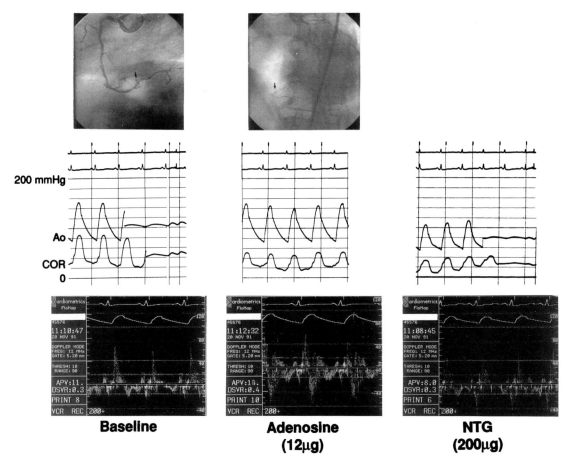

Baseline   **Adenosine**   **NTG**
                      (12μg)   **(200μg)**

Fig. 13. Right coronary collaterals supplied from the left anterior descending artery demonstrating both changes in distal flow and pressure during intracoronary adenosine and intracoronary nitroglycerin. Intracoronary adenosine had minimal effect on collateral flow velocity. The distal coronary pressure was 50 mm Hg. Intracoronary nitroglycerin reduced both the distal pressure and aortic systemic pressure and reduced collateral flow velocity, indicating a pressure-dependent phenomenon that appears to be related to the flow supplied through the contralateral collateral supply vessel. (From Kern et al. [5] with permission.)

Methods of Assessing Collateral Function

In animal models, timed retrograde volume collection and distal coronary pressure have been used to determine the physiology of collateral flow [2]. The deficiencies of this approach for patients are obvious in that distal coronary perfusion pressure can only be obtained during balloon angioplasty, and retrograde collateral flow cannot be collected. Artifacts of animal preparation for the collateral model have left quantitation somewhat in question. There is an absence of coronary resistance during timed retrograde collection, and distal coronary pressure and flow are usable indexes of collateral development only in the presence of maximal coronary vasodilatation and controlled extravascular resistance [3]. In addition, the transmural distribution of coronary collateral perfusion cannot be obtained by this method in animal studies.

Microsphere or diffusible indicator techniques to assess collateral flow have been employed widely [9,10].

However, these techniques are limited by overlap of antegrade and retrograde perfusion within a zone of mixed blood flow due to the contribution of both epicardial and collateral channels. Methods of measuring collateral flow in patients are, in general, qualitative and based on angiographic assessment of collateral density. Gregg et al. [3] indicated that the size of the collateral-dependent zone reflects the adequacy of collateral perfusion. Under some circumstances, collateral connections provide the anatomic substrate to produce a coronary steal phenomena, at times theoretically shunting blood from jeopardized but adequately perfused (at baseline) zones to dependent zones, producing ischemia. In addition, in a single normal vessel providing perfusion to a large collateral-dependent zone, the vasodilator reserve may be mildly impaired for reasons that are unclear by the current models.

Methods of evaluating coronary collateral circulation

in patients have employed, principally, an angiographic approach. However, coronary collaterals of <200 μm are not detectable by angiography. Clinical studies in patients with angiographic high-grade collaterals appear to have increased distal coronary perfusion pressure and retrograde flow in the diseased segment served by these collateral channels [12,13]. Indirect approaches to the assessment of the functional capacity of coronary collaterals have been provided by correlations with left ventricular function, exercise scintigraphy, and exercise wall motion studies, but are of limited value in patients with multivessel coronary disease who have confounding factors of ischemia in regions not subtended by the collaterals of interest.

Our laboratory has used the Doppler guidewire and its ability to interrogate blood flow velocity in the coronary arteries distal to occlusions and/or inflated angioplasty balloons to investigate both the patterns and quantitation of collateral blood flow in patients undergoing coronary angioplasty [5,6,8]. Case studies illustrating some of these observations are presented in this Interventional Physiology. Notably, variability in both phasic pattern and response to pharmacologic or mechanical intervention has been demonstrated.

Major areas of interest with regard to collateral development and clinical significance remain under study. These topics include the rate of coronary collateral development, patient specific factors for the development of collaterals, coexistent atherosclerotic and circulatory disease, and resolution of methodologic limitations to the measurement of collateral flow. Many aspects of the contributors to both native and collateral coronary circulatory dynamics can now be explored during intervention using a Doppler-tipped angioplasty guidewire.

SUMMARY

Antegrade or retrograde collateral flow velocity Doppler signals, acquired with the flowire, permit the quantitation of collateral blood flow and its phasic patterns. The velocity spectra are easily visualized, and reproducible alterations during balloon occlusion may be directly related to coronary collateral flow-dependent variables of ischemia and left ventricular wall motion. The effects of pharmacologic stimulation on collateral flow remain under study.

ACKNOWLEDGMENTS

The authors thank the J.G. Mudd Cardiac Catheterization Laboratory team and Donna Sander for manuscript preparation.

REFERENCES

1. Schaper W (ed): "The Collateral Circulation of the Heart." New York: Elsevier, 1971.
2. Schaper W (ed): Wustern B. Collateral circulation. In "The Pathophysiology of Myocardial Perfusion." Amsterdam: Elsevier/North-Holland Biomedical Press, 1979,
3. Gregg DE: The natural history of coronary collateral development. Circ Res 35:335–344, 1974.
4. Rentrop KP, Cohen M, Blanke H, Phillips RA: Changes in collateral channel filling immediately after controlled coronary artery occlusion by an angioplasty balloon in human subjects. J Am Coll Cardiol 5:587–592, 1985.
5. Kern MJ, Donohue TJ, Bach RG, Aguirre FV, Caracciolo EA, Ofili EO: Quantitating coronary collateral flow velocity in patients during coronary angioplasty using a Doppler guidewire. Am J Cardiol 71(14):34D–40D, 1993.
6. Bach RG, Donohue TJ, Caracciolo EA, Wolford T, Aguirre FV, Kern MJ: Quantification of collateral blood flow during PTCA by intravascular Doppler. In Fleck (ed.): Advances in cardiac ultrasound for the evaluation for coronary artery disease: Stress echo and Intracoronary doppler. Symposia, Berlin, January 21–23, 1994: Harcourt Brace, Eur Heart J 1995.
7. Piek JJ, Koolen JJ, van Rijn ACM, Bot H, Hoedemaker G, David GK, Dunning AJ, Spaan JAE, Visser CA: Spectral analysis of flow velocity in the contralateral artery during coronary angioplasty: A new method for assessing collateral flow. J Am Coll Cardiol 21:1574–1582, 1993.
8. Donohue TJ, Bach RG, Caracciolo EA, Wolford T, Kern MJ, Aguirre FV, Cauley M. Quantitation of coronary collateral flow velocity by anatomic pathway in patients. J Am Coll Cardiol 415A, 1994 (abst).
9. Cibulski AA, Lehan PH, Timmis HH: Retrograde flow technique vs. Krypton-85 clearance technique for estimation of myocardial collaterals. Am J Physiol 223:1081, 1972.
10. Levy MN, Imperial ES, Zieske H Jr: Collateral blood flow to the myocardium as determined by the clearance of $Rb^{86}Cl$. Circ Res 9:1035, 1961.
11. Marcus ML, Kerber RE, Ehrhardt J, Abboud FM: Three dimensional geometry of acutely ischemic myocardium. Circulation 52:254, 1975.
12. Goldstein RE, Stinson EB, Scherer JL, Seningen RP, Grehl TM, Epstein SE: Intraoperative coronary collateral function in patients with coronary occlusive disease: Nitroglycerin responsiveness and angiographic correlation. Circulation 49:298, 1974.
13. Goldstein RE, Michaelis LL, Morrow AG, Epstein E: Coronary collateral function in patients without occlusive coronary artery disease. Circulation 51:118, 1975.

Part VIII

Acute Myocardial Infarction

Chapter 15

Alterations in Coronary Blood Flow Velocity During Intracoronary Thrombolysis And Rescue Coronary Angioplasty for Acute Myocardial Infarction

Michael S. Flynn, MD, Morton J. Kern, MD, Frank V. Aguirre, MD, Richard G. Bach, MD, Eugene A. Caracciolo, MD, and Thomas J. Donohue, MD

INTRODUCTION

Recent reports have identified advantages with direct angioplasty over thrombolytic therapy in patients who present early with acute anterior myocardial infarction [1–3]. These advantages include rapid, early, and complete reperfusion, reduced hemorrhagic complications, and reduced risk of cerebrovascular accident [1,2].

In patients with acute coronary occlusion owing to a large or platelet-rich thrombus, mechanical revascularization may be the only means of coronary recanalization. Although return of adequate coronary flow post-reperfusion is routinely documented angiographically [3–5], no physiologic measurement of coronary blood flow has been reported because of technical limitations. With the use of a Doppler-tipped angioplasty guidewire (FloWire™, Cardiometrics, Inc., Mountain View, CA) [6–8], we report, for the first time, pathophysiologic alterations in coronary blood flow velocity during intracoronary thrombolysis and direct angioplasty for acute myocardial infarction. This methodology has the potential to yield unique diagnostic and therapeutic information during the procedure.

CASE REPORT

A 40-year-old man had the acute onset of severe crushing chest pain radiating to both arms which occurred while smoking a cigarette during his work as a mechanic. Within 30 min he was taken to the emergency department where an electrocardiogram documented an acute anterolateral myocardial infarction. Physical examination was remarkable for a distressed young, diaphoretic, and anxious male. Systolic blood pressure was 80 mm Hg. Heart rate was 95 beats/min. An enlarged dyskinetic apical impulse and summation gallop were noted. The patient was immediately given 325 mg of oral aspirin and 10,000 units of intravenous heparin bolus and transferred to the Cardiac Catheterization Laboratory. Emergent coronary angiography (Fig. 1A,B) revealed complete left anterior descending coronary artery occlusion with an intraluminal filling defect consistent with a large thrombus. The total occlusion in the mid portion of the left anterior descending occurred just after the origin of the first diagonal branch which also had a large portion of the thrombus straddling the take-off of the first diagonal branch and left anterior descending artery. The TIMI grade flow in both the left anterior descending artery and diagonal branch was zero.

In preparation for coronary angioplasty, a 0.018″ Doppler flowire (Cardiometrics, Inc., Mountain View, CA) was advanced into the distal left anterior descending artery (Fig. 1C) with an increase of flow to grade TIMI 1. The validation and method of use of the Doppler flowire has been previously described in detail [6–8]. On initial crossing from the unobstructed to the obstructed portion of the left anterior descending artery, the accelerated flow velocity in the proximal region (>75 cm/s) decreased markedly (<20 cm/s) (Fig. 2, top). Pathophysiologically attenuated phasic flow signals were evi-

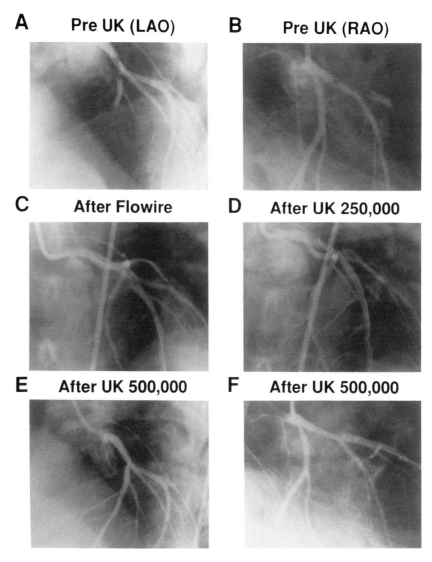

A Pre UK (LAO)

B Pre UK (RAO)

C After Flowire

D After UK 250,000

E After UK 500,000

F After UK 500,000

Fig. 1. A: Left anterior oblique (LAO) angiogram revealing large intracoronary thrombus straddling the proximal left anterior descending coronary artery and large first diagonal branch with absence of distal angiographic flow (TIMI 0). B: Right anterior oblique (RAO) angiogram displaying extent of intracoronary thrombus in the proximal left anterior descending coronary artery and diagonal branch. C: Anteroposterior angiogram of the left anterior descending coronary artery revealing contrast penetration distal to obstructing thrombus after the insertion of intracoronary flowire. D: Anteroposterior cranial angio-gram after intracoronary administration of 250,000 units of uro-kinase revealing some reduction of the thrombus. E: Left ante-rior oblique (LAO) angiogram of the left anterior descending coronary artery after the administration of 500,000 units of in-tracoronary urokinase. F: Right anterior oblique (RAO) angio-gram of the left anterior descending coronary artery after the administration of 500,000 units of intracoronary urokinase re-vealing a marked decrease in intracoronary thrombus as com-pared to B.

dent (Fig. 2, top right). Because of the large thrombus mass, 250,000 units of intracoronary urokinase [9,10] were slowly administered over 15 min with minimal im-provement of coronary flow (angiographic TIMI grade 2) and some resolution of the patient's chest pain. A second bolus of 250,000 units of urokinase was given over another 15–20 min period. Continuous trend anal-ysis of distal flow velocity revealed cyclical flow veloc-ity variations during intracoronary urokinase administra-tion (Fig. 3, period 4, arrow). At the end of the urokinase infusion, during cyclical flow variations, two brief Sal-vo's of premature ventricular contractions were noted with rapidly improved coronary flow velocity.

Because of transient hypotension and the potential to enhance and maintain coronary patency [11–14], an in-tra-aortic balloon pump was inserted with augmented distal coronary flow velocity (Fig. 2, bottom right) [14]. A residual 50% stenosis in the proximal left anterior

A.D. 40 yr old, LAD (IC) Thrombolysis and IABP

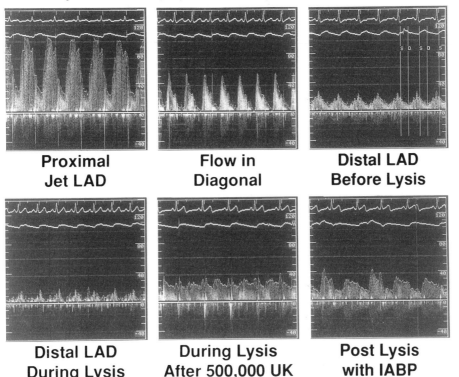

Proximal Jet LAD	Flow in Diagonal	Distal LAD Before Lysis
Distal LAD During Lysis After 250,000 UK	During Lysis After 500,000 UK	Post Lysis with IABP

Fig. 2. Phasic intracoronary flow velocity signals obtained over the course of this study. Upper left: Left anterior descending coronary artery jet lesion flow (average peak velocity 75 cm/s). Upper middle: The diagonal artery (average peak velocity 35 cm/s). Upper right: The distal left anterior descending artery prior to lytic therapy revealing a marked decrease in coronary flow velocity (10 cm/s) in comparison to the proximal left anterior descending coronary artery. The phasic pattern was also markedly abnormal. Bottom left: Distal left anterior descending coronary flow velocity during the administration of 250,000 of intracoronary urokinase. Bottom middle: Flow improvement in coronary flow velocity after 500,000 units of urokinase (average peak velocity 30 cm/s). Bottom right: Flow velocity with intra-aortic balloon pump counterpulsation (2:1 mode). Note distal velocity augmentation of attenuated beats.

descending coronary artery was dilated with a 3.5 mm angioplasty balloon with satisfactory angiographic result without a significant increase in coronary flow. Of special interest, no post-occlusion or adenosine-induced coronary hyperemia was observed.

The continuous trend analysis of coronary flow velocity (Fig. 3) summarizes and demonstrates the coronary flow alterations observed during the various manipulations used to recanalize the thrombotically occluded vessel. On the initial passage of the guidewire through the occlusion (Fig. 3, period 1), a high velocity jet is recorded (Fig. 2, top left). Distal to the thrombus, angiographic TIMI I flow showed an impaired phasic flow velocity pattern with an average velocity of 20 cm/s (Fig. 3, period 2). During the initial 250,000 units of urokinase, coronary flow velocity decreased (presumably as the thrombus began to disintegrate). Continued intracoronary thrombolysis was associated with cyclical flow variations (Fig. 3, period 4) followed by reperfusion ventricular arrhythmias immediately before abrupt increase in coronary flow velocity to 25–30 cm/s (Fig. 3, arrow, period 5). Selected phasic patterns of flow velocity are shown on Figure 2 for these events. Angiography after intracoronary urokinase demonstrated TIMI grade 3 flow with mean velocity 30–35 cm/s. As noted above, neither angioplasty coronary occlusions (Fig. 3, periods 6,7) nor adenosine (Fig. 3, period 8) produced hyperemia.

Final angiography revealed brisk (TIMI 3) flow and minimal residual stenosis (Fig. 1F). Left ventriculography revealed akinetic anterolateral and apical segments with marked recovery of function by surface echocardiography 3 days later.

30 yr old AMI with LAD
(IC) Thrombolysis, IABP, PTCA

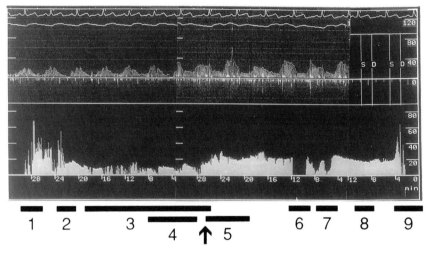

1 Wire advanced past lesion
2 Distal flow with clot
3 UK infusion, (250,00 x 2) = 500,000 units IC
4 Cyclic flow variations, PVC's (↑)
5 IABP
6 PTCA
7 PTCA (no hyperemia)
8 IC Adenosine (18μg) - no effect
9 Wire pull back

Fig. 3. Continuous trend plot of average coronary velocity. Display is divided. Top: Signal displays (top to bottom) electrocardiogram, arterial pressure, and phasic coronary flow velocity. Bottom: Trend velocity plotted in 4 min intervals over 1 hr 15 min. Horizontal numbered bars identify duration of specific interventions enumerated 1–9.

DISCUSSION

This case demonstrates the first continuous coronary flow velocity monitoring during intracoronary urokinase with direct coronary angioplasty and confirms several phenomenon related to thrombotic coronary occlusion and recanalization. The low initial velocity with an impaired phasic pattern in the distal left anterior descending coronary beyond the thrombus corresponded to angiographic low flow grade (TIMI 1). On initiation of clot disruption, cyclical flow variations as noted in the Folts model [15] of thrombotic coronary obstruction were identified. The time at which reperfusion satisfied oxygen demands of ischemic myocardium was associated with both a clinical response and physiologic measure-

ment of increased flow as documented by VPCs and augmented flow velocity seen after 30 min of urokinase (Fig. 3, period 5).

The adequacy of TIMI grade 3 flow, corresponding to a coronary flow velocity 35 cm/s (Fig. 2, lower right), was not significantly changed by angioplasty of the 50% residual stenosis, suggesting that the angiographic lesion may not have been flow-limiting or required mechanical enlargement. Lack of coronary hyperemic responses to both balloon occlusion and intracoronary adenosine documented that coronary vasodilatory reserve was exhausted or significantly impaired.

Trend analysis of continuous flow monitoring with simultaneous recording of mechanical and pharmacologic events may yield important new data contributing to our understanding of coronary recanalization and the response to interventional events [16,17]. Recording the onset of no-reflow and other coronary flow responses documents limitations involved with the illusion of successful reperfusion [18]. Maintenance of adequate flow verified by velocity trending may have clinical utility in decreasing angiographic contrast volume. By using another more objective parameter of flow, the assessment of acute reclosure may be refined, enabling the operator a confident termination of an interventional procedure.

Cyclical flow variations in coronary arteries measured by a Doppler wire during angioplasty has been previously reported [16,17,19]. An association of intracoronary thrombus with cyclical flow variations and the attenuation of this phenomenon with monoclonal antiplatelet antibodies has been demonstrated [17]. Non-selective fibrinolytic therapy has also been implicated in enhancing platelet adhesion and aggregation, thus, exacerbating cyclical flow variation in this patient, even prior to balloon angioplasty. Mechanistic trigger events, such as recent smoking by the patient, is postulated to produce endothelial injury which may have initiated primary platelet activation and subsequent thrombus formation. These activated platelets are released downstream post-lysis and contribute to flow variations, reperfusion arrhythmias, and possibly no re-flow owing to leaching of potent vasoconstrictors and subsequent microvascular constriction [20,22]. Although the no-reflow phenomenon was not demonstrated angiographically in this case, others have postulated that this process may be induced by local effects of acute cellular injury and distal embolization [21]. The severity and duration of impaired reflow and vasodilatory reserve may mirror the severity and duration of acute ischemia and its early complete and sustained relief. By the same mechanism, reperfusion ventricular arrhythmia may be a response to differences in regional flow recovery enhancing macro or micro reentry phenomenon.

Further studies using intracoronary flow velocity and trend monitoring will assist in defining the completeness of early reperfusion and the time course of sustained coronary flow following treatment of acute myocardial infarction and will quantitate results of coronary interventions to restore distal coronary blood flow.

ACKNOWLEDGMENTS

The authors wish to thank the J.G. Mudd Cardiac Catheterization team, Trina Stonner, RN, MSN, Marilyn Cauley, Carol Mechem, RN, Lisa Abbott and Donna Sander for manuscript preparation.

REFERENCES

1. Grines CL, Browne KF, Marco J, et al.: A comparison of immediate angioplasty with thrombolytic therapy for acute myocardial infarction. N Engl J Med 328:673–679, 1993.
2. Mooney MR, Mooney JF, Goldenberg IF, Almquist AK, Van Tassel RA: Percutaneous transluminal coronary angioplasty in the setting of large intracoronary thrombi. Am J Cardiol 65:427–431, 1990.
3. The TIMI Study Group: The thrombolysis in myocardial infarction (TIMI) trial. N Engl J Med 312:932–937, 1985.
4. Topol EJ, Califf RM, George BS, et al.: A randomized trial of activator in acute myocardial infarction. N Engl J Med 317:581–588, 1987.
5. Chesebro JH, Knatterud G, Roberts R, Borer J, Cohen LS, Dalen J, et al.: Thrombolysis in myocardial infarction (TIMI) Trial, Phase 1: a comparison between intravenous tissue plasminogen activator and IV streptokinase. Circulation 76:142–154, 1987.
6. Doucette JW, Corl PD, Payne HM, Flynn AE, Goto M, Nassi M, Segal J: Validation of a Doppler guide wire for intravascular measurement of coronary artery flow velocity. Circulation 85:1899–1911, 1992.
7. Ofili EO, Kern MJ, Labovitz AJ, St. Vrain JA, Segal J, Aguirre F, Castello R: Analysis of coronary blood flow velocity dynamics in angiographically normal and stenosed arteries before and after endoluminal enlargement by angioplasty. J Am Coll Cardiol 21:308–316, 1993.
8. Segal J, Kern MJ, Scott NA, King SB III, Doucette JW, Heuser RR, Ofili E, Siegel R: Alterations of phasic coronary artery flow velocity in man during percutaneous coronary angioplasty. J Am Coll Cardiol 20:276–286, 1992.
9. Morishita H, Hattori R, Aoyama T, Kawai C, Yui Y: The intracoronary administration of urokinase following direct PTCA for acute myocardial infarction reduces early restenosis. Am Heart J 123:1153–1156, 1992.
10. Grill HP, Brinker JA: Nonacute thrombolytic therapy: an adjunct to coronary angioplasty in patients with large intravascular thrombi. Am Heart J 118:662–667, 1989.
11. Ohman EM, Califf RM, George BS, et al., Thrombolysis and Angioplasty in Myocardial Infarction (TAMI) Study Group: The use of intraaortic balloon pumping as an adjunct to reperfusion therapy in acute myocardial infarction. Am Heart J 121:895–901, 1991.
12. Ishihara M, Sato H, Tateishi H, Uchida T, Dote K: Intraaortic balloon pumping as the postangioplasty strategy in acute myocardial infarction. Am Heart J 122:385–389, 1991.
13. Kern MJ, Aguirre FV, Tatineni S, Penick D, Serota H, Donohue T, Walter K: Enhanced coronary blood flow velocity during intra-aortic balloon counterpulsation in critically ill patients. J Am Coll Cardiol 21:359–368, 1993.
14. Kern MJ, Aguirre F, Bach R, Donohue T, Segal J: Augmentation of coronary blood flow by intra-aortic balloon pumping in patients after coronary angioplasty. Circulation 87:500–511, 1993.
15. Folts JD, Crowell EB, Rowe GG: Platelet aggregation in partially obstructed vessels and its elimination with aspirin. Circulation 54:365–370, 1976.
16. Anderson HV, Kirkeeide RL, Stuart RT, Smalling RW, Hibig J, Willerson JT: Coronary artery flow monitoring following coronary interventions. Am J Cardiol 71:62D–69D, 1993.
17. Anderson HV, Levanna M, Rosales O, et al.: Intravenous administration of monoclonal antibody to the platelet GP IIb/IIIa receptor to treat abrupt closure during coronary angioplasty. Am J Cardiol 69:1373–1376, 1992.

18. Lincoff AM, Topol EJ: The illusion of reperfusion. Circulation 88:1361–1374, 1993.

19. Kern MJ, Donohue T, Bach R, Aguirre F, Bell C: Monitoring cyclical coronary blood flow alterations following coronary angioplasty for stent restenosis using a Doppler guidewire. Am Heart J 125:1159–1160, 1993.

20. Wilson RF, Laxson DD, Lesser JR, White CR: Intense microvascular constriction after angioplasty of acute thrombotic coronary arterial lesions. Lancet 1(8642):807–811, 1989.

21. Cobb FR, McHale PA, Rembert JC: Effects of acute cellular injury on coronary vascular reactivity in awake dogs. Circulation 57:962–968, 1978.

22. Golino P, Ashton JH, Buja LM, Rosolowski M, Taylor AL, McNatt J, Campbell WB, Willerson JT: Local platelet activation causes vasoconstriction of large epicardial canine coronary arteries in vivo: thromboxane A_2 and serotonin are possible mediators. Circulation 79:154–166, 1989.

Chapter 16

Coronary Flow Velocity During Coronary Angioplasty in Regions of Myocardial Infarction

Joseph A. Moore, MD, and Morton J. Kern, MD

INTRODUCTION

The measurement of blood flow velocity during coronary interventions permits exploration of human coronary physiology under unusual clinical circumstances and is an important and useful adjunct to angiographic data. The physiologic influences of infarcted myocardium will alter the assessment of coronary flow across lesions before, during, and after interventions [1–3]. With the increasing use of angioplasty in patients with recent myocardial infarction, it is helpful to be able to recognize common flow velocity patterns and understand the implications of changes in coronary flow velocity occurring in abnormal infarcted myocardial regions.

Flow Velocity in an Occluded Right Coronary Artery After Inferior Myocardial Infarction

A 43-year-old man was admitted with an inferior myocardial infarction recently treated with intravenous thrombolytic therapy. The post-infarction hospital course was uncomplicated. Low-level exercise stress testing before discharge revealed inferior ischemic ST changes with a large reversible inferior perfusion defect. Cardiac catheterization demonstrated occlusion of the proximal right coronary artery (Fig. 1A) with prominent distal collateralization via the left anterior descending artery which had a 60% stenosis proximally. The inferior wall was mildly hypokinetic with a global ejection fraction of 55%. Angioplasty of the right coronary artery was performed.

The lesion was initially crossed with a 0.010″ Silk™ guidewire and 0.018″ Tracker™ catheter combination. The Silk guidewire was replaced with a 0.018″ Doppler guidewire (FloWire™, Cardiometrics, Inc., Mountain View, CA). Prior to balloon inflation, reversal of distal flow velocity was easily detected in this collaterally supplied right coronary artery, confirming and quantitating the angiographic findings (Fig. 1B). Note that collateral flow is retrograde, by convention negative on the spectral display, and clearly biphasic with the largest flow component occurring during systole. A limited antegrade distal flow signal occurs only during early diastole with a peak velocity of 20 cm/sec, but extremely small flow velocity integral (3.1). This collateral flow pattern is commonly recorded in the presence of mature epicardial collaterals [4] and will be discussed below.

125

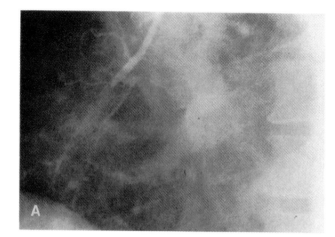

Case 1:
Pre-angioplasty distal flow

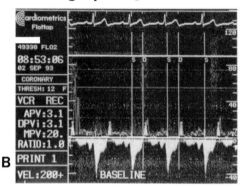

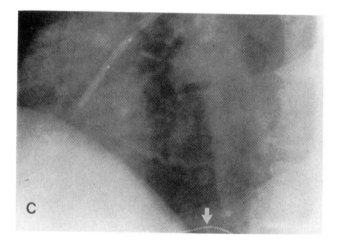

Case 1:
Post-angioplasty distal flow

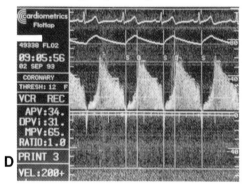

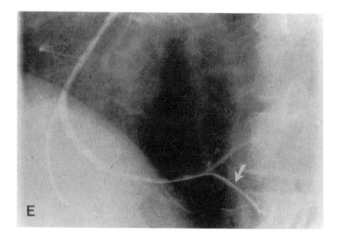

Fig. 1. A: Cineangiogram before angioplasty demonstrating total occlusion of the proximal right coronary artery after myocardial infarction (left anterior oblique projection). B: Following placement of the guidewire in the distal vessel, collateral flow was easily demonstrated by velocity reversal. Inverted velocity spectral below the zero line indicates direction of flow coming toward wire tip. Flow occurs primarily during systole with a peak velocity of 40 cm/sec. The systolic and diastolic phases are noted by vertical lines with S and D denoting the onset of each phase. The velocity scale is 0–200 cm/sec with 1 second time marks at the top of the page. APV, average peak velocity (cm/sec); DPVi, diastolic peak velocity integral (units); MPV,

maximal peak velocity (cm/sec). C: Cineangiogram demonstrating distal position of the Doppler guidewire during balloon inflation (arrow). D: After successful angioplasty, the flow velocity is now antegrade with a significantly increased diastolic flow velocity and normalization of the phasic flow velocity pattern. Note the absence of retrograde (negative) systolic flow velocity consistent with obliteration of collateral flow as seen in Figure 1B. Velocity scale is 0–200 cm/sec. APV, average peak velocity (cm/sec); DPVi, diastolic peak velocity integral (units); MPV, maximal peak velocity (cm/sec). E: Post-angioplasty angiogram reveals a widely patent right coronary artery with TIMI 3 distal flow. The flowire is in the posterior descending branch (arrow).

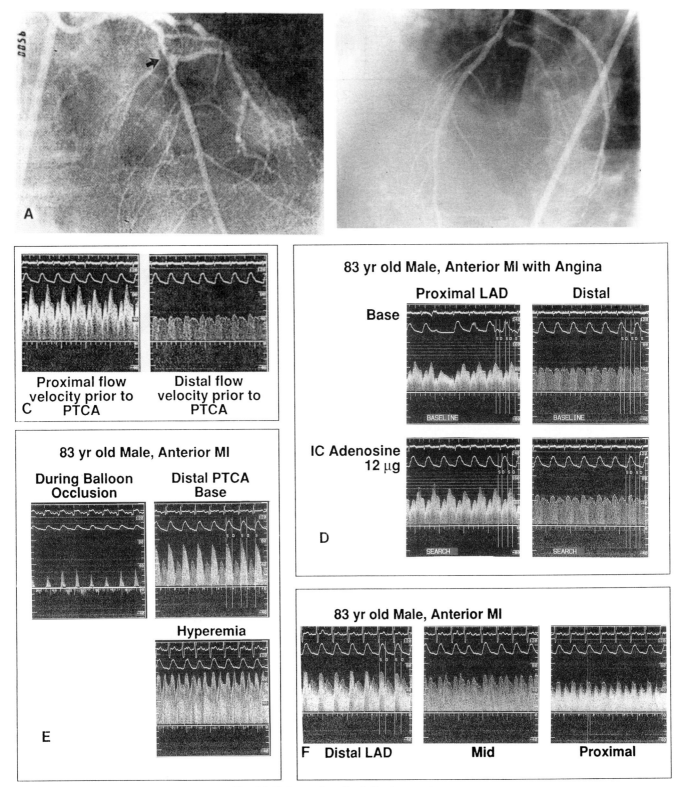

Fig. 2A–F. Legend on the following page.

A 3.0 mm × 30 mm Olympix (Cordis, Corp., Miami, FL) balloon was used over the flowire after exchanging out the tracker catheter (Fig. 1C). Following balloon deflation, the angiographic appearance was satisfactory with a residual stenosis of <25%. Distal antegrade flow was now restored with a return of a normal mean and phasic flow velocity recorded in the posterior descending artery branch (Fig. 1D). The phasic flow is predominantly diastolic (diastolic/systolic flow velocity ratio = 3.0) with a normal small systolic component. The diastolic flow velocity integral was 31 units with a mean velocity of 34 cm/sec. With repeat balloon inflations, rapid recruitment of collateral flow by flow velocity reversal was again observed without further quantitative changes in the flow velocity signal. Likewise, further balloon inflations did not improve distal antegrade flow velocity. The final angiograms demonstrated a widely patent artery with no evidence of dissection or thrombus (Fig. 1E).

Flow During Left Anterior Descending Angioplasty in Anterior Non-Q Wave Myocardial Infarction

An 83-year-old man with known coronary artery disease, hypertension, peripheral vascular disease, and non-

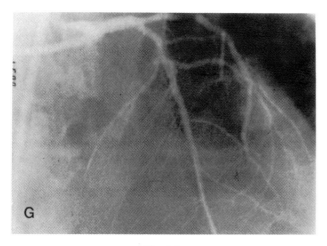

Fig. 2G.

insulin dependent diabetes mellitus was admitted with a non-Q wave myocardial infarction and experienced post-infarction angina. Coronary arteriography demonstrated a severe complex lesion in the mid left anterior descending artery with evidence of thrombus (Fig. 2A,B). An anomalous left circumflex artery with an 80% stenosis arising from the proximal right coronary artery, and occlusion of the right coronary artery just after the origin of the circumflex was also present. Left ventriculography was not performed because of mild renal insufficiency. Two-dimensional echocardiography revealed moderately preserved left ventricular function with anterior akinesis. Because of acute symptoms, angioplasty of the left anterior descending artery lesion was performed.

Proximal left anterior descending flow measurements were obtained using a 0.014″ Doppler angioplasty guidewire (FloWire™, Cardiometrics, Inc., Mountain View, CA) revealing a normal phasic pattern and high velocity flow (maximal and mean velocities were 119 and 83 cm/sec, respectively) (Fig. 2C). Coronary vasodilatory reserve was assessed in this location and later in the distal artery using intracoronary adenosine (12 μg). Proximal flow velocity increased minimally (coronary vasodilatory reserve was 1.4) (Fig. 2D). The lesion was then crossed with the flowire without difficulty. The distal flow velocity pattern prior to balloon inflations was abnormal with attenuation of the phasic pattern with the systolic and diastolic flow velocities equal (diastolic/systolic flow velocity ratio = 1.0). Maximal and mean velocities were reduced (49 and 40 cm/sec, respectively). Coronary vasodilatory reserve was again measured and showed no significant augmentation of distal flow velocity nor a change in the phasic flow pattern (CVR = 1.2). The reduced distal flow, abnormal dia-

Fig. 2. A: Angiographic view of the left coronary artery (right anterior oblique projection), showing a complex, severe lesion in the left anterior descending artery involving the origin of a large diagonal branch (arrow). **B:** Angiographic view of the left coronary artery (left anterior oblique projection) showing a complex, severe lesion in the left anterior descending artery involving the origin of a large diagonal branch (arrow). **C:** Flow velocities recorded in the proximal left anterior descending artery prior to angioplasty (left panel) show high velocity diastolic flow (normal pattern). Distal to the lesion, diastolic flow is attenuated with equalization of systolic and diastolic velocities (right panel). Also note that distal peak flow velocities are half that of the proximal velocities. Velocity scale is 0–200 cm/sec. **D:** Proximal and distal coronary flow velocity reserve (CVR) prior to angioplasty. Intracoronary adenosine (12 μg) produced vasodilation resulting in increased coronary blood flow. Proximal to the lesion (left panel), flow velocity is augmented (75 to 106 cm/sec) to produce a CVR of 1.4 (velocity scale is 0–300 cm/sec). Distal to the stenosis (right panel), similar minimal augmentation is seen (CVR = 1.2; velocity scale is 0–200 cm/sec). Note that systolic and diastolic period markers are not tracking due to poor electrocardiographic signal. The velocity scales have been changed from proximal to distal measurements. **E:** Distal flow velocity during balloon occlusion (top left panel). Small antegrade systolic velocity consistent with immature collaterals (most likely septal collaterals entering the left anterior descending proximal to the wire tip) and ST elevation on electrocardiogram. Top right panel: At baseline after angioplasty, systolic flow is now predominant. This pattern, although abnormal, reveals flow velocities twice those of pre-angioplasty values (Fig. 2D). Bottom right panel: Hyperemic flow following balloon deflation with equal systolic and diastolic peak velocities. **F:** Doppler flow velocity recorded during removal of the guidewire. Distal flow shows persistent systolic predominance (left panel). This pattern continues into the mid (middle panel) and proximal (right panel) regions of the left anterior descending artery. Comparison of the proximal pattern before (Fig. 2D) and after successful angioplasty reveals loss of diastolic predominance (decreased diastolic/systolic flow velocity ratio). **G:** Following angioplasty, cineangiograms demonstrate a hazy result with TIMI 3 distal flow (left and right anterior oblique projections) and probable dissection.

stolic/systolic flow velocity ratio, and impaired vasodilatory response supported the angiographic features of a complex lesion which is hemodynamically significant.

The lesion was crossed with a 2.5 mm balloon. During balloon inflations, distal flow velocity reversal, and persistent antegrade systolic flow velocity was recorded (Fig. 2E). The magnitude of systolic flow reversal was small (<5 cm/sec), consistent with poorly developed, acute recruitable collateral vessels. Immediately following balloon deflation, a striking increase in flow was observed (Fig. 2E). However, the phasic pattern of flow now appeared more abnormal with a marked systolic predominance with diastolic/systolic flow velocity ratio of 0.6 compared to 1.0 before angioplasty. Intracoronary adenosine produced an increase in mean velocity from 41 to 72 cm/sec (coronary vasodilatory reserve = 1.8) with the increase in diastolic flow accounting for most of this flow improvement. The abnormal phasic systolic predominant pattern persisted as the Doppler guidewire was withdrawn into the region proximal to the lesion (Fig. 2F). The post-angioplasty cineangiograms showed a hazy result with probably a limited dissection and angiographic TIMI 3 flow (Fig. 2G). Although the final coronary flow velocity pattern was abnormal, the patient had resolution of ischemic symptoms without clinical evidence of vessel reclosure prior to discharge.

DISCUSSION

These cases illustrate that different patterns of collateral flow velocity reversal may be seen in arteries supplying infarcted myocardial regions and that despite a satisfactory angiographic appearance, phasic flow velocity may be persistently abnormal when myocardial contraction is impaired.

Influence of Lesions on Phasic Coronary Flow Velocity Patterns

In patients, coronary flow velocity patterns show normal phasic variation with diastolic predominance and a systolic peak velocity anywhere from 25–50% that of the diastolic peak velocity [5–7]. The diastolic/systolic flow velocity ratio in the proximal segment of the right coronary artery often approaches 1.0 with nearly equal peak diastolic and systolic peak flow velocity integrals. The proposed mechanisms of the various phasic patterns are centered on contraction related flow modulation. During systole, increasing left ventricular wall tension results in a decreased aorta-intramyocardial pressure gradient and decreased epicardial coronary blood flow. On left ventricular relaxation, this gradient increases potentiating diastolic flow into the myocardium. Hemodynamically significant coronary stenoses with approximately 70% of the lumen cross-sectional area obstructed (45–50% diameter stenosis) maintain resting blood flow by compen-

satory microcirculatory vasodilation [8]. Flow is preserved until approximately 90% of the cross-sectional area is obliterated [9]. The effect of hemodynamically significant stenoses on flow results in an abnormal resting distal phasic flow pattern with decreased diastolic flow velocity due to the preferential effect of stenoses on periods of high flow(diastole). Systolic flow may be unchanged and thus appears to become equiphasic or predominant. Systolic flow velocity is dependent on intramyocardial resistance and is reduced across critical stenosis, resulting in a predominantly systolic distal flow pattern with reduced mean and peak velocities, as seen in the second case [10].

Prior to dilation, distal coronary flow velocity patterns feature predominantly systolic flow with reduced peak and mean velocities. Total or subtotal occlusions generally do not allow antegrade flow. Following successful angioplasty, distal average peak velocity increases an average of 84% [6,7] with a return of the diastolic predominant pattern. This is reflected by an increase in the diastolic/systolic flow velocity ratio of approximately 50%. These patterns were exhibited by the first patient described above who experienced rapid return of high velocity antegrade flow with a normal diastolic/systolic flow ratio (Fig. 1B).

In the second patient, the post-angioplasty angiographic result was adequate and, although average peak velocity was increased, the normal flow pattern was not restored (Fig. 2F). Conversion of the distal flow pattern to the normal diastolic predominance may be seen in 80% of patients and may require up to 10 min post-dilation [7]. It remains to be determined if a persistently abnormal phasic flow velocity pattern is predictive of reduced successful interventional outcomes compared to angiographic endpoints. Physiologically, the restoration of distal flow is critical to recovery of myocardial function and the relief of ischemia.

Collateral Flow

Often collateral flow can be easily detected and quantitated using the Doppler angioplasty wire [11]. In the first case, retrograde collateral flow had a velocity >40 cm/sec beyond the total proximally occluded artery segment. This high velocity flow was indicative of well-developed, mature collateral vessels which can be demonstrated angiographically by significant well opacified epicardial communications. Collateral flow may allow for prolonged balloon inflations. Occasionally, antegrade systolic distal flow is found distal to coronary occlusions, indicating collateral flow entering the native vessel proximal to the Doppler guidewire tip. The phasic pattern and magnitude of collateral flow appears to be related to the anatomic pathway and, in preliminary studies, unresponsive to direct coronary vasodilators [4]. As shown in these two cases, the collateral flow pattern may be minimally affected in some zones after myocardial infarction.

Coronary Flow Velocity in Regions of Myocardial Infarction

Following myocardial infarction, distal coronary flow velocity is often abnormal and depends on a variety of factors. After an infarct-related artery has recanalized, flow will depend, in part, on the residual stenosis and status of the microcirculation in the infarct zone. If collateral supply is present, the jeopardized myocardium may be relatively protected during epicardial vessel occlusion. Depending on the extent and duration of infarction and the degree of sustained or transient ischemic injury involving the macro- and micro-vasculature, the metabolic control of coronary flow will be altered [1]. While basal flow velocity may be relatively well-preserved, vasoregulatory compensatory mechanisms, as assessed using a variety of vasodilating drugs (e.g., intracoronary adenosine) may be strikingly abnormal [1,2].

Abnormal coronary flow regulation and hyperemic responses to vasodilators is well described in infarcted myocardium and appears most likely due to ischemic injury to the microcirculation [1,2]. This impairment may require a prolonged recuperative period before restoration of normal function. The time course of flow normalization in patients is reflected in a number of studies wherein microcirculatory vasoregulatory function was assessed following angioplasty [12–14]. Coronary flow reserve, the ratio of maximal hyperemia to resting flow velocity, obtained immediately after successful angioplasty showed remarkable variations. The wide range of coronary vasodilatory reserve values appears to depend on the status of microcirculatory and vasoregulatory responses in relation to vasoactive drugs, abnormalities of endothelial function, diabetes, hypertension, myocardial hypertrophy, long standing ischemia, or infarction, and the release of local and circulating vasoactive compounds [12,15,16] and the extent of ischemic injury following infarction. Hence, a poor correlation is found between post-angioplasty angiographic stenosis, cross-sectional area, or coronary flow reserve [17]. Distal coronary flow responses depend, in part, on the vasoregulatory capacity of infarcted tissue more than epicardial residual stenosis following successful angioplasty. Conversely, phasic distal flow patterns depend on the hemodynamic effect of residual epicardial stenoses and, as illustrated in the above cases, may normalize or remain abnormal following successful angioplasty.

ACKNOWLEDGMENTS

The authors wish to thank the J.G. Mudd Cardiac Catheterization Laboratory team and Donna Sander for manuscript preparation.

REFERENCES

1. Klein L, Agarwal J, Schneider R, Herman G, Weintraub W, Helfant R: Effects of previous myocardial infarction on measurements of reactive hyperemia and coronary vascular reserve. J Am Coll Cardiol 8:357–363, 1986.
2. Straur B: The significance of coronary reserve in clinical heart disease. J Am Coll Cardiol 15:775–783, 1990.
3. Demer L, Gould KL, Kirkeeide RL: Assessing stenosis severity: coronary flow reserve, collateral function, quantitative coronary arteriography, positron imaging, and digital subtraction angiography: A review and analysis. Prog CV Dis 30:307–322, 1988.
4. Kern MJ, Donohue TJ, Bach RG, Aguirre FV, Caracciolo EA, Ofili EO: Quantitating coronary collateral flow velocity in patients during coronary angioplasty using a Doppler guidewire. Am J Cardiol 71:34D–40D, 1993.
5. Ofili EO, Labovitz AJ, Kern MJ: Coronary flow velocity dynamics in normal and diseased arteries. Am J Cardiol 71:3D–9D, 1993.
6. Ofili EO, Kern MJ, Labovitz AJ, St. Vrain JA, Segal J, Aguirre F, Castello R: Analysis of coronary blood flow velocity dynamics in angiographically normal and stenosed arteries before and after endolumen enlargement by angioplasty. J Am Coll Cardiol 21:308–316, 1993.
7. Segal J, Kern MJ, Scott NA, King SB III, Doucette JW, Heuser RR, Ofili E, Siegel R: Alterations of phasic coronary artery flow velocity in humans during percutaneous coronary angioplasty. J Am Coll Cardiol 20:276–286, 1992.
8. Gould KL, Kelley KO, Bolson EL: Experimental validation of quantitative coronary arteriography for determining pressure-flow characteristics of coronary stenosis. Circulation 66:930–937, 1982.
9. Gould KL, Kelley KO: Physiologic significance of coronary flow velocity and changing stenosis geometry during coronary vasodilation in dogs. Circ Res 50:695–704, 1982.
10. Spaan JAAE, Breuls NPW, Laird JD: Diastolic-systolic coronary flow differences are caused by intramyocardial pump action in the anesthetized dog. Circ Res 49:584–593, 1981.
11. Donohue TJ, Kern MJ, Aguirre FV, Bell C, Penick D, Ofili E: Comparison of hemodynamic and pharmacologic perturbations of coronary collateral flow velocity in patients during angioplasty (Abstr). J Am Coll Cardiol 19:383A, 1992.
12. Wilson RF, Johnson MR, Marcus ML, Aylward PEG, Skorton DJ, Collins S, White CW: The effect of coronary angioplasty on coronary flow reserve. Circulation 77:873–885, 1988.
13. Serruys PW, Julliere Y, Zijlstra F, Beatt KJ, De Feyter PJ, Suryapranata H, van den Branch M, Roelandt J: Coronary blood flow velocity during percutaneous transluminal coronary angioplasty as a guide for assessment of the functional result. Am J Cardiol 61:253–259, 1988.
14. Kern MJ, Deligonul U, Vandormael M, Labovitz A, Gudipati R, Gabliani G, Bodet J, Shah Y, Kennedy HL: Impaired coronary vasodilatory reserve in the immediate post-coronary angioplasty period: Analysis of coronary artery velocity indexes and regional cardiac venous efflux. J Am Coll Cardiol 13:860–872, 1989.
15. Houghton JL, Frank MJ, Carr AA, von Dohlen TW, Prisant M: Relations among impaired coronary flow reserve, left ventricular hypertrophy and thallium perfusion defects in hypertensive patients without obstructive coronary artery disease. J Am Coll Cardiol 15:43–51, 1990.
16. Cannon R, Watson R, Rosing D, Epstein S: Angina caused by reduced vasodilator reserve of the small coronary arteries. J Am Coll Cardiol 1:1359–1373, 1983.
17. White CW: Clinical applications of Doppler coronary flow reserve measurements. Am J Cardiol 71:10D–16D, 1993.

Chapter 17

Alterations of Coronary Flow Velocity During Intervention for Acute Myocardial Infarction:
Responses to Complications of Intracoronary Thrombolysis and Angioplasty

Morton J. Kern, MD, Eugene Caracciolo, MD, Frank V. Aguirre, MD,
Richard G. Bach, MD, and Thomas J. Donohue, MD

INTRODUCTION

Urgent intervention for acute myocardial infarction may require infusion of thrombolytic agents to reduce the occlusive thrombotic burden and permit visualization of arterial pathways before proceeding with angioplasty [1, 2]. After recanalization by thrombolysis, coronary flow is often dramatically improved angiographically, but the quantitative correlations with measured flow velocity have not been reported. With the availability of a Doppler-tipped angioplasty guidewire, coronary flow velocity changes during intracoronary thrombolysis with subsequent angioplasty for treatment of acute myocardial infarction can be studied. Alterations in coronary flow velocity during such procedures permit identification of phenomenology, which may portend favorable or unfavorable outcomes [3, 4]. We present observations in a patient who had an acute inferolateral myocardial infarction due to thrombotic occlusion of the circumflex coronary artery, which was successfully recanalized with intracoronary urokinase and angioplasty. In the course of the procedure, flow velocity was continuously monitored. Cyclical flow velocity variations, as well as flow due to changing arterial vasomotor tone of the instrumented vessel prior to side branch closure, are described. These unique findings promote our understanding of the physiology occurring during coronary interventions for acute myocardial infarction.

CASE REPORT

The patient was 55-year-old and with a history of inferior wall myocardial infarction treated with thrombolytic therapy 2 years prior to current presentation. He had a history of prior smoking and hypercholesterolemia. Two years ago severe angina pectoris occurred associated with a non-Q-wave myocardial infarction. Coronary angiography was performed due to persistent angina in the coronary care unit unrelieved by intravenous nitroglycerin, heparin, and oral calcium channel blockers. Coronary arteriography showed a normal left anterior descending coronary artery, a patent circumflex artery with total occlusion of the proximal first obtuse marginal branch, and serial 40% and 70% diameter narrowings in the distal right coronary artery. Left ventricular systolic function was within normal limits with an ejection fraction of 64%. Medical therapy was maximized and the patient discharged without symptoms. On the current hospitalization, the patient was readmitted with pulmonary edema, episodic bradycardia, and hypotension preceded by increasing exertional angina. A temporary pacemaker was placed and emergent cardiac catheterization performed.

In the cardiac catheterization laboratory, the patient was intubated, mechanically ventilated, and hemodynamically stabilized with intravenous dopamine. The blood pressure was 100/70 mmHg. The electrocardiogram demonstrated complete heart block with a 100% paced rhythm, inferior/posterior myocardial infarction,

60 yr old Male, Inferior Lateral MI

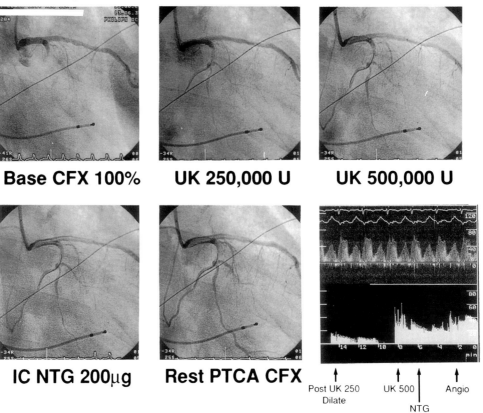

Fig. 1. Top: Left panel: Angiographic frames of the left coronary artery in the right anterior oblique (RAO) projection showing total occlusion of the circumflex artery (arrow). Middle panel: Angiographic appearance after 250,000 units of intracoronary urokinase over 5 min. The flowire is positioned in the midcircumflex artery beyond the first marginal bifurcated branch. Far right panel: Angiographic improvement after additional 250,000 (total 500,000 units) units of urokinase intracoronary. Bottom:Left panel: Narrowed artery diameters associated with increased flow velocity after urokinase immediately before introduction of nitroglycerin (200 μg) into the coronary artery. Middle panel: Coronary artery after coronary angioplasty. Note enlarged distal vessel and the hazy effect at the angioplasty site at the location of previous thrombus. Flowire can be seen within the midcircumflex beyond the large marginal branch takeoff. Right panel: Trend of flow velocity (bottom section, 0–100 cm/sec scale; 15-min recording with 2-min interval markers) showing both the velocity during urokinase (UK) at angioplasty (dilatations) and nitroglycerin (NTG). Cyclical flow variations are identified immediately at the posturokinase 250,000 units mark. After the second administration of urokinase because of diminished artery diameter, coronary flow velocity increased dramatically. NTG normalized flow velocity. Angiography (angio) was taken when flow was improving associated with bottom middle angiogram. For the top section of this panel, the phasic velocity is shown. The velocity scale is 0–200 cm/sec. Intra-aortic balloon pumping (2:1 mode) demonstrates alternating augmentation of arterial pressures associated with augmentation of the flow velocity integral. The alternation of greater and lesser flow velocity signals can be easily seen in the phasic pattern.

and ST depressions in leads V_2-V_4. The chest X-ray was consistent with acute pulmonary edema. An intra-aortic balloon pump was inserted. Coronary arteriography showed total occlusion of the proximal circumflex artery (and non-visualization of the first obtuse marginal branch) and minimal irregularities in the left anterior descending coronary artery (Fig. 1, top left panel). The right coronary artery had serial 70% proximal and mid-vessel stenoses, unchanged from the previous year.

Because of the acute circumflex occlusion with lateral wall infarction and clinical shock, emergent angioplasty was planned. Prior to performance of angioplasty, intracoronary urokinase was administered in an attempt to reduce the thrombus burden and identify the course of the coronary artery. A Doppler flowire was placed in the circumflex artery to quantitate flow changes during thrombolysis. Intracoronary urokinase (250,000 units) was given over 5 min with an improvement in both the angiographic and Doppler coronary flow velocity (Fig. 1, middle and right panels). While intracoronary urokinase was infusing, cyclical variations of the coronary flow velocity pattern could be seen (Fig. 1, bottom right), an event consistent with thrombus resolution as described by Folts et al. [5]. To further reduce coronary obstruction, angioplasty was performed with a 3.0 mm balloon (18K Medtronic) over the 0.018″ flowire that had been placed in the distal circumflex artery before thrombolysis. Multiple balloon inflations were performed, which further improved coronary flow velocity. Because of persistent thrombus after the first series of dilatations, a second bolus of urokinase (250,000 units) was administered. Flow velocity was nearly doubled after 500,000 units of urokinase (Fig. 1, bottom right). The distal vessel appeared to be narrowed with accelerated flow velocity. To reduce potential spasm, intracoronary nitroglycerin was administered. The effect of nitroglycerin on vessel diameter can be identified both by the enlarging angiographic cross-sectional area (Fig. 1, bottom left) as well as the diminishing flow velocity (Fig. 1, bottom right).

Following the initial dilatations, continued monitoring of flow demonstrated initial distal coronary flow increase followed by gradual decrease in flow velocity (Fig. 2, bottom left). Angiography at that time showed occlusion of the previously patent but stenotic obtuse marginal branch (Fig. 2, top left). Administration of a third dose of intracoronary urokinase (250,000 units for a total dose of 750,000 units) produced little improvement in the marginal branch flow (Fig. 2, top middle). Angioplasty of the marginal branch was then performed, noting that the flow velocity had gradually increased in the distal circumflex bed without change in vessel caliber (Fig. 2, middle bottom). Final angiography demonstrated a 30% residual circumflex lesion (Fig. 2, top right) with a satisfactory distal flow velocity (Fig. 2, bottom right) and a mildly dissected marginal branch. Of note, intra-aortic balloon pumping demonstrated improved flow velocity augmentation as previously reported [7] (Fig. 1, alternating phasic pattern, lower right upper section). The balloon pump was maintained in place for 48 hr and removed without complications. The patient had an uneventful recovery in the post-infarction period.

DISCUSSION

This patient demonstrated four features that are remarkable during coronary intervention for acute myocardial infarction: cyclical flow variations, coronary vasoconstriction with flow acceleration, coronary vasodilation with nitroglycerin and flow deceleration with lumen enlargement, and flow velocity augmentation during side branch occlusion. Previously reported in experimental animal and patient studies of thrombolytic oc-

clusions [5,6], cyclical flow variation is evident during recanalization of an artery due to lysis of the thrombotic coronary occlusion. Cyclic flow variation may occur either during thrombolysis or thrombosis, both of which have been known to occur spontaneously or after intravenous or intracoronary urokinase or other thrombolytic agents. The demonstration of cyclical flow variations is associated with both re-establishment of patency, as well as impending vessel closure and indicates unstable coronary flow due to varying luminal impingement [3,4]. In this patient, improving angiographic coronary flow after urokinase was important clinically to relieve symptoms and technically to facilitate the angioplasty. The immediate effects of recanalization with thrombolysis on coronary flow velocity have not been extensively studied.

Coronary spasm was an unexpected complicating factor after angioplasty in the setting of thrombolysis. Coronary vasospasm can result from both humeral factors of thrombolysis and mechanical factors related to balloon or guidewire irritation and trauma of vascular smooth muscle and endothelium, releasing vasoconstricting products such as endothelin-1. Moreover, continued thrombus formation and aggregating platelets, not appreciated angiographically, may release vasoactive products including thrombin and thromboxane associated with vessel narrowing. Some or all of these mechanisms likely contributed to coronary vasospasm observed angiographically and quantitated physiologically with an increased flow velocity during luminal narrowing. After resolution of the thrombotic coronary occlusion and angioplasty, intracoronary nitroglycerin was highly effective in restoring the constricted coronary diameter, promoting improved antegrade coronary flow, and potentially facilitating safe performance of the procedure.

The fourth major finding in this case was the observation that side branch closure was associated with an unanticipated increase in flow velocity in the adjacent circumflex vessel. Diversion of flow previously entering a side branch would be seen as an increase in total flow now entering the remaining patent vessels. This paradoxic increase in flow may also have been due to concurrent vasoconstriction occurring around the flowire with a diminished cross-sectional area. However, this possibility was not demonstrated angiographically.

SUMMARY

Alterations, either an increase or decrease, in the distal flow velocity over time are associated with alterations in vessel diameter and/or unstable flow velocity. Unexplained unstable flow velocity patterns should act as early warning signs to prompt the interventionalist to assess continued coronary patency and need for renewed interventions.

60 yr old Male, Inferior Lateral MI

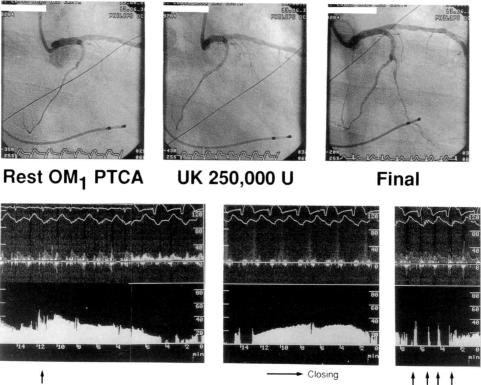

Rest OM₁ PTCA   UK 250,000 U   Final

Fig. 2. Top panel: Angiograms after urokinase and angioplasty with subsequent alterations in the flow velocity with initially increasing and decreasing flow velocity over time (lower panels) was associated with the marginal branch closing. Top middle: Further administration of urokinase failed to recanalize the marginal branch after attempted angioplasty. Lower middle: Distal vessel vasoconstriction resulted in increasing average trend flow velocity. Top right: Angiogram shows result after final angioplasty with restoration of a large marginal branch, but occlusion of the small first branch off this large vessel due to dissection. Multiple dilatations failed to restore this small branch. Lower right: Final flow velocity was satisfactory and stable. Velocity trend scale is 0–100 cm/sec.

ACKNOWLEDGMENTS

The authors thank the J.G. Mudd Cardiac Catheterization Laboratory Team and Donna Sander for manuscript preparation.

REFERENCES

1. Yusuf S, Collins R, Peto R, Furberg C, Stampfer MJ, Goldhaber SZ, Hennekens CH: Intravenous and intracoronary fibrinolytic therapy in acute myocardial infarction: overview of results on mortality, reinfarction and side effects from 33 randomized controlled trials. Eur Heart J 6:556–585, 1985.
2. Kennedy JW, Ritchie JL, Davis KB, Stadius ML, Maynard C, Fritz JK: The Western Washington randomized trial of intracoronary streptokinase in acute myocardial infarction. N Engl J Med 312:1073–1078, 1985.
3. Anderson HV, Kirkeeide RL, Stuart Y, Smalling RW, Heibig J, Willerson JT: Coronary artery flow monitoring following coronary interventions. Am J Cardiol 71(14):62D–69D, 1993.
4. Kern MJ, Aguirre FV, Donohue TJ, Bach RG, Caracciolo EA, Flynn MS: Coronary flow velocity monitoring after angioplasty associated with abrupt reocclusion. Am Heart J 127:436–438, 1994.
5. Folts JD, Crowell EB, Rowe GG: Platelet aggregation in partially obstructed vessels and its elimination with aspirin. Circulation 54:365–370, 1976.
6. Eichhorn EJ, Grayburn PA, Willard JE, Anderson HV, Bedotto JB, Carry M, Kahn JK, Willerson JT: Spontaneous alterations in coronary blood flow velocity before and after coronary angioplasty in patients with severe angina. J Am Coll Cardiol 17:43–52, 1991.
7. Kern MJ, Aguirre F, Bach R, Donohue T, Segal J: Augmentation of coronary blood flow by intra-aortic balloon pumping in patients after coronary angioplasty. Circulation 87:500–511, 1993.

Chapter 18

Assessment of Serial Lesions in the Proximal Right Coronary Artery Following Intracoronary Thrombolysis

Joseph A. Moore, MD, and Morton J. Kern, MD

INTRODUCTION

Coronary angiography imprecisely defines the hemodynamic significance of intermediate coronary lesions [1,2], a situation further complicated by intravascular thrombosis. Pressure and flow relationships derived from experimental animal data [3,4] and human physiologic studies performed under controlled settings have been applied to assess the physiologic significance of coronary artery lesions using direct measurements of translesional pressure gradient and intracoronary Doppler flow velocity with and without pharmacologic hyperemia [5–7]. Although a single coronary stenosis may be easily addressed by translesional pressure and flow velocity measurements, the presence of serial lesions complicates the physiologic impact of these observations. To add an additional confounding factor, consideration of alterations in coronary flow that occur during and after acute coronary thrombosis and pharmacologically stimulated thrombolysis must be made.

RIGHT CORONARY ARTERY THROMBOSIS AFTER RENAL TRANSPLANTATION

A 43-yr-old man with a 2-month history of exertional chest pressure and dyspnea relieved with rest was admitted with crescendo angina pectoris of 2 d duration. The past medical history was significant for renal transplantation 3 yr prior to admission. There was no prior history

of cardiac disease. Cardiac risk factors include hypercholesterolemia, hypertension, smoking, and a family history of coronary artery disease. Medications on admission were cylcosporine A, prednisone, imuran, and mevacor. The admission physical examination was unremarkable. Laboratory data revealed a modest elevation of serum creatinine (3.6 mg/dl) and mild reductions of hemoglobin and hematocrit (8.4 gm/dl and 24.9%, respectively). The electrocardiogram showed normal sinus rhythm, left ventricular hypertrophy, and inferior Q waves consistent with a previous infarction of unknown age. No acute ST and T-wave abnormalities were noted. The patient was treated with intravenous nitroglycerin, packed red cells, heparin, and oral aspirin with prompt resolution of his symptoms.

Diagnostic cardiac catheterization and coronary angiography performed the following day demonstrated a 60% stenosis in the midportion of the right coronary artery with angiographic evidence of intraluminal thrombus (Fig. 1). Moderate inferior hypokinesis was seen on left ventriculography. Intracoronary urokinase (500,000 units) was infused into the right coronary artery over 20 min with minimal angiographic improvement in the appearance of the intraluminal lucency. Intravenous heparin (to maintain aPTT >60 sec) was continued until a repeat catheterization 3 d later, which demonstrated substantially resolved thrombus with sequential, complex lesions in the proximal and midright coronary artery of

LAO   RAO

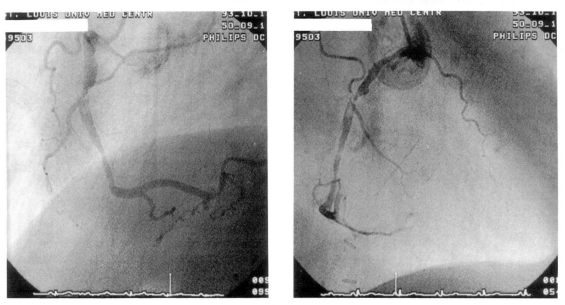

Fig. 1. Right coronary artery (RCA) angiograms in left (LAO) and right anterior oblique (RAO) projections. A complex lesion is seen in the midportion of the vessel with angiographic evidence of thrombus.

moderate severity (Fig. 2). By quantitative angiography, the diameter narrowings were 75% and 61% for the proximal and midright coronary artery lesions, respectively.

Prior to balloon angioplasty, translesional flow velocity was measured with a 0.018″ Doppler angioplasty guidewire (FloWire™, Cardiometrics, Mountain View, CA) and pressure was measured with an end-hole 2.2F infusion catheter (Tracker 18™, Target Therapeutics). Flow velocities recorded proximal to the first stenosis showed a mean velocity of 37 cm/sec (Table I) with diastolic predominance (diastolic/systolic velocity ratio = 1.12) (Fig. 3, top left). Following 8 μg of intracoronary adenosine, flow velocity increased to 68 cm/sec with proximal coronary vasodilatory reserve equal to 1.8 (Fig. 3, bottom left). The Doppler guidewire was advanced across both lesions without difficulty. Distal flow velocities in the midright coronary artery were similar to those recorded proximally (mean velocity = 36 cm/sec, diastolic/systolic velocity ratio = 1.47, coronary vasodilatory reserve = 1.4) (Fig. 3, top and bottom right). On further advancement of the flowire to the distal posterolateral branch, the flow pattern became abnormal with reduced diastolic predominance and mean velocity of 12 cm/sec and no evidence of hyperemia (Fig. 4, top left and middle). The resting translesional pressure gradient was 70 mmHg, which increased to 85 mmHg after 8 μg of intracoronary adenosine (Fig. 4, bottom panels).

Angioplasty was then performed on the midright coronary artery lesion using a fixed-wire system due to inability to cross the lesion with an over-the-wire system. The Doppler guidewire remained in the distal right coronary artery just proximal to several large posterolateral branches during angioplasty. During balloon inflations, low velocity antegrade distal flow was recorded (Fig. 5, lower left). Persistent flow during artery occlusion may have been the result of incomplete occlusion of the vessel by the angioplasty balloon or, more likely, collateral flow entering the vessel proximal to the site of the Doppler guidewire tip. Following successful dilations of the more distal lesion, the distal mean flow velocity was 21 cm/sec with a predominantly systolic flow pattern (Fig. 5, lower right, upper half of panel, trend print). Increased narrowing of the proximal lesion near the guide catheter tip was noted, which remained unchanged with intracoronary nitroglycerin (200 μg). The proximal lesion was then dilated. The flow velocity trend was recorded during balloon inflations and demonstrated stable low flow velocity signals of collateral input during balloon inflations. Hyperemia following balloon deflation is also noted (Fig. 5, lower right, trend plot arrows). Despite repeat balloon inflations, both lesions exhibited a hazy appearance on angiography with TIMI-3 angiographic flow. The distal flow velocity was stable for >5 min following

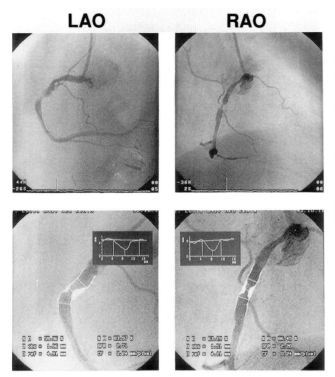

LAO   **RAO**

Fig. 2. Orthogonal views (left anterior oblique, LAO; right anterior oblique, RAO) of the right coronary artery (RCA) after 72 h of intravenous heparin (1,000 units/h) demonstrate a complex lesion (long black arrow) of moderate severity on quantitative coronary angiography (lower panels). A moderate lesion (open arrow, RAO) is also noted in the proximal vessel. Small black arrow denotes region of diffuse nonsignificant narrowing.

TABLE I. Translesional Flow Velocities and Pressure Gradients Before and After Angioplasty*

	APV (cm/sec)	MPV (cm/sec)	DSVR	CVR	Gradient (mmHg)
Pre-PTCA[a]					
Proximal baseline	37	45	1.12	—	—
Proximal adenosine	68	83	0.93	1.8	—
Mid baseline	36	49	1.47	—	70
Mid adenosine	50	61	1.30	1.4	85
Distal baseline	12	20	1.1	—	—
Distal adenosine[b]	12	20	—	1.0	—
Post-PTCA					
Proximal baseline	26	41	—	—	—
Proximal adenosine	—	—	—	—	—
Distal baseline	13	18	1.27	—	25
Distal adenosine	18	25	1.24	1.4	40

*Abbreviations: APV = average peak velocity; MPV = maximal peak velocity; DSVR = diastolic/systolic velocity ratio; CVR = coronary vasodilatory reserve.
[a]Adenosine = 8 μg intracoronary bolus.
[b]Posterolateral branch.

the final balloon dilation. The balloon catheter was withdrawn.

After the final inflation, the mean distal flow velocity

was minimally improved, but the phasic pattern (DSVR) was normalized. There was a reduction of peak flow velocity with retention of the preangioplasty diastolic to systolic flow ratio (Fig. 6, top panels; Table I). The coronary vasodilatory reserve was unchanged from preangioplasty values. The postangioplasty translesional pressure gradient was 25 mmHg, which increased to 40 mmHg during maximal hyperemia with 8 μg of intracoronary adenosine (Fig. 6, bottom panels). The Doppler guidewire was then withdrawn into the proximal right coronary artery (near the more proximal lesion) where flow velocities were slightly increased (Table I). The final angiograms continued to demonstrate an hazy appearance to both lesions with a type A dissection of the proximal lesion (Fig. 7). The final QCA diameters were 45% and 33% for the proximal and midright coronary artery lesions, respectively.

Despite the final angiographic appearance and slightly reduced peak and mean flow velocities following angioplasty, flow remained stable for 10 min postangioplasty. The patient experienced no clinical or laboratory evidence of acute reclosure of the right coronary artery prior to discharge home on routine postangioplasty medications.

DISCUSSION

The assessment of some moderate and severe lesions at the time of diagnostic catheterization remains a difficult problem. Ideally, angiographic information supplements noninvasive measures of ischemia in decisions regarding lesion severity and the need for interventions. This case illustrates several interesting points regarding serial lesion assessment postthrombolysis and angioplasty.

Unstable angina associated with angiographic evidence of intralesional thrombus resolved after intravenous heparin administration. The subsequent repeat coronary arteriography demonstrated a midlesion of obvious (>90%) severity in the right anterior oblique projection with a more proximal lesion of only moderate (50–70%) narrowing. What was not initially appreciated was the mild midvessel narrowing distal to the midlesion, which may, in part, be responsible for the increased flow velocity measured in this region (Fig. 3). Furthermore, velocity in the posterolateral branch (Fig. 4) was decreased and indicated more impaired flow to this distal bed. Thus the summed result of serial lesions in this artery is a loss of distal flow velocity and phasic pattern.

Coronary Flow Velocity Measurements

The phasic pattern of distal right coronary artery flow was abnormal before angioplasty and normalized after angioplasty, despite only a modest increase in mean ve-

Proximal   **Distal**

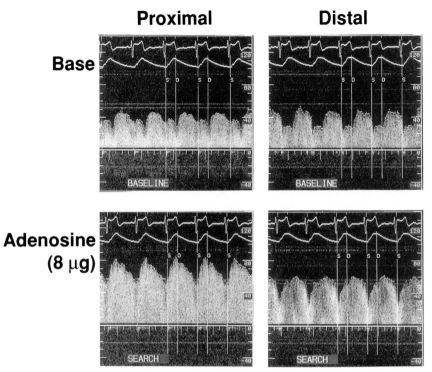

Fig. 3. Before angioplasty, proximal and distal flow velocities at rest and during hyperemia with adenosine (8 μg). Velocity scale 0–200 cm/sec. S,D denote onset of systole, diastole. Electrocardiography and aortic pressure tracings are displayed at top of each panel. Flow velocity values can be found in Table I.

locity (Fig. 6). In the normal left coronary artery, the diastolic/systolic flow velocity ratio is >2.0 [5,8]. The normal right coronary artery diastolic/systolic flow velocity ratio is closer to 1.5 and depends on the extent to which the right coronary artery supplies left ventricular myocardium. Critical stenoses result in diminished distal flow with an abnormal systolic predominant pattern [5,8].

The diastolic/systolic flow velocity ratios distal to the lesions in this patient were ~1.5 in portions of the vessel supplying primarily the right ventricle. When the Doppler guidewire was placed in the posterolateral branches, the flow pattern changed dramatically (Fig. 5, top right). As opposed to a normal diastolic predominant pattern in arteries supplying left ventricular myocardium, the flow is essentially equiphasic with a diastolic/systolic flow velocity ratio of 1.0; a clearly abnormal pattern implying the lesions in the proximal and midright coronary artery are hemodynamically limiting despite the more normal recordings in the mid right coronary artery.

In branching coronary arteries, a proximal to distal flow ratio >1.7 indicates a significant reduction of distal flow and is associated with a translesional pressure gradient >30 mmHg [6]. In the above patient, the proximal to systolic flow ratio was 0.97, despite angiographic and

hemodynamic evidence of a significant stenosis. Flow velocity in normal non-branching right coronary arteries has been found to be similar proximally and distally in accordance with the continuity equation for a uniform diameter tube model. This principle supports data acquired in the midright coronary artery, provided there was no artifact from flow acceleration within the midright coronary artery due to diffuse segmental narrowing (Fig. 2, small arrow). Thus serial narrowings must be considered in the interpretation of proximal to distal flow velocity values when discordant with clinical findings.

Coronary Vasodilatory Reserve After Thrombolysis

Coronary vasodilatory reserve is a measure of the ability of the vasoregulatory microcirculation to respond to various physiologic and pharmacologic influences. The vasoregulatory function of the microcirculation is impaired following myocardial infarction and in the presence of hypertension, diabetes mellitus, hypercholesterolemia, and tobacco smoke exposure [9]. In this patient, coronary vasodilatory reserve measured in both the proximal and distal right coronary artery were initially abnormal (Table I). Although not measured in the posterolateral branches, coronary vasodilatory reserve would also

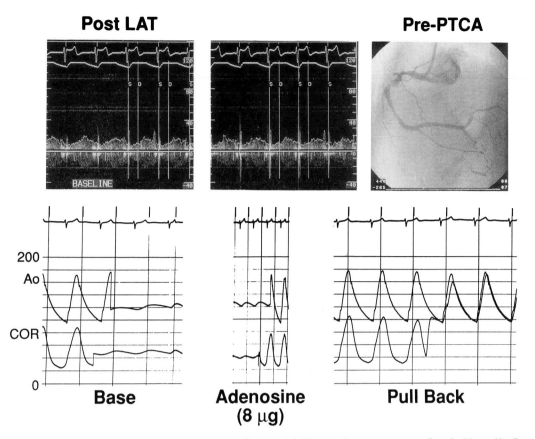

Post LAT   **Pre-PTCA**

Base   **Adenosine**   **Pull Back**
                  (8 μg)

Fig. 4. Distal flow velocity and translesional pressure gradient before angioplasty. The Doppler guidewire is positioned in the large posterolateral (post-LAT) branches (arrow, top right panel). Resting flow velocity is reduced and does not increase after 8 μg intracoronary adenosine (top, left, and middle pan- els). The resting pressure gradient is 70 mmHg (lower left) and increases to 85 mmHg after intracoronary adenosine (lower middle). Pullback through the midright coronary artery (RCA) narrowing documents the location of the pressure gradient (lower right).

likely have been abnormally low due to the presence of infarcted or stunned myocardium as evidenced by ventriculography. Infarcted tissue may or may not have vasoregulatory competence as a result of ischemic injury to the vascular endothelium depending on the duration of ischemia prior to reperfusion and other factors [9,10]. For this reason, coronary vasodilatory reserve measurements performed following thrombolytic therapy and angioplasty yield variable results and are not predictive of the hemodynamic severity of coronary lesions, as evident in this patient. As noted by Wilson et al. [11], coronary vasodilatory reserve is often reduced immediately following coronary angioplasty and may not return to normal until several months following intervention.

Quantitative Coronary Angiography and Hemodynamics

Computer-assisted quantitative coronary angiography accurately measures ex vivo coronary artery cast dimensions but is less precise for in vivo measurements of hemodynamic severity. It is difficult to define both the angiographic and hemodynamic lesion severity of eccentric lesions, long lesions, and those with complex geometry, particularly if the lesion in question is not examined in orthogonal views with the imaging camera perpendicular to the long axis of the vessel. The presence of intraluminal thrombus, motion artifact, changes in contrast mixing, injection rate and pressure, camera height, magnification, differences between systolic and diastolic coronary dimensions, perfusion pressure, and variability of coronary vasomotor tone introduce further error into the angiographic estimation of lumen cross-sectional area. The influence of many of these variables can be reduced by careful attention to angiographic technique, however, the total variability of quantitative coronary angiography remains 8–15% [1,2].

Coronary Flow Velocity After Coronary Angioplasty

Following angiographically successful coronary interventions, distal average peak velocity increases an average of 84% [8] with a return to a normal diastolic pre-

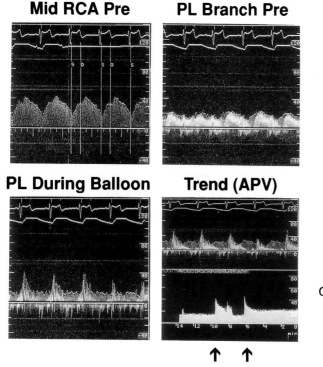

Fig. 5. (Top row): Flow velocities recorded in the midright coronary artery (RCA) and posterolateral (PL) branches show markedly different flow patterns. Flow in the mid RCA is predominantly diastolic with an average velocity of 36 cm/sec (Table I). In the posterolateral branches flow velocity is diminished with average peak velocity (APV) of 15 cm/sec with loss of diastolic predominance. (Bottom): During balloon inflations, antegrade collateral flow is noted in the posterolateral branches (lower left). Note flow is primarily systolic. The average flow velocity trend (0–100 cm/sec scale over 15 mins) reveals stable low velocity flow during balloon inflation and moderate postocclusive hyperemia (arrows).

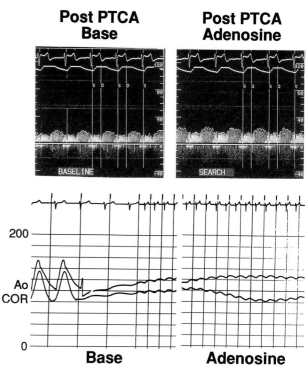

Fig. 6. Postangioplasty flow velocities recorded in the distal right coronary artery (RCA) reveal reduced resting and hyperemic flow (Table I). Note that flow is predominantly diastolic. The translesional pressure gradient is improved. The rest gradient of 25 mmHg (lower left) increases to 40 mmHg following intracoronary adenosine (lower right). Ao = guide catheter; cor = coronary pressure. (Pressure scale 0–200 mmHg, velocity scale 0–200 cm/sec.).

dominant pattern, which may require several minutes. Occasionally, however, an abnormal systolic predominant pattern may persist or average peak velocities may remain reduced. In this patient, the flow velocity pattern was unchanged following successful coronary angioplasty (Fig. 6). Peak flow velocities measured distally were reduced when compared to proximal values (Table I). Several factors may account for these findings: (1) the flow velocity measured in the proximal artery may have been artifactually elevated by an high intralesional jet velocity, (2) following angioplasty, a dissection at the proximal lesion was present, contributing to suboptimal flow despite a low residual gradient, and (3) despite adequate anticoagulation, thrombus and platelet aggregates released from the site of dissection may release powerful vasoconstrictors, which may influence downstream flow.

Translesional Pressure Gradients

Translesional pressure gradients have been evaluated as a means of assessing intermediate lesions and, in branching artery systems, found to correlate well with distal coronary flow velocity measurements [6]. For branching coronary arteries, a pressure gradient >30 mmHg is highly correlated with a proximal to distal flow velocity ratio >1.7 [6]. The measured gradient, however, does not always correlate with angiographic percent diameter stenosis, particularly in intermediate lesions. During pharmacologic stimulation of maximal coronary flow, translesional pressure gradients may increase substantially depending on the arterial cross-sectional lesion area. The hemodynamic impact is thus the net relationship of pressure and flow. As seen in this case, the final resting pressure gradient of 25 mmHg, which increased to 45 mmHg after intracoronary adenosine-induced hyperemia, indicates a steep slope of the pressure-velocity relationship and important physiologic severity of these lesions despite their intermediate angiographic appearance. Consideration of stent placement

LAO   RAO

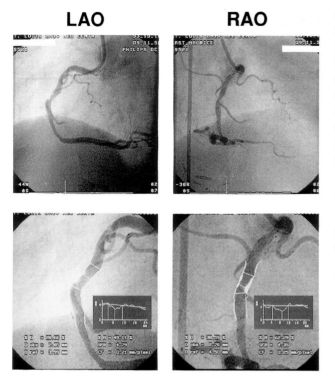

Fig. 7. Postangioplasty cineangiograms (top) and quantitative coronary angiography (bottom). The lesion in the midright coronary artery (RCA) has been reduced to 39% residual stenosis in the right anterior oblique (RAO) view. The proximal lesion appears hazy with a dissection plane (most evident in RAO view [arrow]).

may have been appropriate given the final angiographic and pressure/flow responses.

Persistent translesional pressure gradients >20 mmHg often indicate hemodynamic compromise despite a satisfactory angiographic appearance. How best to approach lesions in which the gradient is improved to a high normal range (i.e., 20 mmHg resting gradient) with normalization of phasic distal flow as seen in this patient in unclear. In this patient the final flow velocities were only minimally improved from the preangioplasty values. Thus it remains to be seen if translesional pressure or flow velocity become more predictive than angiographic endpoints of short- and long-term clinical success of coronary interventions.

Summary

Assessment of angiographically serial coronary lesions at the time of diagnostic catheterization remains a difficult clinical problem. Doppler flow velocity data is easily obtainable and allows physiologic interrogation of the distal coronary microcirculation, but has limitations in the detection of some flow-limiting stenoses. In cases of serial lesions or distal arterial disease, particularly after thrombolysis, flow velocity data may be insufficient to identify the hemodynamic significance of the coronary lesions. Translesional pressure measurements may be combined with flow velocity data to support an appropriate physiologically based therapeutic approach.

ACKNOWLEDGMENTS

The authors thank the J.G. Mudd Cardiac Catheterization Laboratory Team and Donna Sander for manuscript preparation.

REFERENCES

1. Zir LM, Miller SW, Dinsmore RE, Gilbert JP, Hawthorne JW: Interobserver variability in coronary angiography. Circulation 53: 627–632, 1976.
2. DeRouen TA, Murray JA, Owen W: Variability in the analysis of coronary angiograms. Circulation 55:324–328, 1977.
3. Gould KL, Lipscomb K, Hamilton GW: Physiologic basis for assessing critical coronary stenosis. Am J Cardiol 33:87–94, 1974.
4. Gould KL, Kelley KO, Bolson EL: Experimental validation of quantitative coronary arteriography for determining pressure-flow characteristics of coronary stenosis. Circulation 66:930–937, 1982.
5. Ofili EO, Kern MJ, Labovitz AJ, St. Vrain JA, Segal J, Aguirre F, Castello R: Analysis of coronary blood flow velocity dynamics in angiographically normal and stenosed arteries before and after endolumen enlargement by angioplasty. J Am Coll Cardiol 1993;21:308–316.
6. Donohue TJ, Kern MJ, Aguirre FV, Bach RG, Wolford T, Bell CA, Segal J: Assessing the hemodynamic significance of coronary artery stenoses: Analysis of translesional pressure-flow velocity relationships in patients. J Am Coll Cardiol 1993;22:449–458.
7. Wilson RF, Laughlin DE, Ackell PH, et al: Transluminal, subselective measurement of coronary artery blood flow velocity and vasodilator reserve in man. Circulation 72:82–92, 1985.
8. Segal J, Kern MJ, Scott NA, King SB III, Doucette JW, Heuser RR, Ofili E, Siegel R: Alterations of phasic coronary artery flow velocity in humans during percutaneous coronary angioplasty. J Am Coll Cardiol 1992;20:276–286.
9. White CW, Marcus ML, Wilson RF: Methods of measuring coronary flow in humans. Prog Cardiovasc Dis 31:79–94, 1988.
10. Marcus ML, Harrison DG, White CW, Hiratzka LF: Assessing the physiologic significance of coronary obstruction in man. Can J Cardiol 2 (suppl A):195A–199A, 1986.
11. Wilson RF, Marcus ML, White CW: Effects of coronary bypass surgery and angioplasty on coronary blood flow and flow reserve. Prog Cardiovasc Dis 31:95–114, 1988.

Chapter 19

Translesional Pressure and Flow Velocity After Thrombolysis: Assessment of Suboptimal Angioplasty for Serial Lesions

Joseph A. Moore, MD, Thomas J. Donohue, MD, and Morton J. Kern, MD

INTRODUCTION

Variations in vascular lumen dimensions directly influence pressure and flow velocity relationships. The angiographic characteristics of a coronary artery occluded with thrombus may suggest multiple organic stenosis, some or all of which can improve after thrombolysis. In the course of treating a patient with post-infarction angina, translesional flow and pressure data were obtained across serial lesions in a large, partially thrombosed right coronary artery. Abnormal variations in expected flow across significant lesions in the right coronary artery were encountered. This case emphasizes the contribution (or lack thereof) of right coronary marginal side branches and unsuspected luminal narrowings which can accelerate flow velocity. These data may be helpful in the assessment of suboptimal angioplasty results.

CASE REPORT

A 54-year-old man had an acute inferior myocardial infarction and received intravenous tissue plasminogen activator (t-PA) within 6 hr of the onset of symptoms. Because of continued intermittent chest pain, the patient was transferred for evaluation and treatment. The physical examination and laboratory data were within normal limits. The electrocardiogram showed inferior Q waves with T wave abnormalities of a myocardial infarction in evolution.

Coronary arteriography was performed with 6 French Judkins catheters and demonstrated minimally narrowed left anterior descending and circumflex arteries. The right coronary artery had intraluminal lucencies classically associated with intracoronary thrombus (Fig. 1). In the left anterior oblique projection, a proximal >75% diameter narrowed ulcerated lesion (number 1) with Ambrose type IIb morphology (overhanging shelf, irregular edges) could be seen. Immediately distal to this stenosis a large intravascular lucency (thrombus) surrounded by contrast (lesion number 2) was clearly visible. A more distal lesion (number 3) of ≤60% was also present. The posterior descending artery was occluded with an abrupt cut-off at the branch origin (Fig. 1, white arrow). The right anterior oblique projection confirmed the proximal and mid vessel lesions with thrombotic involvement and also revealed an ostial 40% tubular narrowing.

Because of the large thrombus burden, intracoronary urokinase (500,000 units × 20 minutes) was infused through the right coronary artery diagnostic catheter. Intravenous heparin was maintained to establish an ACT >300 sec. Intracoronary urokinase reduced the thrombus and improved TIMI flow from grade 1 to grade 2. The patient was returned to the coronary care unit on intravenous nitroglycerin, heparin, and oral calcium channel blockers. Angioplasty was to be re-considered 24 hr later.

On return to the catheterization laboratory the following day, repeat right coronary arteriography showed complete thrombus resolution and TIMI grade 3 flow (Fig. 2). The proximal stenosis (number 1) was now converted to a more benign appearance with an eccentric configuration of 70% diameter narrowing without the shelf-like configuration. The thrombus (lesion number 2) was not evident. The distal mid vessel lesion (number 3) had a more mild tapering appearance before the crux and

Acute Inferior MI

LAO   RAO

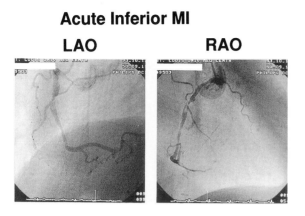

Fig. 1.   Cineangiographic frames of right coronary artery in patient M.E. before thrombolysis. Lesions are labelled number 1 proximal, number 2 thrombotic lesion below number 1, and number 3 mid right coronary artery. White arrow denotes location of occluded posterior descending branch. (LAO, left anterior oblique projection; RAO, right anterior oblique projection).

Pre PTCA

LAO   RAO

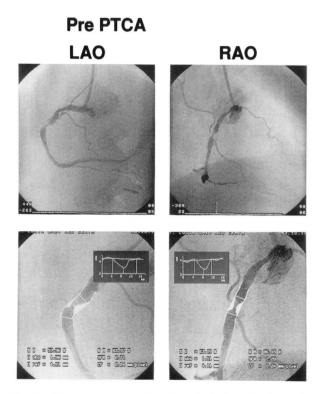

Fig. 2.   Cineangiograms after thrombolysis prior to angioplasty. Note improvement in lesions number 2 and number 3, but more prominent appearance of an ostial lesion in the right anterior oblique (RAO) projection. Lower panels show a 63% diameter narrowing by quantitative angiographic analysis. LAO, left anterior oblique projection.

Pre-PTCA

Proximal   Distal

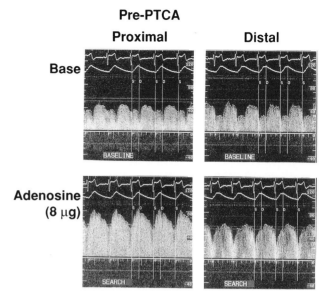

Fig. 3.   Flow velocity spectral signals proximal to lesion number 1 and distal to lesion number 2. Top Left: Normal proximal right coronary artery velocity with nearly normal hyperemia response to intracoronary adenosine (bottom left). Top right: Distal to lesion number 1 flow is also normal in phasic pattern with minimally reduced hyperemic response (bottom left). EKG, aortic pressure, and flow velocity are displayed from top to bottom on each panel. S,D mark onset of systole and diastole, respectively. Velocity scale is 0–200 cm/sec.

posterior descending branch occlusion. The ostial tubular lesion was unchanged.

Because of the previous unstable presentation, balloon angioplasty was performed. A 0.018″ FloWire (Cardio-metrics, Inc., Mountain View, CA) and 2.2F tracking catheter (Target Therapeutics) were used to evaluate the lesions before dilation as previously described [1–3]. Average flow velocity proximal to the first stenosis beyond the ostial narrowing was unusually high for a right coronary artery. The average peak velocity was 31 cm/sec with a diastolic/systolic velocity ratio of 1.3 (normal right coronary artery diastolic/systolic velocity ratio >1.2) (Fig. 3). In this location, intracoronary adenosine (8 μg) increased the basal average peak velocity to 62 cm/sec for a coronary flow reserve (hyperemic/basal average peak velocity ratio) of 2.0 (normal >2.0).

The flowire was advanced distal to the proximal stenosis in the mid right coronary artery after lesion number 2. The average flow velocity was nearly unchanged (24 cm/sec) with a slightly higher diastolic to systolic velocity ratio of 1.4. Intracoronary adenosine elicited a coronary flow reserve of 1.8 (42 cm/sec). The proximal to distal velocity ratio over the first lesion was (38/24) 1.5, which suggests a translesional gradient <30 mm Hg [4]. However, as the flowire was advanced more distally beyond the posterior descending and lateral branch arteries, the flow velocity was markedly reduced (Fig. 4). The average peak velocity was 18 cm/sec with a diastolic to systolic velocity ratio of 1.2, and a proximal to distal ratio now of >2.0. Intracoronary adenosine produced no

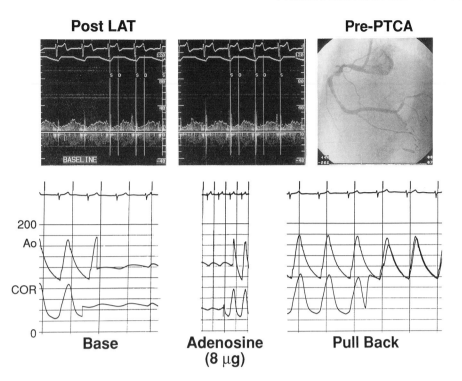

Fig. 4. Top left, middle: Flow velocity in the posterior descending artery (arrow on angiogram) beyond lesion number 3 shows markedly impaired flow velocity signal, no phasic pattern, and abnormal coronary vasodilatory reserve (1.0). Lower panels: Translesional pressure gradient measured with the guiding catheter (Ao, aortic pressure) and tracker catheter (COR) in the location shown on the angiogram (arrow). Base and hyperemic flow had similar pressure gradients which were caused exclusively by lesion number 1. Velocity scale as in Figure 3. Pressure scale is 0–200 mm Hg.

hyperemia yielding a coronary flow reserve of 1.0. A corresponding translesional pressure gradient between the aortic pressure in the guiding catheter and the posterolateral branch location was 70 mm Hg. The gradient increased to 80 mm Hg during the maximal hyperemia after intracoronary adenosine. The catheter pullback to the region proximal to lesion number 1 but distal to the ostial narrowing demonstrated the gradient was produced exclusively by the severe proximal lesion and not the ostial or more distal narrowings (Fig. 4, bottom right).

Angioplasty was performed with a 3.5 mm balloon catheter. During coronary balloon occlusion, persistent antegrade flow velocity was recorded indicating recruitable collateral flow from left-to-right with source vessels entering proximal to the flowire tip position (Fig. 5). Viability of the distal microcirculatory response was suggested by post-occlusive reactive hyperemia (Fig. 5, bottom right). Balloon inflations were also performed at the right ostial location because of a guide catheter-induced angiographic irregularity. Following ostial dilation, a dissection at this location was evident without flow impairment. Angiographic improvement in the proximal lesion (number 1) was present with a residual stenosis of 35% (QCA) diameter narrowing (Fig. 6). The ostial tubular narrowing was unchanged with a small

linear dissection. These suboptimal angiographic findings were associated with minimal improvement in average peak velocity (19 cm/sec) with a diastolic to systolic velocity ratio of 1.3 and a coronary flow reserve of 1.5 (26/19). The final resting translesional gradient was 20 mm Hg due to ostial and proximal lesion residual narrowing. The hyperemic gradient response was 40 mm Hg (Fig. 7).

Because of the recent thrombus in these activated lesions, a conservative approach was adopted. Consideration to stent and/or rotablator ablation for potential ostial restenosis was discussed. The patient was discharged after 48 hr of heparin on the fourth post-procedure day.

DISCUSSION

Alterations of angiographic characteristics after thrombolysis has important implications for the interpretation and strategy for angioplasty and flow velocity and pressure data.

Proximal to Distal Flow Velocity Ratio and Diffuse Luminal Disease

Flow velocity measured along the course of a coronary artery is influenced by the cross-sectional area in which

Mid RCA Pre **PL Branch Pre**

PL During Balloon **Trend (APV)**

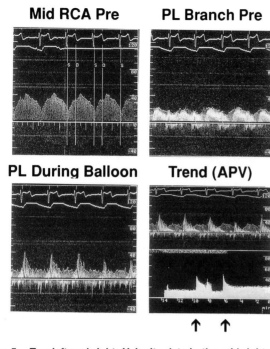

↑ ↑

Fig. 5. Top left and right: Velocity data in the mid right coronary artery at lesion number 3 and in the posterolateral (PL) branch prior to angioplasty (pre). Bottom left: Velocity during balloon occlusion in lesion number 1, representing persistent antegrade collateral flow. Velocity spectral format as in Figure 3. Bottom right: Trend of average peak velocity (APV) during right coronary artery angioplasty on lower half of panel. Two arrows indicate hyperemic responses after balloon deflation. APV scale is 0–100 cm/sec.

Post PTCA

LAO **RAO**

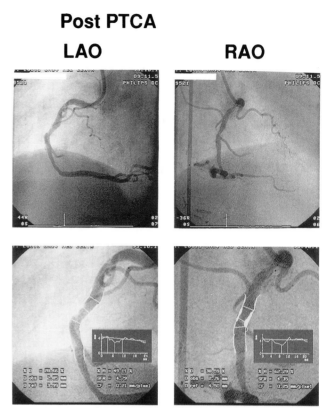

Fig. 6. Cineangiographic frames after angioplasty. Lesion number 1 is 38% diameter narrowed by quantitative coronary angiography. Note ostial lesion dissection.

the velocity is sampled [5]. In this patient, flow velocity proximal to the first lesion demonstrated a high value and probably reflected some acceleration due to the unappreciated ostial narrowing at the time of the first measurements. Flow velocity along the course of the right coronary artery did not fall until after the posterolateral branch origin, indicating that the tubular narrowing in region number 3 caused a secondary flow velocity acceleration and thus no fall in velocity which is usually associated with high translesional gradients in branching systems [4]. Limitations of the proximal to distal flow velocity ratio in the right coronary artery are well known due to the complex contribution of branch flow, location of measurements, ostial lesions, and distal disease. In general, the proximal to distal flow velocity ratio may be a specific but not a sensitive indicator of translesional pressure gradients. The velocity ratio value is most often helpful in the left coronary artery where branches serve to divert flow to regions of lower resistance. However, as noted before [5], for ostial lesions in the left coronary artery, measurements of the proximal to distal velocity ratio to reflect an accurate gradient may not be suitable. The lesion significance in this case was confirmed by

lack of distal hyperemia, impairment of the diastolic/systolic velocity ratio at the posterolateral location, and the translesional pressure gradient.

Coronary Flow Reserve: Variance in Locations Relative to the Target Lesion

Coronary flow reserve was greater in the proximal than the distal regions in a stepwise fashion as measurements were made across the first three lesion zones. Coronary reserve reflects both the contribution of branch flow at each location and the distal coronary bed flow. In this individual after acute myocardial infarction, there was a significantly impaired distal flow response relative to more proximal locations and right ventricular branches. It is important to note that after reduction of the translesional gradient from 70 mm Hg to 20 mm Hg, distal hyperemia (1.5 × basal flow) increased the resting translesional pressure gradient. The impaired reserve was higher than that prior to intervention. The routine measurement of coronary reserve along the course of coronary arteries has not been routinely studied. Variance in coronary vasodilatory reserve in several locations relative to branch points would suggest that diffuse distal disease unappreciated by angiography may be responsi-

Post PTCA Base   Post PTCA Adenosine

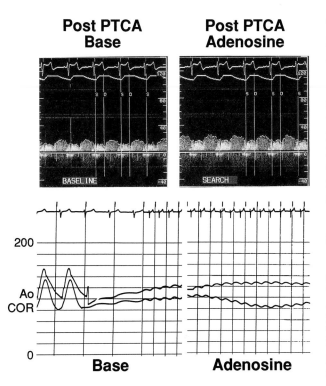

Fig. 7. Post-angioplasty flow velocity (Top) and translesional pressure (Bottom) at rest (left) and during hyperemia (right). Phasic flow has improved but coronary vasodilatory reserve is only minimally increased. The pressure gradient is 20 mm Hg at rest and 40 mm Hg during peak flow. Format as in Figure 4.

ble [6]. Coronary flow reserve in the distal right coronary artery should only reflect the responses of branches supplying the left ventricular inferior wall. Proximal right coronary flow reserve reflects both the distal bed and the contributions from right ventricular branches. Because, as shown in this patient, flow velocity measurements in different locations along the course of the coronary artery may be subject to variations due to diffuse disease, a translesional pressure gradient is used to assess serial lesions. In this case, a pullback of the pressure gradient catheter demonstrated a significant pressure gradient only across lesion number 1 with no contribution from the ostial lesion or the second and third lesions.

Collateral Flow and Post-Occlusive Hyperemia in Patients With Acute Infarction

Angiographic collaterals were not evident on the diagnostic study. Acutely recruitable collateral flow was identified in this individual by the persistence of antegrade flow velocity in the posterolateral branch during coronary balloon occlusion in the proximal lesion (number 1). As shown in Figure 5 (lower left panel), the velocity signal was predominantly systolic with a low velocity flat monophasic diastolic flow contribution.

This flow pattern suggests recruited collateral flow via intraseptal or intramyocardial channels [7].

Viability and Flow Responses

The hyperemic response after balloon occlusion was equal to post-procedural coronary vasodilatory reserve with adenosine. Coronary hyperemia following transient ischemia suggests that the collateral flow was likely sufficient to maintain some myocardial viability [8]. This common finding after angioplasty for acute myocardial infarction has not yet been prospectively examined as an assessment of myocardial viability.

Distal Flow and Pressure Data After Suboptimal Angioplasty

Finally, the suboptimal angioplasty result was associated with a translesional pressure gradient of 20 mm Hg. The distal flow velocity signal was also minimally improved and hyperemia remained impaired. The pressure-flow relationship was improved despite only a minimal increase in flow. Owing to the recent thrombosis in the proximal lesions, stent placement was deferred. Under routine circumstances, a suboptimal angiographic result coupled with a residual translesional pressure gradient of 20 mm Hg and suboptimal distal flow would be addressed by stenting. The patient did well clinically and did not require re-intervention by 4 months of follow-up.

Summary

Translesional pressure and flow velocity observations in the right coronary artery remain among the most difficult data to interpret because of variation in the location and relative size of branches, and unsuspected diffuse disease. Use of distal hyperemic response and translesional pressure gradients provides the most accurate assessment of serial lesions in such patients. In addition, the use of intracoronary thrombolysis can improve the angiographic appearance of lesions and facilitate later successful interventions. The post-infarction distal microvascular responsiveness may be impaired and, thus, abnormal coronary reserve values in this particular setting should be considered with lesion specific indicators of successful recanalization.

ACKNOWLEDGMENTS

The authors thank the J.G. Mudd Cardiac Catheterization Laboratory Team and Donna Sander for manuscript preparation.

REFERENCES

1. Kern MJ, Aguirre FV, Bach RG, Caracciolo EA, Donohue TJ: Translesional pressure-flow-velocity assessment in patients. Cathet Cardiovasc Diagn 31:49–60, 1994.

2. Kern MJ, Aguirre FV, Bach RG, Caracciolo EA, Donohue TJ, Labovitz AJ: Fundamentals of translesional pressure-flow velocity measurements. Cathet Cardiovasc Diagn 31:137–143, 1994.

3. Flynn MS, Kern MJ, Aguirre FV, Bach RG, Caracciolo EA, Donohue TJ: Alterations in coronary blood flow velocity during intracoronary thrombolysis and rescue coronary angioplasty for acute myocardial infarction. Cathet Cardiovasc Diagn 31:219–224, 1994.

4. Donohue TJ, Kern MJ, Aguirre FV, Bach RG, Wolford T, Bell CA, Segal J: Assessing the hemodynamic significance of coronary artery stenoses: analysis of translesional pressure-flow velocity relations in patients. J Am Coll Cardiol 22:449–458, 1993.

5. Kern MJ, Donohue TJ, Flynn MS, Aguirre FV, Bach RG, Caracciolo EA: Limitations of translesional pressure and flow velocity for long ostial left anterior descending stenoses. Cathet Cardiovasc Diagn 33:50–54, 1994.

6. Gould KL, Goldstein RA, Mullani NA, Kirkeeide R, Wong G, Smalling R, Fuentes F, Nishikawa A, Matthews W. Non-invasive assessment of coronary stenoses by myocardial perfusion imaging during pharmacologic coronary vasodilation. VIII. Clinical feasibility of positron cardiac imaging without a cyclotron using generator-produced rubidium-82. J Am Coll Cardiol 7:775–789, 1986.

7. Kern MJ, Donohue TJ, Bach RG, Aguirre FV, Caracciolo EA, Ofili EO. Quantitating coronary collateral flow velocity in patients during coronary angioplasty using a Doppler guidewire. Am J Cardiol 71:34D–40D, 1993.

8. Schelbert HR, Wisenberg G, Phelps ME, Gould KL, Henze E, Hoffman EJ, Gomes A, Kuhl DE: Noninvasive assessment of coronary stenoses by myocardial imaging during pharmacologic coronary vasodilation. VI. Detection of coronary artery disease in human beings with intravenous N-13 ammonia and positron computed tomography. Am J Cardiol 49:1197–1207, 1982.

Part IX

Intra-Aortic Balloon
Counterpulsation

Chapter 20

Influence of Intra-Aortic Balloon Counterpulsation and Collateral Flow Reversal During Multivessel Angioplasty

Bassam Al-Joundi, MD, Morton J. Kern, MD, Frank V. Aguirre, MD, Thomas J. Donohue, MD, Joseph A. Moore, MD, and Michael S. Flynn, MD

INTRODUCTION

During multivessel angioplasty, transient ischemia may be hemodynamically tolerated, despite severe diffuse disease, through several mechanisms [1–5]. One intrinsic mechanism available to the myocardium is collateral blood flow [5–9]. An example of an extrinsic mechanism is intra-aortic balloon pumping, which reduces myocardial demand and augments coronary flow [6–8]. Both mechanisms may be active simultaneously. Ischemia during an angioplasty procedure may occur despite optimal results with balloon recanalization due to coronary spasm complicating an initially satisfactory angiographic result [10]. The flow limitation caused by coronary spasm is nearly always improved with intracoronary nitroglycerin, but the identification and management of spasm-induced ischemia can prolong what may already be an extended and difficult procedure. In this discussion of Interventional Physiology, we examine the perturbations of coronary blood flow associated with intra-aortic balloon pumping, coronary spasm, and collateral flow during a complex, high risk, sequential multivessel coronary angioplasty of an occluded left anterior descending coronary artery with right-to-left collateral supply from a stenosed right coronary artery after recent myocardial infarction.

CASE REPORT

A 67-year-old man with a history of hypertension presented to the Veterans' Administration Hospital with the acute onset of severe substernal pain and pressure associated with diaphoresis. Episodes of chest pressure with moderate exercise began approximately 3–4 weeks earlier. An electrocardiogram (ECG) performed for evaluation of those episodes revealed normal sinus rhythm and poor R wave progression in the anterior leads (Fig. 1, ECG A). The chest pain increased in frequency and intensity and began occurring at rest during the week prior to admission. The patient was taking no medications. His risk factors for coronary artery disease included hypertension and cigarette smoking. In the hospital, he was treated with intravenous heparin and nitroglycerin, beta blockers, and aspirin. The electrocardiogram on presentation showed an acute anterolateral myocardial infarction (Fig. 1, ECG B). Admission laboratory data revealed elevated creatine-phosphokinase (CPK) to 600 units with a positive CK-MB fraction. The postmyocardial infarction course was complicated by angina on a daily basis which resolved with additional intravenous nitroglycerin. On the morning of the 5th hospital day, severe substernal chest pain recurred. These symptoms were similar to the initial chest pain syndrome. An ECG at that time revealed further ST-segment elevation in the precordial leads (4–5 mm) with hyper-acute ST-T wave changes and inferolateral reciprocal changes (Fig. 1, ECG C). The patient was transferred to another Veterans' Administration Hospital for emergency cardiac catheterization, where complete left anterior descending artery occlusion and high-grade serial lesions in the right coronary artery were demonstrated. The anterior wall was akinetic with an ejection fraction of 0.32. The patient was subsequently transferred to St. Louis University Hospital for coronary revascularization.

In the Coronary Care Unit, the patient was stable,

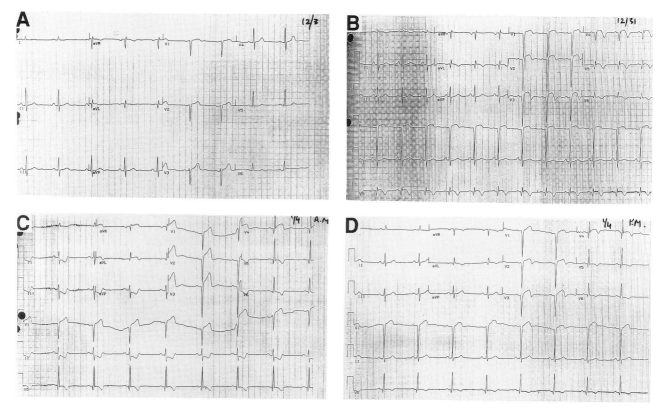

Fig. 1.   Serial 12-lead electrocardiograms. A: Baseline electrocardiogram on 12/3/93. B: ECG on presentation to the VA Hospital on 12/31/93. C: ECG on transfer, 1/4/94. D: ECG on arrival, 1/4/94.

receiving oral metoprolol (25mg bid), enteric-coated aspirin (325 mg qd), intravenous heparin, and nitroglycerin. The blood pressure was 160/90 mm Hg, pulse 60/min and regular, and respirations 16/min. There were no carotid bruits or jugular venous distension. Chest examination was normal. Cardiac examination revealed a regular rate and rhythm, normal S_1 and S_2, and no gallops or murmurs. Examination of the abdomen and extremities were also normal with 2+ arterial pulses throughout. An ECG revealed improvement in ST-T-wave changes (Fig. 1, ECG D). Because of the extensive anterior akinesis with decreased ejection fraction, multivessel coronary artery disease, and recent myocardial infarction, medical therapy was increased and a cardiothoracic surgical consultation was obtained.

The coronary angiograms obtained at the Veterans' Hospital showed total occlusion of the mid left anterior descending artery with high grade single mid right coronary artery narrowing, but because of technical difficulties, right-to-left collateral supply could not be detected. In view of the ECG changes occurring in the anterior leads, it was presumed that the left anterior descending coronary occlusion was a recent event. Alternatively, ischemia could be occurring from variable flow

through the right coronary artery collaterals (if any) to the left anterior descending aretry with a similar presentation.

The patient continued to have angina and, following discussions with the patient and surgeons, angioplasty of the occluded left anterior descending was planned. If successful, angioplasty of the right coronary artery would be performed in a staged, second procedure. For better identification of the collateral supply to, and occlusion length of, the left anterior descending artery, right coronary arteriography was repeated and revealed serial severe mid and distal right coronary artery narrowings and mature grade 2–3 collateral filling of the left anterior descending through both septal and apical epicardial pathways (Fig. 2). The length of the left anterior descending occlusion was estimated to be >8 mm. In view of the high risk nature of an angioplasty, an abdominal aortogram was performed to identify significant peripheral vascular disease prior to intra-aortic balloon pump insertion, if needed. Immediately after aortography, the patient complained of chest pressure and had a systolic blood pressure of 60 mm Hg, and a heart rate of 60/min. Intravenous fluids, atropine (1 mg IV) and aramine (1 mg) were given. An intra-aortic balloon

Pre-PTCA

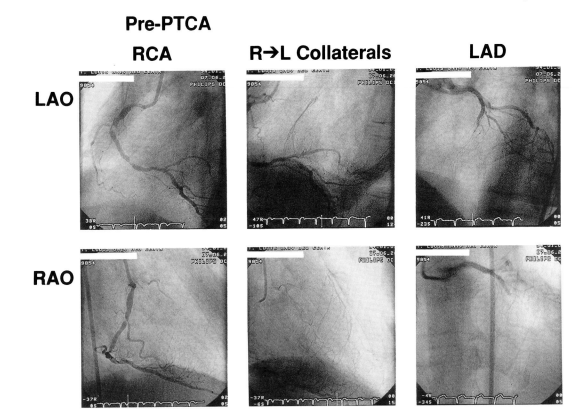

Fig. 2. Selected frames from a cineangiogram of the right coronary artery and left anterior descending artery in the left anterior oblique and right anterior oblique views. Right coronary artery angiogram shows serial 90% and 60% diameter narrowings (arrows) in the left anterior oblique projection. Late cineframes of the right coronary artery shows collateral filling of the left anterior descending through the septal artery and apical pathways. The left anterior descending angiogram demonstrated 100% occlusion (arrow) prior to the first septal artery.

pump was inserted via the left femoral artery with re-establishment of hemodynamic stability and resolution of his chest pain. A subsequent electrocardiogram showed no significant changes. Dilating the left anterior descending coronary artery lesion as a first procedure was considered a rational approach in order to achieve reperfusion of the presumed infarct artery and to permit collateral blood flow to the right coronary artery through a reversal of septal collaterals prior to right coronary artery angioplasty at this or a subsequent setting.

Left Anterior Descending Artery Angioplasty

An 8F 4-cm left Judkins guiding catheter (Cordis, Miami, FL) was placed in the left main coronary artery. A 3.0-mm balloon and a 0.018-inch flowire were advanced into the proximal left anterior descending artery. Coronary blood flow velocity was measured with and without intra-aortic balloon pumping (Fig. 3, bottom). The flowire failed to cross the mid left anterior descending occlusion and was exchanged for a 0.014-inch standard guidewire (USCI) which crossed the occlusion with

some difficulty. A 3.0-mm angioplasty balloon catheter (Intrepid, Baxter) was then advanced across the occlusion. To confirm an intraluminal position, the guidewire was withdrawn and radiographic contrast was injected through the lumen of the balloon with faint opacification of the distal left anterior descending artery (Fig. 3, top). The flowire was re-advanced through the balloon lumen into the distal left anterior descending and distal blood flow velocity was measured again during intra-aortic balloon pumping. Distal left anterior descending artery flow velocity beyond the occlusion demonstrated a biphasic signal with both antegrade and retrograde flow components consistent with collateral flow input both proximal and distal to the guidewire tip. The proximal collateral input was through septal collaterals and flow was predominantly systolic and monophasic. The distal collateral input was from apical epicardial collaterals and was predominantly diastolic. Intra-aortic balloon pumping did not significantly improve right-to-left collateral flow velocity. Multiple balloon dilatations were performed in the mid left anterior descending coronary segment. After

LAD

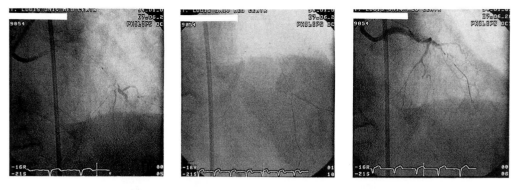

Proximal   **Distal**

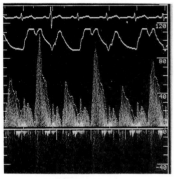

IABP 2:1   **IABP 2:1**

Fig. 3. Top, left to right: Cineangiographic frames demonstrate contrast injection through the angioplasty catheter filling the septal artery (left) and distal apical left anterior descending (middle). Right: Contrast did not opacify the distal left anterior descending with the guidewire distal to the lesion. Bottom: Left: Coronary flow velocity signal in the proximal left anterior descending during 2:1 intra-aortic balloon pumping. The mean velocity is 30 cm/sec which is augmented to 42 cm/sec during intra-aortic balloon pumping. Right: Biphasic collateral flow signal. The upright component is antegrade flow during systole (12 cm/sec) with a small retrograde diastolic flow velocity (<5 cm/sec). Intra-aortic balloon pumping did not change this flow pattern. Velocity scale is 0–160 cm/sec. The ECG and aortic pressure tracing are displayed at the top of the frames.

dilations, coronary flow velocity was poor and the vessel appeared diffusely narrowed. Two doses of intracoronary nitroglycerin (200 μg) were given with enlargement of the lumen and improvement in distal blood flow velocity. The mid left anterior descending was now patent with a small dissection and good distal blood flow (Fig. 4). Distal mean coronary flow velocity increased to 30 cm/sec after angioplasty. Postangioplasty antegrade flow velocity was augmented 10–15% during intra-aortic balloon pumping. The ostium of the septal artery supplying proximal collateral flow could now be visualized by antegrade contrast and appeared to be severely narrowed. As the flowire was withdrawn, flow velocity reversal was noted near the ostium of the septal perforator branch of the mid left anterior descending artery. This retrograde biphasic signal obtained during intra-aortic balloon pumping has a larger systolic component with a mean systolic velocity of −15 cm/sec and a diastolic velocity

of <5 cm/sec (Fig. 5). This collateral flow was detected, despite what angiographically appeared to be a widely patent left anterior descending.

Electrocardiograms before and during balloon inflation are shown in Figure 6 (ECG E,F), demonstrating the ischemic response to left anterior descending artery occlusion and reperfusion.

Angioplasty of the Right Coronary Artery

In view of the ECG changes observed during left anterior descending angioplasty and the now recognized more chronic nature of the left anterior descending occlusion, the right coronary artery took on a more critical significance. After successful left anterior descending angioplasty, a discussion ensued regarding whether to proceed with a sequential procedure or to defer one day for a staged procedure. In support of the staged approach would be the limitation of further contrast media, stabi-

LAD

Post PTCA   Post NTG

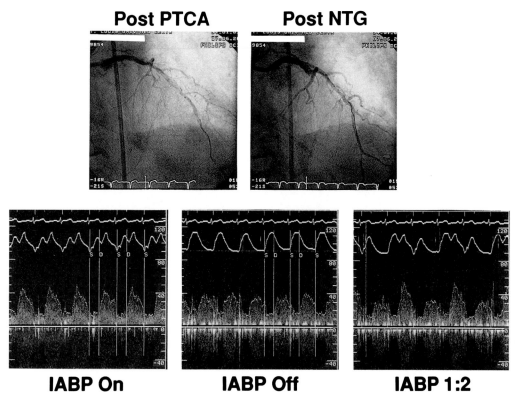

IABP On   IABP Off   IABP 1:2

Fig. 4. Top: Cineangiographic frames after coronary angioplasty (left), which demonstrated a patent left anterior descending angioplasty site with narrowed vessel around the guidewire. Both angiographic and Doppler flow were poor during vessel spasm. After nitroglycerin (NTG) (right), the distal left anterior descending dilated with improved flow as noted in the three panels on the bottom. Velocity signal format as in Figure 2. Note that the origin of the septal artery is severely narrowed (arrow).

lization of flow through the left anterior descending and recovery of anterior ventricular function (if any). Factors in favor of an immediate approach were the stable hemodynamics, intra-aortic balloon pump support, and desire to treat what may have been the culprit lesion. Should angioplasty need to be performed on the right coronary artery in the next 72 hr, the intra-aortic balloon pump would likely require reinsertion through recently instrumented and diseased femoral arteries. Prolonged heparin infusion after the left anterior descending angioplasty was planned, given the chronic nature of the occlusion and might defer further invasive procedures.

The patient had tolerated the left anterior descending angioplasty with satisfactory angiographic and flow results, and thus angioplasty of the right coronary artery was then performed.

An 8F 0.084-inch large-lumen right Judkins guiding catheter (Cordis, Miami, FL) was placed without difficulty. A 0.018-inch flowire inside a 3.5-mm balloon catheter (Spirit, Medtronic) balloon was advanced into the proximal then distal right coronary artery where blood flow velocity was measured (Fig. 7). Proximal right coronary artery mean flow velocity was 45 cm/sec, which augmented to 60 cm/sec during intra-aortic balloon pumping, a 33% increase. These were high values for the right coronary artery. The flow velocity measured in the posterior descending artery was reduced, with an average peak velocity of only 25 cm/sec and minimal (<10%) augmentation with intra-aortic balloon pumping.

Initial balloon dilations resulted in suboptimal angiographic results, but a significant increase in distal blood flow velocity. The balloon was then advanced into the more distal stenosis (Fig. 7). Balloon inflation showed a prominent mid balloon narrowing (waist) which was eliminated at 6 atm. (Serial ECG during RCA angioplasty are shown in Fig. 8.) The 3.5-mm balloon was exchanged for a 4.0-mm balloon and repeat dilation resulted in minimal residual stenosis (Fig. 9). During balloon inflation, retrograde collateral flow was detected in the distal right coronary artery, most likely from the apical collateral vessels. Post-angioplasty distal flow was normalized.

Electrocardiograms during right coronary artery occlusion (Fig. 6, ECG H; Fig. 8, ECG I) demonstrated ST-

LAD, Post PTCA

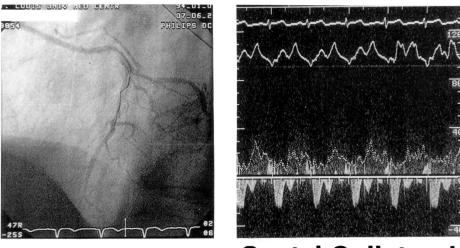

Septal Collateral Inflow

Fig. 5. Left: Left anterior oblique cineangiographic frame showing the flowire positioned toward the septal artery. Right: Flow velocity reversal of septal input flow. Mean retrograde systolic flow is −15 cm/sec and diastolic flow is <5 cm/sec. Velocity signal format as in Figure 2.

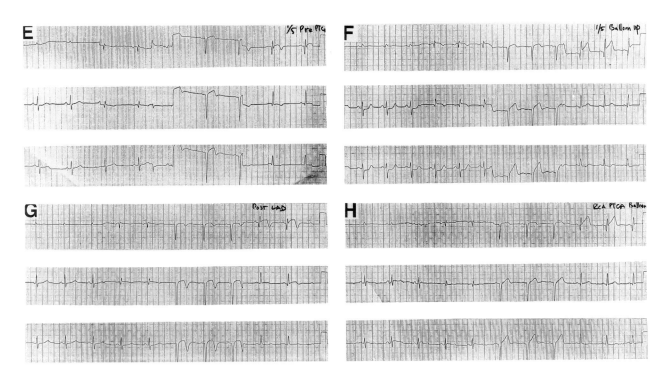

Fig. 6. Serial 12-lead electrocardiograms. E: ECG before angioplasty of the left anterior descending artery. F: ECG during balloon inflation across the mid left anterior descending stenosis. G: ECG after angioplasty of the left anterior descending artery. H: ECG during balloon inflation across the mid-right coronary artery stenosis (cf. ECG F).

Pre PTCA

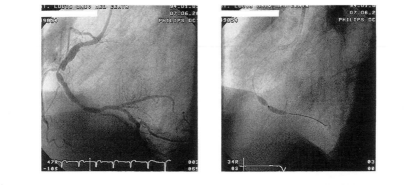

Proximal   Distal   Balloon Occlusion

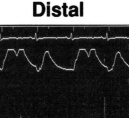
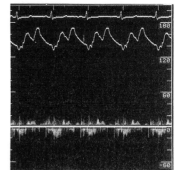

IABP 1:2

Fig. 7. Top: Left: Cineangiographic frames of the right coronary artery before angioplasty. The location of the proximal and distal flowire measurements are indicated by the arrows. Right: Partially inflated 3.5-mm angioplasty balloon in the distal right coronary artery lesion. Note that the position of the flowire during balloon occlusion is where the left-to-right collateral flow velocity signal is recorded. Bottom: Left: Coronary flow velocity during 1:2 intra-aortic balloon pumping in the proximal right coronary artery. Middle: Flow velocity in the posterior descending artery. Right: Flow velocity during balloon occlusion. Mean retrograde signal is biphasic systolic and diastolic <5 cm/sec.

segment elevation with T-wave pseudonormalization in the precordial leads. ECG changes during distal right coronary artery occlusion were very similar to those seen with both the initial presenting episode of chest pain and with postinfarction anginal episodes.

The post-angioplasty proximal and distal right coronary artery stenoses were 30% and 15% diameter narrowing, respectively. Distal flow velocity increased to a mean of 40 cm/sec with a normal phasic pattern. Proximal flow velocity was also increased by 25%. Final coronary angiography demonstrated no opacification of the right-to-left collaterals to the distal left anterior descending. Faint collaterals through the septal perforator to the mid left anterior descending coronary were still observed (Fig. 10).

The initial postangioplasty course in the coronary care unit was unremarkable. Heparin was to be continued for 48 hrs. The intra-aortic balloon pump and femoral arterial and venous sheaths were removed the next morning. Three hours later the patient complained of chest pain.

The ECG showed anterolateral ST elevation and T-wave pseudonormalization similar to that seen during balloon inflation (Fig. 8, ECG K). The patient was brought back to the catheterization laboratory emergently where coronary angiography revealed significant vessel re-narrowing at the midleft anterior descending angioplasty site. The right coronary artery angioplasty sites were unchanged. Repeat mid left anterior descending angioplasty was performed with a 3.0-mm Rx perfusion balloon. A 30-min balloon inflation resulted in an excellent angiographic result. The patient was discharged 3 days later and has remained stable.

DISCUSSION

Decisions to perform multivessel angioplasty in patients with a recent myocardial infarction can be especially difficult when trying to assess risk and identify the culprit vessel. This patient presented with ischemia resulting from abnormal coronary flow due either to jeop-

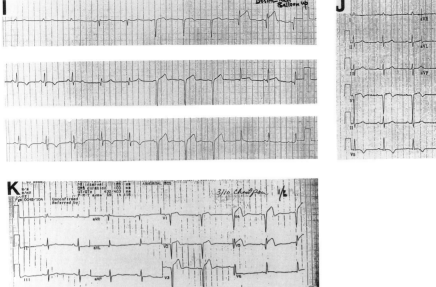

Fig. 8.   Serial 12-lead electrocardiograms. I: ECG during balloon inflation across the distal right coronary artery stenosis. J: ECG after angioplasty of the right coronary artery. K: ECG during recurrence of chest pain 24 hrs postangioplasty.

RCA, Post PTCA

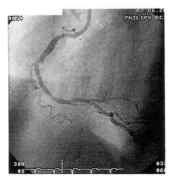

Proximal   **Distal**

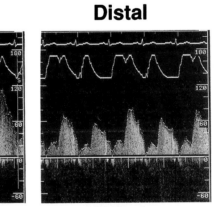

IABP On   **IABP 2:1**

Fig. 9.   Top: Cineangiogram of the right coronary artery after serial angioplasty. Bottom: Proximal and distal flow velocity after right coronary artery angioplasty. Velocity signal format as in Figure 2.

Post-PTCA

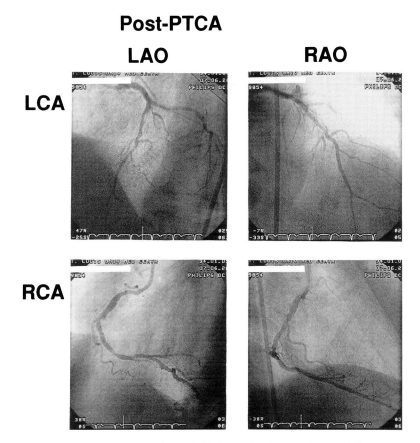

Fig. 10.   Cineangiographic frames after serial left anterior descending and right coronary artery angioplasty. The left anterior descending septal artery origin remains severely narrowed and is faintly filled during right coronary artery angiography. Format as in Figure 1.

ardized right collateral supply to a remote left anterior descending region or acute occlusion of the left anterior descending. The right-to-left collateral supply to the left anterior descending artery was not seen on the initial study due to limited angiographic technique. This resulted in the erroneous assumption that the left anterior descending was the acutely occluded culprit vessel and was responsible for the clinical presentation. Mature angiographic collaterals, visualized prior to left anterior descending angioplasty, were more consistent with either a longstanding total occlusion or high-grade stenosis [11]. Distal left anterior descending opacification via collaterals also suggested that the lesion was longer than one might anticipate for a more acute thrombotic occlusion. Two features of collateral flow were of particular interest in this case. Collateral supply through the septal perforator was still present to some degree despite reestablished antegrade left anterior descending flow. The stenosis at the origin of the septal perforator prevented adequate antegrade filling and thus right-to-septal collateral flow persisted despite excellent left anterior descending revascularization. Apical epicardial collaterals were eliminated by left anterior descending angioplasty.

The second observation on collateral flow is the left-to-right collateral flow signal seen during distal right coronary artery occlusion. Providing an open left anterior descending artery with the potential to reverse collateral flow to the contralateral artery has been previously demonstrated [12]. Theoretically, this approach may provide a margin of safety when performing multivessel angioplasty. In this patient, distal right coronary artery collaterals were provided through apical channels since the septal artery had a significant stenosis as its origin.

Ischemic Electrocardiographic Findings in a Culprit Lesion

Ischemic electrocardiographic findings of a culprit lesion are often difficult to obtain prior to performance of angioplasty. The ECG changes in this case suggested that the ischemia was predominantly due to the right coronary artery stenoses compromising left anterior descending coronary collateral supply. However, ischemic ECG changes were also present during left anterior descending coronary angioplasty and with postangioplasty left anterior descending restenosis. These changes may have been due to septal collateral flow impairment from the inflated balloon. The ECG findings during right coronary artery dilatation of anterior ST-segment changes, suggested impairment of collateral supply to the anterior wall and reflected the ischemic potential of the right coronary artery lesion.

Effects of Intra-Aortic Balloon Pump on Collateral Flow

A previous study of the effect of intra-aortic balloon pumping on collateral flow suggested that angiographically mature collaterals with grade 3 angiographic filling could be augmented by intra-aortic balloon pumping, whereas blood flow through acutely recruitable collaterals were not affected [13]. In this patient, the apical epicardial and transseptal coronary collateral circulation was minimally augmented by intra-aortic balloon pumping, suggesting a diastolic pressure independent mechanism influencing collateral supply. The effect of intra-aortic balloon pumping promoting antegrade flow has been previously demonstrated to assist in promoting patency of recently dilated coronary arteries [14].

Coronary Spasm After Coronary Angioplasty

Coronary spasm after coronary angioplasty produced a characteristic decrease in flow with severe coronary narrowing and was reversed with intracoronary nitroglycerin. The flow velocity changes during coronary spasm in this case indicated the luminal narrowing was such that flow was markedly impaired. In some individuals, flow velocity may initially increase and then decrease due to a narrowing of the cross-sectional area at the region of flow measurements. Coronary spasm proximal to the guidewire tip will result in decreasing flow due to decreasing luminal area. Recognition of flow velocity changes with coronary spasm may be important in the management of patients undergoing multivessel angioplasty such as this [15].

SUMMARY

Flow velocity changes during multivessel angioplasty suggests that collateral flow has an important role in determining safety and ischemic threshold during these procedures. The physiology of collateral flow with and without intra-aortic balloon pumping has been demonstrated in this individual and provides insight into the mechanisms of reduced ischemia during high-risk coronary interventions.

ACKNOWLEDGMENTS

The authors thank the J.G. Mudd Cardiac Catheterization Laboratory Team, and Donna Sander for manuscript preparation.

REFERENCES

1. Kern MJ, Deligonul U, Labovitz A: Influence of drug therapy on the ischemic response to acute coronary occlusion in man: Supply side economics. Am Heart J 118:361–380, 1989.
2. Cohen M, Rentrop KP: Limitation of myocardial ischemia by collateral circulation during sudden controlled coronary artery occlusion in human subjects: A prospective study. Circulation 74: 469–476, 1986.
3. Schwartz H, Leiboff RH, Bren GB, Wasserman AG, Katz RJ, Varghese PJ, Sokil AB, Ross AM: Temporal evolution of the human coronary collateral circulation after myocardial infarction. J Am Coll Cardiol 4:1088–1093, 1984.
4. Pellinen TJ, Virtanen KS, Toivonen L, Heikkila J, Hekali P, Frick MH: Coronary collateral circulation. Clin Cardiol 14:111–118, 1991.
5. Rentrop KP, Cohen M, Blanke H, Phillips RA: Changes in collateral channel filling immediately after controlled coronary artery occlusion by an angioplasty balloon in human subjects. J Am Coll Cardiol 5:587–592, 1985.
6. Szatmary LJ, Marco J: Haemodynamic and antiischaemic protective effects of intraaortic balloon counterpulsation in high risk coronary heart patients undergoing percutaneous transluminal coronary angioplasty. Cor Vasa 29:183–191, 1987.
7. Kern MJ, Aguirre F, Bach R, Donohue T, Siegel R, Segal J: Augmentation of coronary blood flow by intra-aortic balloon pumping in patients after coronary angioplasty. Circulation 87: 500–511, 1993.
8. Kahn JK, Rutherford BD, McConahay DR, Johnson WL, Giorgi LV, Hartzler GO: Supported "high risk" coronary angioplasty using intraaortic balloon pump counterpulsation. J Am Coll Cardiol 15:1151–1155, 1990.
9. Hansen JF. Coronary collateral circulation: Clinical significance and influence on survival in patients with coronary artery occlusion. Am Heart J 117:290–295, 1989.
10. Conti CR. Large vessel coronary vasospasm: Diagnosis, natural history and treatment. Am J Cardiol 55:41B–49B, 1985.
11. Stone GW, Rutherford BD, McConahay DR: Procedural outcome of angioplasty for total coronary artery occlusion: An analysis of 971 lesions in 905 patients. J Am Coll Cardiol 15:849–856, 1990.
12. Ofili E, Kern MJ, Tatineni S, Deligonul U, Aguirre F, Serota H, Labovitz AJ: Detection of coronary collateral flow by a Doppler-tipped guidewire during coronary angioplasty. Am Heart J 122: 221–225, 1991.
13. Flynn MS, Kern MJ, Donohue TJ, Aguirre FV, Bach RG, Caracciolo EA: Alterations of coronary collateral flow velocity during intra-aortic balloon pumping in patients. Am J Cardiol 71: 1451–1454, 1993.
14. Ohman EM, Califf RM, George BS, Quigley PJ, Kereiakes DJ, Harrelson-Woodlief L, Candela RJ, Flanagan C, Stack RS, Topol EJ: Thrombolysis and Angioplasty in Myocardial Infarction (TAMI) study group: The use of intra-aortic balloon pumping as an adjunct to reperfusion therapy in acute myocardial infarction. Am Heart J 121:895–901, 1991.
15. Donohue T, Kern MJ, Wolford T, Bach R, Aguirre F, Miller L: The effects of epicardial coronary spasm on intracoronary flow velocity and pressure gradient in a patient after cardiac transplantation. Am Heart J 124:1645–1648, 1992..

Part X

Transplant Coronary Physiology and Endothelial Function

Chapter 21

Assessment of Transplant Arteriopathy by Intracoronary Two-Dimensional Ultrasound Imaging and Coronary Flow Velocity

Thomas Wolford, MD, and Morton J. Kern, MD

INTRODUCTION

Transplant coronary arteriopathy is the major impediment to the long-term survival of cardiac allografts. The recognition that arteriopathy could present, within the first year post-transplantation, with an insidious onset prompted the clinical practice of yearly catheterizations. However, two-dimensional intravascular imaging [1] and pathologic studies [2] revealed the insensitivity of angiography in detecting coronary disease with its associated poor prognosis [3].

The advent of intracoronary two-dimensional echocardiographic imaging and Doppler flow velocity techniques have revolutionized the assessment of transplant arteriopathy. Information on endovascular arterial morphology that previously could be obtained only by a pathologist now can be readily obtained by the interventional cardiologist. The consequences of these findings will have critical importance for the future management and treatment of transplant patients. This interventional physiologic discussion addresses methods and preliminary findings using two-dimensional imaging and Doppler flow in assessing transplant coronary arteriopathy.

INTRAVASCULAR ULTRASOUND

High frequency intravascular ultrasound imaging (IVUS) has been used for over half a decade [4–6]. The types of available catheters and technical descriptions are provided elsewhere [7,8]. Only recently, however, have the devices reached a size (2.9–4.3 French) that has allowed routine intracoronary use. The ultrasound imaging frequency (20–30 MHz) of the catheters has likewise reached a point that fine detail of the coronary architecture could be routinely obtained. This technological advancement has particular usefulness in the transplant population. St. Goar and his colleagues [1,9] initially showed the utility of intravascular ultrasound in transplant arteriopathy. Beyond 1 year, nearly every patient, including those with normal coronary angiograms, had evidence of myointimal proliferation with two-thirds having moderate to severe endoluminal thickening with preservation of nearly concentric lumina.

CORONARY IMAGING METHODOLOGY

A common protocol for imaging coronary arteries in our laboratory follows the technique of St. Goar et al. [1,9]. After the patient undergoes standard selective coronary angiography, an 8F guiding catheter is placed in the left or right coronary ostium. The patient then receives 10,000 units of Heparin by intravenous bolus. Instrumentation of the coronary artery is not performed until an activated clotting time (ACT) of >300 is achieved. After adequate anticoagulation is confirmed, the artery is traversed with a 0.014″ angioplasty or Doppler flow guidewire. The guidewire is placed as far distally as possible to permit sufficient echo catheter movement. If a floppy guidewire is used, the ultrasound device should not be manipulated onto the soft part of the guidewire. The IVUS catheter is then advanced to the tip of the guiding catheter. To prevent spasm, intracoronary nitroglycerin (200 μg) is administered. If sublingual nitroglycerin is preferred, 5 minutes should elapse before entering the coronary artery to permit adequate coronary vasodilatory effects [10]. Additionally, for patients with low right-sided filling pressures, saline (200–500 mL) prior to nitroglycerin is helpful to avoid hypotension. After nitrate administration, the IVUS catheter is turned on and advanced slowly into the left main artery segment. Imaging settings [gain, zoom, compression, and time gain compensation (TGC)] are optimized to enhance vessel wall and lumen contrast and to minimize image artifacts (from blood speckle). After the initial settings are chosen and recorded, they should not be changed during the study. The IVUS catheter is then advanced into the proximal artery. In the left anterior descending, the circumflex artery usually will be visualized as an additional circular lumen in the far field. Using the ''rotate'' control on the video imaging unit, the circumflex vessel is positioned to the 3:00 o'clock location on the video screen. This orientation allows plaque or other landmarks to be evaluated in a standard manner in follow-up studies. Once these preliminary procedures are completed, the IVUS catheter is advanced as far distally as the vessel size will allow. However, caution is needed since the incidence of vasospasm increases as the catheter is advanced distally. There always should be a blood lumen visible on the video screen. The absence of a lumen indicates the catheter is obstructing the vessel. In this situation, image quality is generally poor and the risk of spasm increases. A further confounding technical factor is vessel tortuosity. IVUS catheters have relatively stiff tips. Negotiating sharp bends in vessels can be difficult and generally should not be attempted if resistance to catheter movement is encountered. After obtaining distal vessel images, the catheter is slowly pulled back. Four to six sites are examined to assess the amount of plaque present. Sites are also selected based on the quality of the image and the ability to identify the position with echo landmarks (i.e., side branches). Once an imaging site is chosen, an angiogram documents this location on film for future review. To obtain an overall assessment of the entire artery, the IVUS catheter is then placed distally and is slowly pulled back into the guide catheter over 25–30 seconds, continuously recording the images on video tape. This imaging pullback, essential to assess the overall extent of disease, generally gives the best images as the vessel tends to straighten upon pullback, allowing the catheter to assume an axial position. After imaging of the left anterior descending artery, the circumflex and right coronary arteries can be imaged in a similar fashion.

INTRACORONARY DOPPLER FLOW VELOCITY FOR THE MICROCIRCULATION

Intracoronary Doppler flow is used to assess the resistance bed of the microcirculation. The methodology of the intracoronary Doppler flowire has been detailed previously in this series and elsewhere [11,12]. It is postulated that transplant arteriopathy affects the length of the artery including intramyocardial branches beyond the resolution of angiography (i.e., <400 microns). If distal disease is significant, then a diminishment in coronary flow reserve (ratio of hyperemic to resting blood flow velocity) also should be present.

To measure blood flow velocity, the Doppler flowire is manipulated into the proximal right coronary, left anterior descending, and circumflex vessels. Nitroglycerin (200 μg intracoronary bolus) is given prior to flow velocity measurements. In each vessel, resting flow velocity is recorded. Intracoronary adenosine (8–18 μg intracoronary bolus) is given and the maximal flow response is recorded at 15–40 seconds [12]. In our experience, intracoronary adenosine in doses of 30 μg have not produced hyperemic responses greater than that observed with 12 μg in the allograft circulation. After proximal flow velocity is obtained, the flowire is directed distally past the last marginal or diagonal branch and basal and hyperemic flow are again recorded. In general, the flowire is positioned preferably in straight segments so that a fully developed parabolic flow profile can be assumed. By interrogating all three major epicardial vessels, the heterogeneity of microvascular function can be assessed. In addition to coronary flow reserve, by combining the two-dimensional echo measurement of vessel diameter, flow velocity allows determination of volumetric blood flow for each vessel [13].

CASE EXAMPLES
Case #1

A 50-year-old man underwent study for the second annual cardiac transplant evaluation. He was asymptomatic and free of acute rejection at the time of the study. Routine angiography revealed no evidence of significant epicardial disease. Compared to his film from the previous year, no evidence of tertiary vessel occlusion or distal vessel tapering was present. Figure 1 shows the intravascular ultrasound images obtained with two types of IVUS catheters (Sonicath, Boston Scientific and CVIS, Mountain View, CA) in the proximal and midleft anterior descending artery.

This patient illustrates that the IVUS images do not

LAD   2D ECHO₁
Proximal   ECHO₂

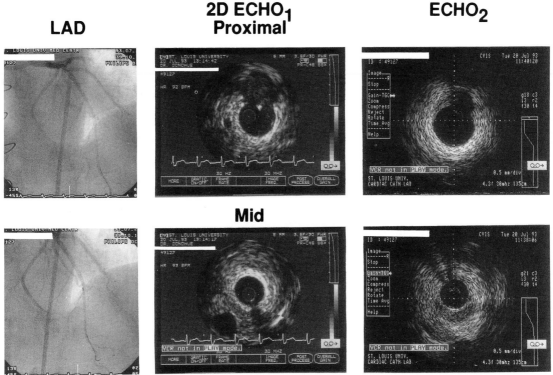

Mid

Fig. 1. Top left: Coronary angiogram of the left anterior descending artery (LAD). A guidewire is seen in the distal vessel. Bottom left: Two-dimensional echo catheter transducer is positioned at midvessel location. Right: Two echocardiographic imaging catheters were used to compare image differences at each location. No evidence of atherosclerotic disease was found with either machine.

always show the trilaminar appearance previously described as "normal" in human muscular arteries [14–16]. This finding is likely due to the fact that the intima is beyond the resolution of the ultrasound imaging capabilities. It is difficult to say no intimal thickening is present, but only that the intima is <140 μm thick, within the theoretical axial resolution of the ultrasound image device. Depending on the age of the donor heart, the level of intimal thickening will vary. With advancing age, the intima thickens [16]. This patient's donor was <30 years of age. One would expect no evidence of myointimal proliferation to be seen. At 24 months, this coronary artery was free of either angiographic or ultrasound evidence of transplant arteriopathy.

Case #2

A 49-year-old male presenting for his first annual posttransplant cardiac evaluation had selective coronary angiography that revealed no discernible disease. Comparison with his cineangiograms of a year prior revealed no evidence of distal vessel occlusion or abnormal tapering. In contrast to the previous patient, there is no evidence of transplant arteriopathy. Figure 2 displays the resting and hyperemic blood flow response in the left

anterior descending artery with ultrasound imaging of myointimal proliferation.

The IVUS images, obtained with a 4.3F 30 MHz probe (CVIS), reveal myointimal proliferation in the proximal vessel. The full circumference of the vessel wall is symmetrically involved. The thickness of the abnormal myointima appears uniform.

Evaluation of the coronary flow reserve in this patient was normal and revealed an ability nearly to triple a normal resting flow velocity, suggesting no loss of resistance vessel function. Measurable proximal myointimal proliferation appeared to occur in the absence of any evidence of distal vessel dysfunction, raising the possibility that in certain patients, transplant arteriopathy does not progress in a distal to proximal fashion.

This patient illustrates two further points about evaluating transplant coronary disease. This patient's donor was in his late forties and had a history of hypertension. The discernable intimal thickness on IVUS may actually represent native disease and simply be secondary to the heart age [16,17]. In this patient, one cannot automatically assume the IVUS abnormality is secondary to transplant arteriopathy. Second, this patient's ventricle was hypertrophied and yet his coronary flow reserve was

Normal LAD Transplant

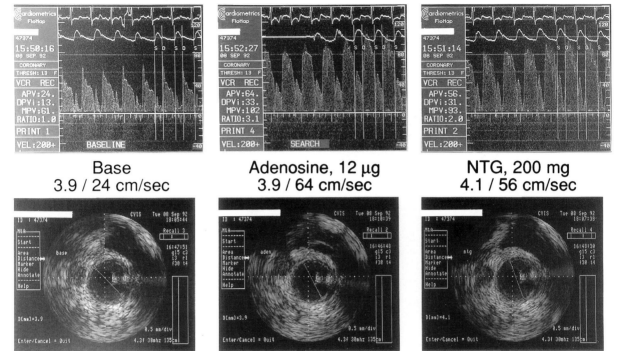

| Base | Adenosine, 12 µg | NTG, 200 mg |
| 3.9 / 24 cm/sec | 3.9 / 64 cm/sec | 4.1 / 56 cm/sec |

Fig. 2. Simultaneous two-dimensional echo coronary imaging and flow velocity spectra in patient #2 after transplant demonstrating normal hyperemic response to intracoronary adenosine and nitroglycerin. Alterations in diameter of the vessel with mild coronary transplant artery disease shown on the lower panels by echocardiography indicates normal conductance and resistance vessel function [16,17]. The numbers above the two-dimensional images indicate mm diameter during flow measurements (in cm/sec).

well within normal limits for patients in our laboratory. This finding suggests that cardiac innervation may mitigate some of the flow abnormalities that accompany left ventricular hypertrophy.

The normal angiographic appearance of this patient's distal vasculature (i.e., free of the Type B lesions described by Gao et al. [20]) and the normal coronary flow reserves indicates that the resistance microcirculation is functioning normally at 12 months posttransplant.

Case #3

A 50-year-old male presenting for second annual posttranslant catheterization is the subject of this study. The patient was asymptomatic and free of acute rejection at the time of the examination. Routine coronary angiography was interpreted as normal. In the interim from the time of his initial annual catheterization, no evidence of distal vessel occlusion or tapering had developed. Figure 3 shows the intravascular ultrasound images with a 4.3F 30 MHz probe (CVIS) in the proximal left anterior descending coronary artery. Figures 4, 5, and 6 demonstrate the resting and hyperemic flows in the diagonal, proximal left anterior descending, and mid left anterior descending coronary arteries.

The inadequacy of angiography for determination of endovascular intimal proliferation is readily demonstrated. In a retrospective review, mild angiographic luminal irregularities were felt to be evident, but there were no indicators to suggest the exuberant myointimal proliferation that was found on IVUS. The myointima approaches 1.0 mm in thickness, involving the entire vessel circumference. This distribution suggests that hemodynamic factors may also play a role in the course of the disease. Complete interrogation of the proximal two-thirds of the vessel revealed more aggressive thickening in the proximal portion of the left anterior descending coronary artery.

It is important to note that the hyperemic coronary flow (reserve) in this patient exceeded 3.0 times basal values in all vessels studied. Basal flow in the proximal left anterior descending artery increased from 38 cm/sec to 125 cm/sec (Fig. 2) for a coronary flow reserve of 3.3. Similar coronary flow reserve values were obtained in the midleft anterior descending and diagonal branches

50 yr old Male, 2 yr s/p Heart Transplant Proximal LAD IVUS

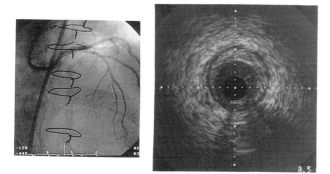

Fig. 3. Left: Coronary angiogram of the left coronary artery in the right anterior oblique projection showing position of the echo catheter transducer in the proximal portion of the left anterior descending artery. Right: Corresponding image of the left anterior descending artery demonstrating a circular lumen with a crescent-shape atherosclerotic plaque and a lucent adventitial ring. This is a typical image for transplant coronary arteriopathy. The scale markers are 0.5 mm.

(Figs. 3,4). The proximal myointimal proliferation did not appear to interact with normal coronary flow reserves.

This study also illustrates the variability of coronary flow velocity. Coronary flow reserves measured in the proximal and midleft anterior descending, and diagonal are nearly identical. However, the absolute magnitude of the flow velocity in the different vessels is variable, related to the cross-sectional area of the coronary conduit. Basal average velocity was 38 cm/sec, 23 cm/sec, and 18 cm/sec in the proximal and midleft anterior descending, and diagonal branches, respectively (Figs. 2–4). Serial studies require care in positioning the Doppler wire in the same location. This methodology is particularly important if measures of regional blood flow using velocity and cross-sectional area product method [13,17] are to be obtained.

DISCUSSION

Transplant arteriopathy is presumed to be a process that afflicts the distal vasculature first with an incidence of 10% per year [18,20,21].

Role of Angiography

Angiography is used as the principle risk stratifier of transplant coronary disease. Once angiographic disease is evident, survival is diminished. In the absence of symptoms or left ventricular dysfunction, the clinical significance of angiographically evident disease is less certain [20]. In fact, routine angiography has been

50 yr old Male, 2 yr s/p Heart Transplant Proximal LAD Flow

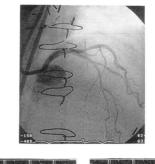

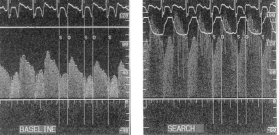

Fig. 4. Top left: Coronary angiogram with flowire in the proximal left anterior descending artery (arrow). Flow velocity on lower left demonstrates a normal phasic pattern with diastolic predominance. The flow velocity is ~38 cm/sec. S and D represent systolic and diastolic periods, respectively, obtained from the electrocardiographic algorithm. Velocity scale is 0–160 cm/sec. Bottom right: Hyperemic response to intracoronary adenosine increasing flow >3 times basal values. Note both systolic and diastolic flow velocity increases. The velocity scale is 0–240 cm/sec.

eclipsed by IVUS as a diagnostic modality for this entity. An asymptomatic patient can develop a significant arteriopathy without showing angiographic evidence of plaque as demonstrated in case #3. The mere appearance of angiographic luminal irregularity, however, changes the prognosis of the individual patient [20]. It is likely that angiographic luminal irregularities indicates a change not only in the volume, but also in the *character* of the plaque mass.

Ultrasound Plaque Characterization

At present, only modest qualitative IVUS tissue characterization is possible [14,15]. Future IVUS refinements may allow quantitative assessment of plaque morphology and confirmation of this hypothesis [20]. Four basic tissue plaque types are discernable by IVUS: fibrous, calcific, lipid, and fibrocellular [19]. With quantitative image refinements, tracking of changes in the content of the myointima and gauging, which changes in the myointima, increase the risk for thrombosis will provide critically important diagnostic information.

50 yr old Male, 2 yr s/p Heart Transplant Mid LAD Flow

50 yr old Male, 2 yr s/p Heart Transplant Diagonal Branch Flow

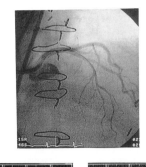

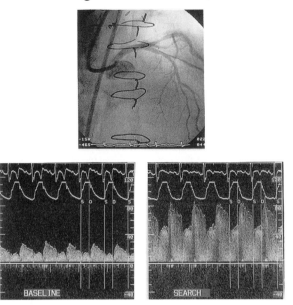

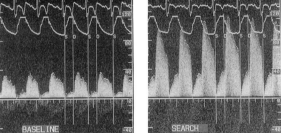

Fig. 5. Top: Coronary angiogram showing flow velocity guidewire in the midleft anterior descending artery beyond the first diagonal branch with corresponding flow velocity at baseline and during hyperemia shown on bottom left and right panels, respectively. Velocity format as in Figure 1. Velocity scale is 0–160 cm/sec (both panels). Flow velocity increases >threefold basal value. Note the decline in absolute magnitude of the flow velocity at baseline.

Fig. 6. Flow velocity in a large diagonal branch demonstrating similar coronary reserve with slightly different measurement of flow velocity basal values. Coronary reserve remains >3 for this location.

Assessment of Microcirculatory Function and Small Vessel Disease

The distal small vessel circulation can be only assessed qualitatively using the standard approach of Gao et al. [18]. It is postulated that transplant arteriopathy is diffuse, inevitably involving the small distal vessels, and thus surgical or nonsurgical conduit revascularization is futile [21]. If, however, IVUS/Doppler flow evaluation of transplant arteriopathy confirms that distal disease is not a necessary concomitant component of proximal epicardial artery disease, then a subset of patients could be identified who may benefit from coronary revascularization. In light of the scarcity of organs and the controversy over diminished survival after a second transplant, identifying a more effective palliative therapy could prolong the useful life of an allograft and be an obvious major therapeutic advance.

Risk of Intravascular Assessment

Patient risk and comfort must be addressed during intravascular evaluation. In our experience with over 120 transplant patients who have undergone right ventricular biopsy, right heart catheterization, selective coronary angiography, IVUS imaging, and multivessel coronary Doppler flow evaluation at the same setting, no major complications (death, myocardial infarction) have occurred. Only two studies were terminated prematurely, one due to proximal vessel spasm (when intracoronary nitroglycerin had not been given) and another due to formation of clot on a guiding catheter (this despite 10,000 units of intravenous heparin). The latter episode justifies documenting an adequate anticoagulation by ACT prior to intravascular instrumentation. Some posttransplant patients may have hemostatic abnormalities [28]. The average time of this procedure is 150 minutes by a single operator, and if two experienced operators are involved, the average time is 120 minutes. These risks are similar to those reported by the IVUS Registry [29].

Preliminary Experience

Previous studies using Doppler catheters and PET scans [22–27] have failed to demonstrate significant microvascular abnormalities. Preliminary experience in our laboratory found that normal coronary angiography predicted a normal coronary flow reserve (2.6±0.5 in 41 patients) compared to coronary flow reserve of 1.9±0.5 (P<0.01) in 11 patients with angiographically apparent irregularities. Based on current observations, we speculate that when proximal myointimal proliferation is present, coronary flow reserve may be unimpaired. These findings stimulate questions regarding the mechanism of a preferentially obliterative process involving the distal vascular bed would leave coronary flow reserve unaffected. It can be hypothesized that transplant coronary disease may thus present in two forms: a distal immuno-obliterative form and a proximal atheromatous form. Intravascular physiology and two-dimensional imaging will assist in resolving this dilemma.

The study of endothelial function, using acetylcholine and other endothelial-dependent and independent vasodilators, in transplant arteriopathy remains controversial [30–35] and will be addressed in future interventional physiology rounds.

Summary

The evaluation of transplant arteriopathy involves determination of endoluminal morphologic abnormalities and functional response of the microcirculation by intracoronary flow velocity reserve measurements. Establishment of the relationship between conductance and resistance vessel disease with immunologic markers will focus future avenues of therapies to prolong patient survival.

The combined use of intravascular imaging and Doppler flow velocity may identify patients suitable for coronary revascularization interventions and allow reliable testing of the efficacy of various pharmacologic agents proposed to be effective in limiting transplant coronary arteriopathy.

ACKNOWLEDGMENTS

The authors thank the J.G. Mudd Cardiac Catheterization Laboratory team and Donna Sander for manuscript preparation.

REFERENCES

1. St. Goar FG, Pinto FJ, Alderman EL, Valantine HA, Schroeder JS, Gao S, Stinson EB, Popp RL: Intracoronary ultrasound in cardiac transplant recipients: In vivo evidence of "angiographically silent" intimal thickening. Circulation 85:979–987, 1992.
2. Johnson DE, Alderman EL, Schroeder JS, Gao S, Hunt S, DeCampli WM, Stinson E, Billingham M: Transplant coronary artery disease: Histopathologic correlations with angiographic morphology. J Am Coll Cardiol 17:449–457, 1991.
3. Keogh AM: Proximal and mid-vessel coronary artery disease in the transplanted heart. J Heart Transplant 11:S87, 1992.
4. Pandian NG, Kreis A, Brockway B, et al.: Ultrasound angioscopy: Real-time, two-dimensional, intraluminal ultrasound imaging of blood vessels. Am J Cardiol 62:493–494, 1988.
5. Yock PG, Linker DT, Angelsen BAJ: Two-dimensional intravascular ultrasound: Technical development and initial clinical experience. J Am Soc Echo 2:296–304, 1989.

6. Yock PG, Linker DT, White NW, et al.: Clinical applications of intravascular ultrasound imaging in atherectomy. Int J Card Imag 4:117–125, 1989.
7. Cavaye DM, White RA (eds): Intravascular ultrasound imaging. New York: Raven Press, 1993, pp 1–38.
8. Higano ST, Nishimura RA (eds): Current problems in cardiology. St. Louis: Mosby-Year Book, 1994, pp. 1–42.
9. St. Goar FG, Pinto FJ, Alderman EL, Fitzgerald PJ, Stinson EB, Billingham ME, Popp RL: Detection of coronary atherosclerosis in young adult hearts using intravascular ultrasound. Circulation 86:756–763, 1992.
10. Pinto FJ, St. Goar FG, Fischell TA, Stadius ML, Valantine HA, Alderman EL, Popp RL: Nitroglycerin-induced coronary vasodilation in cardiac transplant recipients: evaluation with in vivo intracoronary ultrasound. Circulation 85:69–77, 1992.
11. Ofili EO, Labovitz AJ, Kern MJ: Coronary flow velocity dynamics in normal and diseased arteries. Am J Cardiol 71(14):3D–9D, 1993.
12. Donohue TJ, Kern MJ, Aguirre FV, Bach RG, Wolford T, Bell CA, Segal J: Assessing the hemodynamic significance of coronary artery stenoses: Analysis of translesional pressure-flow velocity relations in patients. J Am Coll Cardiol 22:449–458, 1993.
13. Sudhir K, MacGregor JS, Barbant SD, Foster E, Fitzgerald PJ, Chatterjee K, Yock PG: Assessment of coronary conductance and resistance vessel reactivity in response to nitroglycerin, ergonovine and adenosine: In vivo studies with simultaneous intravascular two-dimensional and Doppler ultrasound. J Am Coll Cardiol 21:1261–1268, 1993.
14. Gussenhoven EJ, Essed CE, Lancée CT, Mastik F, Frietman P, Van Egmond FC, Reiber J, Bosch H, Van Urk H, Roelandt J, Bom N: Arterial wall characteristics determined by intravascular ultrasound imaging: An in vitro study. J Am Coll Cardiol 14:947–952, 1989.
15. Tobis JM, Mallery J, Mahon D, Lehmann K, Zalesky P, Griffith J, Gessert J, Moriuchi M, McRae M, Dwyer M, Greep N, Henry WL: Intravascular ultrasound imaging of human coronary arteries in vivo: Analysis of tissue characterizations with comparison to in vitro histological specimens. Circulation 83:913–926, 1991.
16. Fitzgerald PJ, St. Goar FG, Connolly AJ, Pinto FJ, Billingham ME, Popp RL, Yock PG. Intravascular ultrasound imaging of coronary arteries: Is three layers the norm? Circulation 86:154–158, 1992.
17. Sudhir K, MacGregor JS, Gupta M, Barbant SD, Redberg R, Yock PG, Chatterjee K: Effect of selection angiotensin II receptor antagonism and angiotensin converting enzyme inhibition on the coronary vasculature in vivo: Intravascular two-dimensional and Doppler ultrasound studies. Circulation 87:931–938, 1993.
18. Gao S, Alderman EL, Schroeder JS, Silverman JF, Hunt SA: Accelerated coronary vascular disease in the heart transplant patient: coronary arteriographic findings. J Am Coll Cardiol 12:334–340, 1988.
19. Linker DT, Kleven A, Gronningsaether A, Yock PG, Angelsen BAJ: Tissue characterization with intra-arterial ultrasound: Special promise and problems. Inter J Cardiac Imaging 6:255–263, 1991.
20. Keogh AM, Valantine HA, Hunt SA, Schroeder JS, McIntosh N, Oyer PE, Stinson EB: Impact of proximal or midvessel discrete coronary artery stenoses on survival after heart transplantation. J Heart Lung Transplant 11:892–901, 1992.
21. Billingham ME: Histopathology of graft coronary disease. J Heart Lung Transplant 11:(3)S38–S44, 1992.
22. McGinn AL, Wilson RF, Olivari MT, Homans DC, White CW: Coronary vasodilator reserve after human orthotopic cardiac transplantation. Circulation 78:1200–1209, 1988.

23. Senneff MJ, Hartman J, Sobel BE, Geltman EM, Bergmann SR: Persistence of coronary vasodilator responsivity after cardiac transplantation. Am J Cardiol 71:333–338, 1993.

24. Krivokapich J, Stevenson LW, Kobashigawa J, Huang S, Schelbert HR: Quantification of absolute myocardial perfusion at rest and during exercise with positron emission tomography after human cardiac transplantation. J Am Coll Cardiol 18:512–517, 1991.

25. Rechavia E, Araujo LI, De Silva R, Kushwaha SS, Lammertsma AA, Jones T, Mitchell A, Maseri A, Yacoub MH: Dipyridamole vasodilator response after human orthotopic heart transplantation: quantification by oxygen-15-labeled water and positron emission tomography. J Am Coll Cardiol 19:100–106, 1992.

26. Nitenberg A, Tavolaro O, Loisance D, Foult J, Benhaiem N, Cachera J: Severe impairment of coronary reserve during rejection in patients with orthotopic heart transplant. Circulation 79:59–65, 1989.

27. Wolford R, Wolford T, Ast M, Flynn M, Jennison S, Cauley M, Miller L: Angiographic appearance of coronary arteries from transplanted hearts predict coronary flow reserve [abstr]. Circulation 88:I-420, 1993.

28. Hunt BJ, Segal H, Yacoub M: Haemostatic changes after heart transplantation and their relationship to accelerated coronary sclerosis. Transplant Proceed 23(1):1233–1235, 1991.

29. Hausmann D, Erbel R, Alibelli-Chemarin MJ, Boksch W, Caracciolo E, Cohn JM, Culp SC, Daniel WG, De Scheerder I, DiMario C, Ferguson JJ III, Fitzgerald PJ, Friedrich G, Ge J, Görge G, Hanrath P, Hodgson JM, Isner JM, Jain S, Maier-Rudolph W, Mooney M, Moses JW, Mudra H, Pinto FJ, Smalling RW, Talley JD, Tobis JM, Walter PD, Weidinger F, Werner GS, Yeung AC, Yock PG: The safety of intracoronary ultrasound: A multicenter survey of 2207 examinations. Circulation 91:623–630, 1995.

30. Nitenberg A, Benvenuti C, Aptecar E, Antony I, Deleuze P, Loisance D, Cachera J: Acetylcholine-induced constriction of angiographically normal coronary arteries is not time dependent in transplant recipients: Effects of stepwise infusion at 1, 6, 12 and more than 24 months after transplantation. J Am Coll Cardiol 22:151–158, 1993.

31. Rowe SK, Kleiman NS, Cocanougher B, Smart FW, Minor ST, Raizner AE, Henry PD, Roberts R, Pratt CM, Young JB: Effects of intracoronary acetylcholine infusion early versus late after heart transplant. Transplant Proceed 23(1):1193–1197, 1991.

32. Mügge A, Heublein B, Kuhn M, Nolte C, Haverich A, Warnecke J, Forssmann W, Lichtlen PR: Impaired coronary dilator responses to substance P and impaired flow-dependent dilator responses in heart transplant patients with graft vasculopathy. J Am Coll Cardiol 21:163–170, 1993.

33. Kushwaha SS, Crossman DC, Bustami M, Davies GJ, Mitchell AG, Maseri A, Yacoub MH: Substance P for evaluation of coronary endothelial function after cardiac transplantation. J Am Coll Cardiol 17:1537–1544, 1991.

34. Yeung AC, Anderson T, Meredith I, Uehata A, Ryan TJ Jr, Selwyn AP, Mudge GH, Ganz P: Endothelial dysfunction in the development and detection of transplant coronary artery disease. J Heart Lung Transplant 11(3):S69–S73, 1992.

35. Fish RD, Nabel EG, Selwyn AP, Ludmer PL, Mudge GH, Kirshenbaum JM, Schoen FJ, Alexander RW, Ganz P: Responses of coronary arteries of cardiac transplant patients to acetylcholine. J Clin Invest 81:21–31, 1988.

Part XI

Normal Coronary Flow Velocity Patterns: Consideration of Artifacts, Arrthythmias, and Anomalies

Chapter 22

Normal Coronary Flow Velocity Patterns:
Considerations of Artifacts, Arrhythmias, and Anomalies

Christophe Tron, MD, Thomas J. Donohue, MD, and Morton J. Kern, MD

INTRODUCTION

Intracoronary flow velocity measurements using a small Doppler-tipped angioplasty guidewire (FloWire, Cardiometrics, Mountain View, CA) permits accurate measurement of phasic coronary blood flow velocity along the course of coronary arteries and distal to luminal stenoses [1]. As demonstrated in previous studies [2–11] and earlier interventional physiology presentations, coronary flow velocity is currently used to assess the functional significance of coronary stenoses [2,3], to detect coronary collateral flow [4], to measure coronary flow reserve beyond the stenosis [5,6], and to study the effects on coronary blood flow of various mechanical [6–9] and pharmacologic interventions [10]. Given the large spectrum of clinical situations and variety of research applications, variations in normal flow velocity patterns may appear. The purpose of this Interventional Physiology section is to review the patterns of normal coronary flow velocity and examine some variations, artifacts, and anomalies of flow velocity measurements. Identification of these variations will assist in separating normal variations from pathophysiologic events which may be encountered in clinical practice.

NORMAL CORONARY BLOOD FLOW VELOCITY

The method of use of the Doppler angioplasty guidewire for the recording of coronary flow velocity has been extensively described elsewhere [1–3]. In brief, the most common method involves placement of the FloWire after diagnostic angiography. The Doppler guidewire is passed through a standard angioplasty Y-connector attached to a standard angiographic or guiding coronary catheter (5–8F). The guidewire is then advanced into the artery and the blood flow velocity is measured in proximal and distal locations and in selected branches. Continuous flow velocity profiles, using an on-line spectral

velocity analyzer, electrocardiographic and aortic pressure tracings are simultaneously displayed. A typical example of coronary flow velocity obtained in a normal proximal segment of the left anterior descending artery demonstrates the features of the classical coronary diastolic predominant pattern with a small but evident systolic component (Fig. 1). The velocimetry for the Doppler FloWire uses an electrocardiogram-based algorithm to establish markers for the systolic and diastolic periods used in the automatic calculation of peak, mean, and integral values of flow velocity. A positive intracoronary flow signal by convention indicates flow away from the wire tip. For comparison to another Doppler technique, the lower panel of Figure 1 shows the left anterior descending coronary artery flow velocity measured by transesophageal Doppler echocardiography. In this system, flow going away from the transducer is indicated by a negative signal below the zero line. Note the similarities of phasic and mean flow velocity.

VARIATIONS IN PHASIC DIASTOLIC PREDOMINANT FLOW VELOCITY AMONG THE MAJOR CORONARY ARTERIES

As described for many years in animal experiments, coronary flow velocity is similar in normal human arteries and demonstrates a classic diastolic predominant phasic flow pattern. The flow velocity measured in both proximal and distal epicardial artery locations is nearly the same when the arterial segment is >2.0 mm in diameter [6,7]. The diastolic to systolic velocity ratio (DSVR) is usually >2.0 for the left coronary artery, but variability in this pattern often occurs in the proximal right coronary artery where the mean DSVR is only 1.4 [12]. The difference in the patterns of the left and right coronary arteries has been postulated to occur due to a lower right ventricular contractile force and, thus, less impairment of the systolic fraction of flow in the right coronary artery. It is important to note that the DSVR increases when flow is measured in the posterior descending artery or posterolateral branches beyond the crux [13] (Fig. 2). Considerable overlap in DSVR is found between normal and mildly diseased vessels, probably related to the severity of the flow limitation. A majority of angiographic severe lesions studied by Segal et al. [7] had impaired DSVR (1.3 ± 0.5) which increased toward normal (1.8 ± 0.5) after angioplasty.

CORONARY VASODILATORY RESERVE

Coronary vasodilatory reserve, the ratio of hyperemia/ basal mean flow velocity is assessed after recording baseline velocity, then producing coronary hyperemia with intracoronary administration of adenosine (12–18 μg bolus for the left and 6–8 μg for the right coronary artery) [14]. Hyperemic responses are obtained both in the proximal and distal locations to assess branch flow contribution to coronary flow reserve. Adenosine-induced hyperemia augments total flow by increasing both systolic and diastolic flow velocity integrals (Fig. 3). The phasic flow pattern during hyperemia is highly variable but, in general, has minimal influence on normal diastolic/systolic velocity ratios in regions of normal myocardial contractility. In an unselected population of more than 250 patients with normal coronary arteriograms in our laboratory, the mean coronary vasodilatory reserve in men was 2.8 ± 0.6 and in women was 2.5 ± 0.8 undergoing diagnostic angiography. A coronary flow reserve >2 in patients with coronary artery disease correlates with normal thallium scintigraphy in 90% of studies [15]. An abnormal coronary flow reserve can be found in both severe epicardial lesions, as well as in

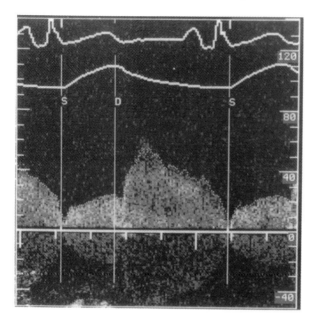

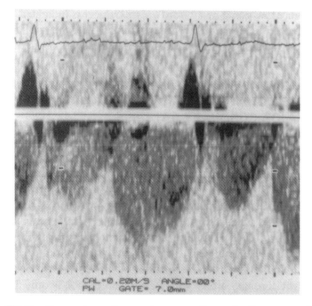

Fig. 1. Comparison of normal coronary flow velocity measured with Doppler FloWire (top) and transesophageal Doppler (bottom). By convention, flow going away from the transducer is positive with the Doppler FloWire and negative with transesophageal Doppler echocardiography. Note the similarities in flow velocity integrals for both systole and diastole and peak velocity responses. For the Doppler FloWire signal, the electrocardiogram and aortic (uncalibrated) pressure signals are displayed at the top of the tracing. The large timing marks are 1 sec. The velocity scale is 0–200 cm/sec. The scale for the transesophageal signal is 0–60 cm/sec. Each calibration mark is 20 cm/sec.

Abbreviations

APV	average peak velocity
ADPV	average diastolic peak velocity
ASPV	average systolic peak velocity
DSVR	diastolic/systolic velocity ratio
SNR	signal to noise ratio
PVi	peak velocity integral
DPVi, SPVi	diastolic, systolic velocity integral
DSiR	diastolic/systolic velocity integral ratio
MPV	maximal peak velocity

Fig. 2. Normal coronary flow velocity obtained in a patient in the proximal and distal right (RCA), circumflex (CFX), and left anterior descending (LAD) coronary arteries. Small arrows on the angiograms indicate location of the proximal and distal flow velocity signals. Basal flow velocity is shown for each artery in both locations. In general, the distal velocity is equal or slightly lower than the proximal velocity. Depending on the diameter of the vessel, the proximal flow velocity integral may also be lower. Note, the slightly lower proximal diastolic flow velocity integral for the right coronary artery compared to the distal segment. Note also that the DSVR is increased in the distal posterior descending artery segment of the right coronary artery compared to the proximal right segment. Velocity format as in Figure 1.

RCA **CFX** **LAD**

Proximal

Distal

LAD

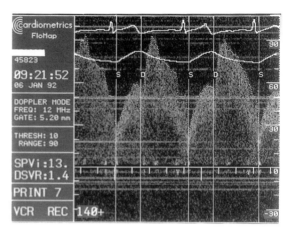

Base

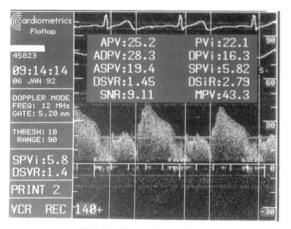

Adenosine, 12μcg

Fig. 3. Normal baseline (left) and hyperemic (right) coronary flow velocity in the left anterior descending (LAD) coronary artery. Hyperemic flow velocity is obtained after adenosine (12 μg intracoronary). Hyperemic flow achieves a 2.4 × basal increase in average peak velocity. Velocity scale is 0–140 cm/sec.

normal epicardial arteries in patients with an impaired microcirculation due to diabetes, hypertension, myocardial infarction, cardiomyopathy, left ventricular hypertrophy, or syndrome X [5,16–18]. Abnormal distal hyperemia is frequently associated with abnormal thallium scintigraphy [15].

ARTIFACTS AND TECHNICAL PROBLEMS

Various technical problems of spectral velocity signal acquisition or analysis may be encountered which can usually be easily corrected. A poor transducer beam angle may yield an unsatisfactory velocity envelope. Optimal placement of the transducer angle as nearly parallel to blood flow as possible will permit acquisition of peak velocities accurately. By directing the distal tip of the FloWire in several different orientations, the maximal spectral flow velocity tracing can be identified (Fig. 4). In contrast to other Doppler catheter systems, a relative position insensitivity for signal acquisition and analysis with the FloWire has been achieved by three features: a wide beam angle (27°), spectral velocity signal analysis, and use of a peak velocity automatic tracking algorithm. For most FloWire tip configurations, the velocity envelope is strong enough to be identified and quantitated. At times, when the beam is directed into the vessel wall, the broken edge of the velocity spectral envelope is easily appreciated. A small adjustment of the guidewire can restore the signal to yield an accurate measurement of flow velocity.

Position Insensitivity

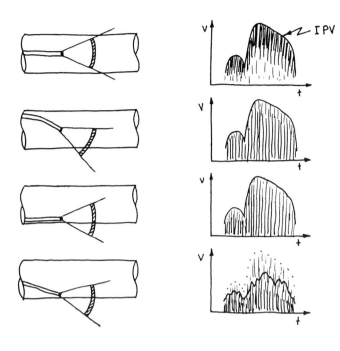

o Wide Beam

o Spectral Analysis

o Peak Velocity Tracking

Fig. 4. Diagram of FloWire and ultrasound beam to demonstrate relative position insensitivity of the FloWire. This feature is attributed to the wide beam angle, the spectral analysis, and the peak velocity tracking algorithm. It is only when the Doppler tip is directed toward the vessel wall (bottom) that the signal is not satisfactory for analysis. V, velocity; t, time; IPV, instantaneous peak velocity.

Erroneous tracking of the Doppler signal may occur due to artifacts of the velocity spectra or a poor electrocardiographic signal. Background electromagnetic radiation from various pieces of catheterization laboratory equipment including the fluoroscopy monitors, physiologic recorders, or other imaging devices may cause noise on the spectral display (Fig. 5). At times this noise prohibits authentic signal analysis, but does not interfere with the more dense flow velocity envelope. In cases with an inverted or wide QRS complex, there may be failure to track the systolic and diastolic portions of the flow velocity envelope accurately such as in Figure 6. The tracking of systolic/diastolic periods based on timing from the QRS is lost. This error can easily be corrected by switching the monitoring electrode leads to those which provide an upright QRS complex.

The direction of the FloWire tip transducer will indi-

cate when blood flow is antegrade (positive signal) or retrograde (negative signal). If the tip is deflected, flow direction can change as emphasized in Figure 7, which shows the flow velocity recorded during an angioplasty of the circumflex artery. Proximal to the lesion, the flow velocity is normal (Fig. 7A), while it is markedly decreased distal to this hemodynamically significant stenosis (Fig. 7B). A reverse flow is recorded because the wire is turned back on itself pointing toward the normal antegrade source (Fig. 7C). This artifact is identified by fluoroscopy and should not be mistaken for collateral flow velocity reversal. The operator only has to straighten the wire tip to obtain the true antegrade flow. The velocity instrument has the ability to invert the signal if required. Figure 7D shows the restoration of a normal flow velocity distal to the lesion after successful angioplasty.

ARRHYTHMIAS

Perturbations of coronary blood flow caused by arrhythmias can be studied with the Doppler FloWire. The pattern of coronary flow velocity during junctional rhythm is not different from that observed during normal sinus rhythm, since the A wave contributes little to coronary filling (Fig. 8). The effect of a short diastole as provoked by a premature ventricular beat limits diastolic more than the systolic component of coronary blood flow. In Figure 8 (right), the diastolic flow velocity integral is markedly decreased relative to an unchanged systolic flow velocity integral. A minimal reduction in mean coronary flow is thus produced. However, the prolonged RR interval after the premature ventricular beat permits a longer diastolic flow period, more than compensating for reduced coronary perfusion.

What happens to coronary flow during ventricular tachycardia? Depending on the etiology and left ventricular function during ventricular tachycardia, coronary flow may or may not be critically compromised. An example of the decrease in coronary flow velocity observed during an episode of ventricular tachycardia is shown in Figure 9. Note the poor tracking of the electrocardiogram (ECG) during the arrhythmia.

CORONARY FLOW RESPONSES TO EXTRINSIC DIASTOLIC PRESSURE AUGMENTATION: FLOW VELOCITY IN TWO HEARTS

A unique study of coronary blood flow velocity in the 2 left anterior descending coronary arteries of a patient who had a heterotopic heart transplant demonstrated the influence of extrinsic pressure effects on coronary flow velocity (Fig. 10). Coronary flow was measured serially in both the donor and native left anterior descending

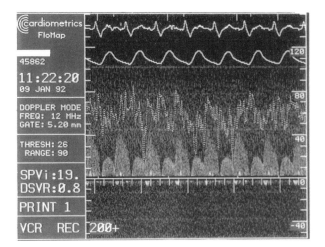

Distal LAD
Post PTCA

Distal LAD
Post Air Bubble

Fig. 5. Flow velocity signal recorded after an angioplasty of the left anterior descending coronary (LAD) artery. Note the failure to track the correct velocity signal (left and right) due to background interference. Right: Flow velocity is markedly decreased due to the passage of an air bubble in the artery. No clinical sequelae occurred. Velocity format as in Figure 1.

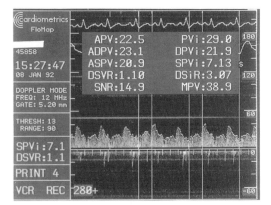

EKG LBBB
Switch Leads
(Upright ORS)

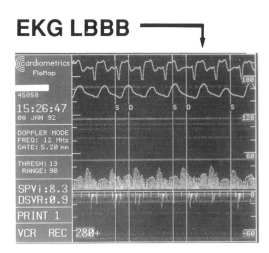

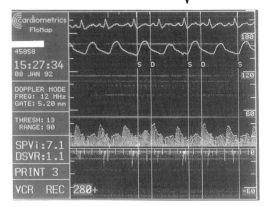

Tracking Off
Good Tracking

Fig. 6. Flow velocity signals with systolic and diastolic position tracking based on electrocardiographic configuration (left). Note the failure to track normally when the electrocardiogram shows an inverted QRS complex, such as obtained during left bundle branch block (LBBB). Right: the ECG is switched to an upright QRS and tracking proceeds normally to identify systolic and diastolic intervals. Velocity scale is 0–280 cm/sec.

Proximal CFX

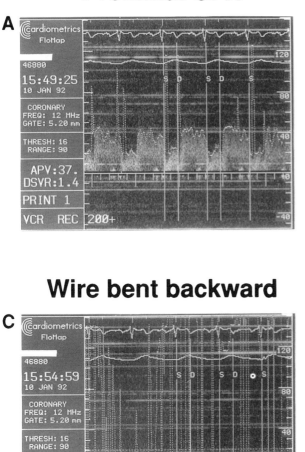

A

Distal CFX
(75% narrowing)

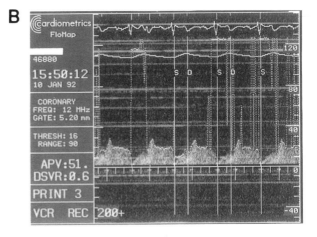

B

Wire bent backward

C

Distal CFX
(15% narrowing)

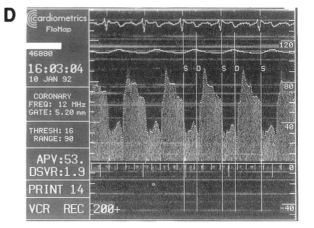

D

Fig. 7. Proximal and distal flow velocity in a circumflex artery with a 75% narrowing before angioplasty and again after angioplasty. **A:** Normal proximal velocity. **B:** Distal velocity with a proximal to distal flow velocity ratio >2 and impaired DSVR, indicating hemodynamic significance. **C:** Velocity after angioplasty when the wire is turned back toward the normal ante-grade coronary flow. This reverse flow pattern is not collateral flow, but indicates that flow is directed toward the wire tip which is bent backward. The wire was straightened out, and the final flow velocity result (**D**) shows normalization of distal flow velocity. Velocity format as in Figure 1.

arteries at rest and during intracoronary adenosine to determine coronary vasodilatory reserve. In this patient, most of the aortic pressure was due to the vigorous contraction of the donor heart. The native heart systole was generally weaker than that of the donor heart. The copulsation and counterpulsation of the systole of the two hearts determines the magnitude of aortic pressure and of diastolic flow velocity in the native heart. The flow velocity in the left anterior descending of the donor heart shows the classic diastolic predominant pattern (Fig. 10,

left). By contrast, in the native heart, the coronary flow is irregular both at rest and during hyperemia, depending on the timing of the contraction of the donor heart (Fig. 10, right). As can be seen on the electrocardiogram and aortic pressure tracings, the contractions of the native and donor hearts are not synchronous. The coronary flow in the native heart is, thus, increased when the contraction of the donor heart occurs during the diastole of the native heart, thus, augmenting the aortic pressure during maximal coronary filling. From the coronary flow view-

Junctional Rhythm

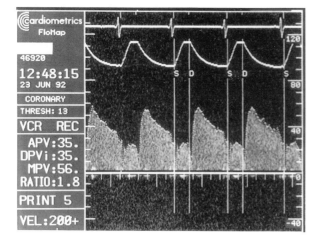

Premature Beat

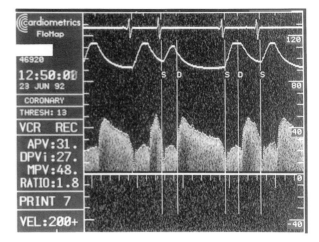

Fig. 8. Coronary flow velocity patterns occurring in a patent distal artery after successful left anterior descending (LAD) stent placement in a patient with junctional rhythm and during premature ventricular beat. Note the effect of the premature ventricular contraction on the intracoronary diastolic flow velocity integral and the increased flow velocity on the following beat. Velocity format as in Figure 1.

Sinus Tach

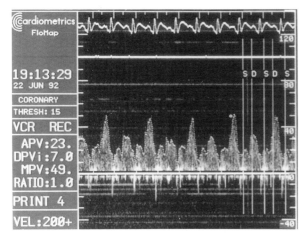

V. Tach

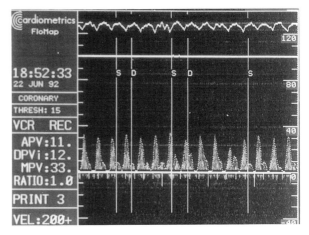

Fig. 9. Left: Coronary flow velocity in a circumflex artery during emergency rescue coronary angioplasty. An intra-aortic balloon pump was functioning in a 2:1 mode. Note alternating accentuation of diastolic flow velocity. Sinus tachycardia demonstrated preservation of normal flow velocity integral. Right: During a brief episode of ventricular tachycardia, coronary flow was diminished but not totally abolished, despite the fact that hypotension occurred. The intra-aortic balloon pump may have contributed to flow maintenance.

Fig. 10. Coronary flow velocity measured in a heterotopic heart transplant patient. The donor and native hearts both have flow velocity measured in the left anterior descending coronary artery. The donor heart is the predominant contractile force and demonstrates a regular coronary flow velocity pattern, despite an altered aortic pressure waveform. The native heart flow pattern is irregular and is dependent on the timing of pressure delivered by the donor heart during native heart diastole. During hyperemia (adenosine), the flow velocity is augmented to a normal degree with nearly doubling of the average peak velocity (shown on the trend plot below). By contrast, the native heart has coronary flow velocity which is altered by the assistance of the donor systole. The flow velocity waveform is irregular both at rest and during coronary hyperemia, but the hyperemic flow velocity response is preserved. Velocity format as in figure 1. The trend of flow velocity is displayed for the adenosine hyperemic period over 90 sec. The average peak velocity scale is 0–50 cm/sec on the lower part of the velocity display.

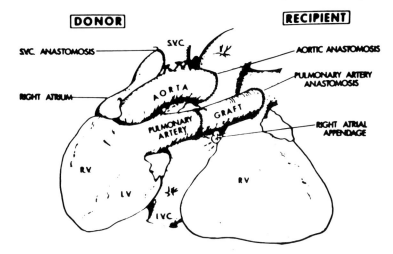

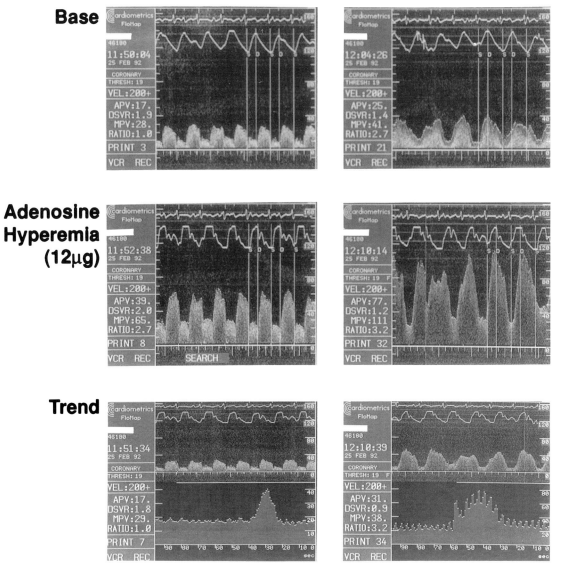

Fig. 10.

point, the donor heart acts as a diastolic counterpulsation, similar to that observed with intra-aortic balloon pumping [8,9].

SUMMARY

During normal flow velocity recording, various physiologic or technical problems may appear which can produce confusing flow signals. This section of Interventional Physiology reviews the patterns of normal coronary flow velocity and examines several artifacts and other features encountered in clinical practice. Recognition of these variations will help the interventional cardiologist to differentiate between physiologic and pathologic events.

ACKNOWLEDGMENTS

The authors thank the J.G. Mudd Cardiac Catheterization Laboratory Team and Donna Sander for manuscript preparation. Dr. Christophe Tron is the recipient of a Lavoisier Grant from the French Ministère des Affaires Etrangères.

REFERENCES

1. Doucette JW, Corl PD, Payne HM, Flynn AE, Goto M, Nassi M, Segal J: Validation of a Doppler guide wire for intravascular measurement of coronary artery flow velocity. Circulation 85: 1899–1911, 1992.
2. Donohue TJ, Kern MJ, Aguirre FV, Bach RG, Wolford T, Bell CA, Segal J: Assessing the hemodynamic significance of coronary stenoses: Analysis of translesional pressure–flow velocity relations in patients. J Am Coll Cardiol 22:449–458, 1993.
3. Kern MJ, Anderson HV (eds): A symposium: The clinical applications of the intracoronary Doppler guidewire flow velocity in patients: Understanding blood flow beyond the coronary stenosis. Am J Cardiol 71(14):1D–86D, 1993.
4. Kern MJ, Donohue TJ, Bach RG, Aguirre FV, Caracciolo EA, Ofili EO: Quantitating coronary collateral flow velocity in patients during coronary angioplasty using a Doppler guidewire. Am J Cardiol 71(14):34D–40D, 1993.
5. White CW: Clinical applications of Doppler coronary flow reserve measurements. Am J Cardiol 71(14):10D–16D, 1993.
6. Ofili E, Kern MJ, Labovitz AJ, St Vrain JA, Segal J, Aguirre F, Castello R: Analysis of coronary blood flow velocity dynamics in angiographically normal and stenosed arteries before and after endolumen enlargement by angioplasty. J Am Coll Cardiol 21: 308–316, 1993.
7. Segal J, Kern MJ, Scott NA, King SB III, Doucette JW, Heuser RR, Ofili E, Siegel R: Alterations of phasic coronary flow velocity in humans during percutaneous coronary angioplasty. J Am Coll Cardiol 20:276–286, 1992.
8. Kern MJ, Aguirre F, Tatineni S, Penick D, Serota H, Donohue T, Walter K: Enhanced coronary blood flow velocity during intra-aortic balloon counterpulsation in critically ill patients. J Am Coll Cardiol 21:359–368, 1993.
9. Kern MJ, Aguirre F, Bach R, Donohue T, Segal J: Augmentation of coronary blood flow by intra-aortic balloon pumping in patients after coronary angioplasty. Circulation 87:500–511, 1993.
10. Al-Joundi B, Kern MJ, Donohue T, Bach R, Aguirre FV, Chaitman BR, Miller DD: Is intravenous dipyridamole coronary hyperemia reversal by aminophylline equivalent to adenosine cessation? Comparison using continuous intracoronary spectral flow velocity measurements. J Am Coll Cardiol 21:420A, 1993 (abst).
11. Labovitz AJ, Anthonis DM, Cravens TL, Kern MJ: Validation of volumetric flow measurements by means of a Doppler-tipped coronary angioplasty guide wire. Am Heart J 126:1456–1461, 1993.
12. Ofili EO, Labovitz AJ, Kern MJ: Coronary flow velocity dynamics in normal and diseased arteries. Am J Cardiol 71(14):3D–9D, 1993.
13. Heller LI, Silver KH, Villegas BJ, Balcom SJ, Weiner BH: Change in coronary blood flow following RCA PTCA. Circulation 88:I-204, 1993 (abst).
14. Wilson RF, Wyche K, Christensen BV, Zimmer S, Laxson DD: Effects of adenosine on human coronary arterial circulation. Circulation 82:1595–1606, 1990.
15. Miller DD, Donohue TJ, Younis LT, Bach RG, Aguirre FV, Wittry MD, Goodgold HM, Chaitman BR, Kern MJ: Physiologic correlation of hyperemic technetium-99m sestamibi myocardial perfusion imaging with post-stenotic intracoronary flow velocity reserve in patients with coronary artery stenoses of angiographically intermediate severity. Circulation May, 1994.
16. Gould KL, Kirkeeide RL, Buchi M: Coronary flow reserve as a physiologic measure of stenosis severity. J Am Coll Cardiol 15: 459–474, 1990.
17. Gould KL: Functional measures of coronary stenosis severity at cardiac catheterization. J Am Coll Cardiol 16:198–199, 1990.
18. Laarman GJ, Serruys PW, Suryapranata H, Brand MVD, Jonkers PR, de Feyter PJ, Roelandt JRTC: Inability of coronary blood flow reserve measurements to assess the efficacy of coronary angioplasty in the first 24 hours in unselected patients. Am Heart J 122:631–639, 1991.

Part XII

Coronary Bypass
Graft Conduit Flow

Chapter 23

Role of Large Pectoralis Branch Artery in Flow Through A Patent Left Internal Mammary Artery Conduit

Morton J. Kern, MD, Richard G. Bach, MD, Thomas J. Donahue, MD, Eugene A. Caracciolo, MD, Thomas Wolford, MD, and Frank V. Aguirre, MD

Blood flow within a left internal mammary artery (LIMA) conduit can reverse and become retrograde, flowing into the subclavian artery when proximal subclavian stenosis limits flow and reduces subclavian pressure relative to aortic pressure, creating a "steal" phenomenon [1,2]. It has been postulated that large proximal LIMA branches to pectoralis muscle that have not been ligated may divert LIMA flow and could possibly contribute to diminished LIMA flow or myocardial ischemia. Conceptually, flow to the coronary circulation occurs predominantly in diastole, while flow to skeletal muscle occurs predominantly during systole. Mean flow may vary, depending on the distribution of flow over each phase.

Can systolic flow to the pectoralis muscle from a large patent LIMA branch compromise normal LIMA flow to the left anterior descending coronary? To answer this question, we measured flow velocity and computed volumetric flow in a branching LIMA.

CASE EXAMPLE

A 50-year-old man had angina pectoris 7 years after a coronary artery bypass grafting with a LIMA to the left anterior descending artery and a saphenous Y vein graft to the first diagonal and obtuse marginal coronary artery branches. Thallium perfusion imaging suggested anterior, as well as anterolateral, reversible perfusion defects. The electrocardiogram demonstrated an old septal myocardial infarction. The physical examination was unremarkable. Cardiac catheterization demonstrated nor-

mal left ventricular function and severe narrowing of the left main (99%), circumflex (100%), and first diagonal branch (100%) with a 90% narrowing beyond the Y branch of the saphenous vein graft to the first diagonal. The right coronary artery has serial 50% and 60% narrowings in the mid and distal segments.

Coronary arteriography of the LIMA demonstrated a large patent proximal pectoralis branch originating approximately 15–20 mm from the subclavian origin of the LIMA (Fig. 1, upper panels). The distal LIMA anastomosis was patent with good angiographic runoff to the left anterior descending artery beyond the more proximal diseased and bypassed segment (Fig. 1, lower panels) without angiographically visible collateral flow to the distal left anterior descending coronary artery.

Using a 0.018 in. Doppler-tipped flowire through a 6F LIMA catheter as previously described [3,4], flow velocity was measured in the main LIMA before the pectoralis branch, in the proximal LIMA after the branch, and in the pectoralis branch 15 mm after the branch origin. The flow velocity findings are summarized in Table I. Resting flow velocity in the main LIMA was predominantly systolic, with a diastolic/systolic velocity ratio of 0.62 and a mean velocity of 15.2 cm/sec (Fig. 2). During hyperemia, induced with intra-LIMA adenosine bolus (18 μg), both the systolic and diastolic flow velocity increased approximately two and three times the basal values, respectively. As the flowire was advanced into the LIMA beyond the pectoralis branch bifurcation, the systolic predominant LIMA flow pattern was shifted to diastolic predominant with a diastolic/systolic velocity

Branching LIMA
LAO   RAO

**Upper
LIMA**

**LIMA +
Anastomois
to LAD**

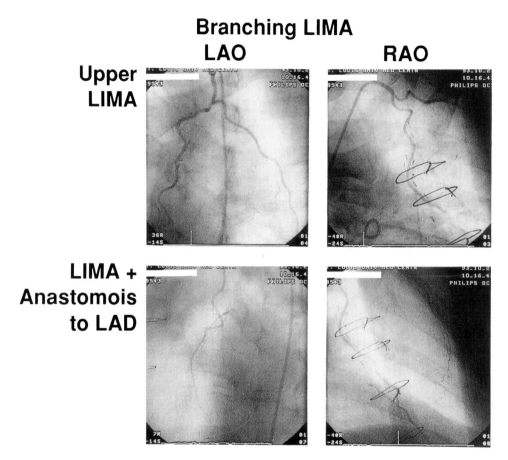

Fig. 1.   Coronary angiography in the left anterior oblique (LAO) and right anterior oblique (RAO) projections of a left internal mammary artery (LIMA). A large patent pectoralis branch can be seen immediately after the origin of the LIMA from the subclavian artery. The top panels indicate the arrangement of the left anterior descending (LAD) portion of the LIMA and its pectoralis branch. The lower two panels indicate the patent LAD coronary artery and distal portions of the anastomosis to the LAD.

ratio of 1.25 and a mean flow velocity 11.1 cm/sec. Adenosine-induced hyperemia again increased diastolic flow 3.5-fold compared with a 2.5-fold increase in systolic flow. Systolic flow increased from 9.7 cm/sec to 26.0 cm/sec. Diastolic flow increased from 12 cm/sec to 40.2 cm/sec with a diastolic predominant pattern relative to the more proximal location (Fig. 3).

The flowire was withdrawn from the LIMA and redirected into the pectoralis branch (Fig. 4). Flow in this branch was systolic predominant, with a diastolic/systolic velocity ratio of 0.4 and a mean velocity of 21.3 cm/sec. Adenosine increased both systolic (34.2–47.6 cm/sec) and diastolic flow (13.8–24.8 cm/sec) components in the pectoralis branch, but to a lesser extent than the increases observed in the main LIMA or left anterior descending LIMA branch. Vasodilatory reserve, the hyperemic/basal average peak velocity, in each measured region was 2.5, 3.1, and 1.6 for the main LIMA, left

anterior descending LIMA, and pectoralis branch, respectively.

This case demonstrates interesting findings of LIMA coronary flow and branch physiology. Normal phasic blood flow velocity characteristics in arterial conduits are different from those identified in venous coronary artery bypass conduits [4,5] and vary in pattern from the proximal to distal regions. Previous work from our laboratory [4] has quantitated the phasic blood flow velocity pattern using the intravascular Doppler spectral analysis signal in coronary bypass conduits during diagnostic cardiac catheterization. Spectral phasic blood flow velocity was characterized in the proximal, mid, and distal segments of 18 internal mammary artery conduits and 11 saphenous vein conduits in 27 patients. In situ internal mammary artery conduits demonstrated a gradual longitudinal transition in the phasic flow with a predominantly systolic velocity ratio proximally (0.6), as was noted in

Main LIMA

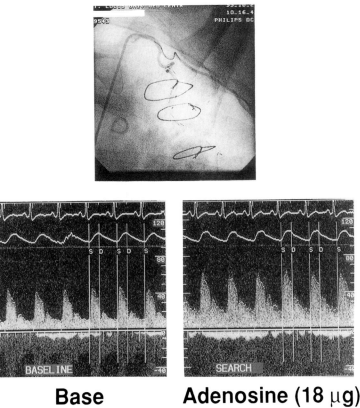

Base   Adenosine (18 μg)

Fig. 2. Top: Angiographic frame indicating the location of the flowire proximal to the bifurcation of the pectoralis and left anterior descending (LAD) left internal mammary artery (LIMA) branch. Bottom: Basal flow velocity obtained in the proximal portion of the main LIMA (left) and hyperemic flow velocity at this location (right). The flow velocity scale is 0–160 cm/sec.

The tracings on the flow panels indicate the electrocardiogram, aortic pressure, and spectral flow velocity from top to bottom. The vertical lines indicate the time between the systolic (S) and diastolic (D) periods. Intragraft adenosine (18 μg) was given and hyperemia is evident, increasing both systole and diastole.

the current case, which transitions to a predominantly diastolic/systolic velocity ratio (DSVR = 1.4). In contrast, saphenous vein graft flow showed a consistently diastolic predominance with diastolic/systolic velocity ratios of 1.4 and 1.5 in the proximal and distal portions, respectively. The mean velocity and total velocity integrals in internal mammary arteries were all significantly higher than those in similar regions within saphenous vein grafts.

These patterns of phasic flow velocity differed between the conduit type, most likely due to arterial compliance and location within the arterial tree. It is interesting to note that at the time of the initial study, no patients were identified with large proximal chest wall branches to provide comparisons to the current observations [6–8]. The coronary steal syndrome may occur through several mechanisms, including medications, surgical reconstruction, fistulas, or subclavian artery steno-

sis, none of which have been implicated in this patient. One potential mechanism related to branch flow diversion was a LIMA artery-pulmonary vein fistula producing postoperative coronary steal [8]. The role of flow diversion due to the pectoralis branch appears minimal and, as shown in Table I, diastolic flow increases in the main LIMA to 103 ml/min, of which 70% is attributed to the coronary artery connection. Of interest is the stimulated flow to the pectoralis branch, increasing 180% in diastole and 140% in systole compared with the left anterior descending artery LIMA flow increases of 335% and 139%, respectively.

There are few reports measuring quantitative flow velocity and angiographic findings in LIMA arteries. Reis et al. [8] report the hemodynamic significance of a LIMA to pulmonary artery fistula in a post-bypass patient with angina. The quantitation by angiography and flow velocity demonstrated that flow through the proxi-

LAD LIMA Branch

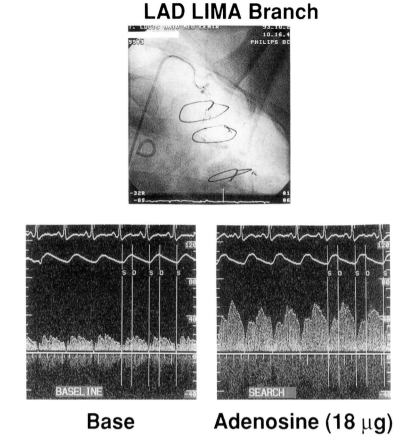

Base   Adenosine (18 μg)

Fig. 3.   Format as in Figure 2 for the location of the flowire in the left anterior descending (LAD) left internal mammary artery (LIMA) branch beyond the bifurcation of the pectoralis muscle. Note the difference in the phasic pattern of basal flow at this location for both the resting and hyperemic states.

TABLE I. Blood Flow Data in a Branching Left Internal Mammary Artery

Location	Arterial diameter (mm)	CSA	CBF$_{dia}$	APV	ADV	DVi	ASV	SVi	DSVR	CVR
Main LIMA	2.72	5.8	B 36	15.2	12.4	5.9	19.8	5.6	0.62	—
			H 103	35.9	35.9	17.0	35.8	10.0	1.00	2.5
LAD branch	2.14	3.6	B 22	11.1	12.0	5.7	9.7	2.7	1.25	—
			H 72	34.9	40.2	18.9	26.0	7.3	1.54	3.1
Chest wall branch	1.97	3.0	B 21	21.3	13.8	6.7	34.2	9.6	0.40	—
			H 37	33.1	24.8	12.1	47.6	13.3	0.52	1.6

ADV = average diastolic velocity (cm/sec); APV = average peak (mean) velocity (cm/sec); ASV = average systolic velocity (cm/sec); B = base; CBF$_{dia}$ = average diastolic velocity × cross-sectional area × 0.5 (ml/min); CSA = cross-sectional area (mm^2); CVR = coronary vasodilatory reserve; DSVR = diastolic/systolic velocity ratio; DVi = diastolic velocity integral (units); H = hyperemia; LAD = left anterior descending coronary artery; LIMA = left internal mammary artery; SVi = average systolic velocity integral (units).

mal LIMA of 14 ml/min was similar to the distal LIMA flow at 15.6 ml/min, indicating a nonsignificant contribution of such a fistula. Similar data, available in our current study, indicate that the chest wall branch has a minimal contribution to flow diversion during the diastolic phase of the cardiac cycle.

In summary, measuring flow velocity in individual branches to assess the physiologic impact of various phasic patterns of flow is a methodology that may reveal the underlying mechanisms and their contribution to ischemic syndromes attributed to the diversion of flow through various vascular beds.

Chest Wall LIMA Branch

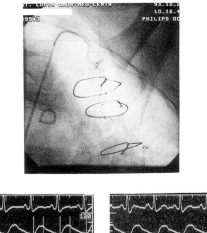

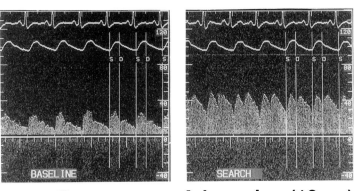

Base   Adenosine (18 μg)

Fig. 4. Same format as in Figure 2 with the flowire located within the pectoralis left internal mammary artery (LIMA) branch. Note that the flow velocity is predominantly systolic in both the basal and hyperemic states. The spectral pattern below the gray line indicates some turbulence located near the distal tip of the flowire.

REFERENCES

1. Brown AH: Coronary steal by internal mammary graft with subclavian stenosis. J Thorac Cardiovasc Surg 73:690–693, 1977.
2. Tyras DH, Barner HB: Coronary subclavian steal. Arch Surg 112:1125–1127, 1977.
3. Doucette JW, Corl PD, Payne HM, Flynn AE, Goto M, Nassi M, Segal J: Validation of a Doppler guide wire for intravascular measurement of coronary artery flow velocity. Circulation 85:1899–1911, 1992.
4. Bach RG, Kern MJ, Donohue TJ, Aguirre FV, Caracciolo EA: Comparison of phasic blood flow velocity characteristics of arterial and venous coronary artery bypass conduits. Circulation 88[part 2]:133–140, 1993.
5. Fusejima K, Takahara Y, Sudo Y, Murayama H, Masuda Y, Inagaki Y: Comparison of coronary hemodynamics in patients with internal mammary artery and saphenous vein coronary artery bypass grafts: A noninvasive approach using combined two-dimensional and Doppler echocardiography. J Am Coll Cardiol 15:131–139, 1990.
6. Samoil D, Schwartz JL: Coronary subclavian steal syndrome. Am Heart J 126:1463–1466, 1993.
7. Valentine RJ, Fry RE, Wheelan RK, Fisher DF Jr, Clagett CG: Coronary subclavian steal from reversed flow in an internal mammary artery used for coronary bypass. Am J Cardiol 59:719–720, 1987.
8. Reis SE, Gloth ST, Brinker JA: Assessment of the hemodynamic significance of a left internal mammary artery graft-pulmonary artery shunt in a post-bypass patient using a Doppler-tipped guide wire. Cathet Cardiovasc Diagn 29:52–56, 1993.

Part XIII

Variants of Normal Coronary Physiology: Spasm and Muscle Bridging

Intramyocardial Muscle Bridging of the Coronary Artery: An Examination of a Diastolic "Spike and Dome" Pattern of Coronary Flow Velocity

Michael S. Flynn, MD, Morton J. Kern, MD, Frank V. Aguirre, MD, Richard G. Bach, MD, Eugene A. Caracciolo, MD, and Thomas J. Donohue, MD

INTRODUCTION

Intramyocardial coursing of a coronary artery has been classified both as an anomaly [1] and considered a normal variant depending on its location [2]. Systolic compression of the arterial lumen, termed muscle bridging, has been considered of relatively minor clinical significance. The transient systolic compression of the coronary artery has been implicated in chest pain syndromes and sudden death [3], but its physiologic effects have been rarely demonstrated. Recently, Jain et al. [4] described the coronary flow velocity pattern, intracoronary two-dimensional ultrasonic luminal changes, and alterations of angiographic appearance of a coronary muscle bridge in a patient 2 years after cardiac transplantation. We also identified this variant angiographically in two patients and documented the coronary flow velocity patterns and intravascular ultrasound characteristics. Imaging confirmed luminal obliteration with each systole. These unique findings corroborate those of Jain et al. [4] and characterize a novel coronary flow velocity pattern of intramyocardial bridging.

PATIENT 1

A 47-year-old white man who underwent repeat orthotopic heart transplantation in May 1993 for accelerated immunologic coronary arteriopathy was referred for coronary angiography 1 month after transplantation recovery. Intracoronary two-dimensional ultrasound imaging and coronary flow velocity reserve assessments were made under an Institutional Review Board-approved protocol.

During coronary angiography in the right anterior oblique projection (Fig. 1), the mid left anterior descending coronary artery exhibited significant luminal narrowing during systole consistent with myocardial bridging. A 0.018 in. Doppler-tipped guidewire (Flowire, Cardiometrics, Inc., Mountain View, CA) was advanced into the distal vessel with flow velocity signal obtained 1 cm proximal and distal to the bridging segment (Fig. 1, bottom panels). The systolic flow velocity appeared blunted. An exaggerated and increased upstroke of the initial diastolic flow velocity pattern and a decreased systolic-to-diastolic flow velocity ratio were also observed. The hyperemic response to intracoronary adenosine [coronary flow reserve (CFR)] was within normal limits.

Intravascular ultrasound imaging (CVIS, Palo Alto, CA) identified complete luminal obliteration during systole (Fig. 2). This luminal obliteration occurred at the site of systolic coronary narrowing and was not altered by intracoronary nitroglycerin (200 mcg) or intracoronary adenosine (18 mcg) administration.

PATIENT 2

A 58-year-old white man was referred for diagnostic cardiac catheterization because of atypical chest pain.

Myocardial Bridging in LAD

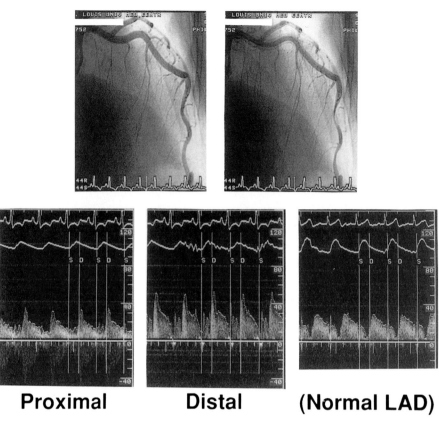

Proximal   Distal   (Normal LAD)

Fig. 1. Angiography during diastole (top left) and systole (top right) showing marked systolic narrowing of the mid left anterior descending (LAD) artery (arrow). The intracoronary flow velocity patterns proximal (bottom left) and distal (bottom middle) to the stenosis show the attenuated systolic component and abnormal diastolic flow velocity pattern with the exaggerated early acceleration, a diastolic "spike and dome" shape of coronary flow. The phasic flow velocity pattern in a normal LAD artery is also shown (bottom right).

Coronary angiography revealed normal coronary arteries with a discrete area of mid left anterior descending coronary artery myocardial bridging.

Intracoronary Doppler flow velocity identified a flow pattern nearly identical to patient 1 with impaired systolic flow and early accelerated diastolic flow velocity pattern. Administration of intracoronary adenosine (18 mcg) yielded normal CFR (3.1, normal using Doppler flowire >2.5) [5].

An intravascular ultrasound (IVUS) catheter was introduced across the left anterior descending coronary artery muscle bridge with images again depicting near intraluminal cavitary obliteration with relaxation in diastole as in Figure 2. Table I summarizes the flow velocity and vessel cross-sectional area changes at the site of coronary muscle bridging.

DISCUSSION

Although usually considered a cause of myocardial ischemia, intramyocardial muscle bridges are found not uncommonly during diagnostic angiography. The prevalence in patients undergoing diagnostic cardiac angiography is 0.7–4.5% [6]. Myocardial bridges are most frequently reported to occur in the proximal portion of the left anterior descending artery. This finding was so consistent in one study [8] that it was interpreted as a normal variant. The significance of systolic bridging in association with and without an obstructive coronary lesion has not been definitively determined. Pathologic descriptions of this anomaly have been reported. The vessel structure has been noted to appear protected by a lack of atherosclerosis at the site of bridging [7]. This finding was not consistent across other studies [6]. Intravascular two-dimensional ultrasound imaging and flow velocity add to our understanding of the quantitative severity of systolic luminal encroachment and allow correlation with the flow velocity changes during the different phases of the cardiac cycle. Angiographic narrowing correlated with two-dimensional echocardiographic images, showing a striking 25–57% systolic reduction of vessel cross-sec-

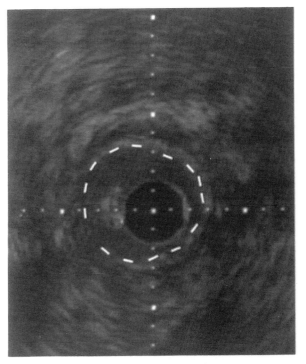 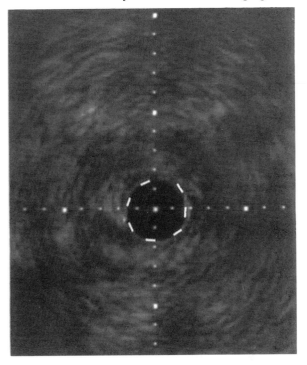

Diastole   Systole

Fig. 2. Left, right: Two-dimensional intracoronary ultrasound imaging of the segment of myocardial bridging. Note the luminal reduction to cavity obliteration during systole. The luminal areas are outlined by white dashed lines.

TABLE I. Intracoronary Flow Velocity and Two-Dimensional Ultrasound Imaging Data*

Patient	Artery segment	Mean velocity (cm/sec)	Flow velocity integral (cm^2) Diastolic	Flow velocity integral (cm^2) Systolic	Peak diastolic "spike" (cm/sec)	CFR	IVUS cross-sectional area (mm^2) Systole	IVUS cross-sectional area (mm^2) Diastole	% Difference
1	Bridge	22	12	3	39	—			
	Normal	17	9	2	28	3.0	3.0	7.0	57
2	Bridge	24	15	3	43	3.1			
Jain et al. [4]	Bridge	40	25	5	85	—	6.0	8.0	25
	Normal	19	12	3	35				

*CFR = coronary flow reserve (hyperemic/basal mean velocity); IVUS = intravascular ultrasound.

tional area [4,6,7]. Although postulated by Angelini et al. [6] to be predominantly eccentric, the systolic reduction of vessel cross-sectional area occurred in a concentric manner in the current two cases. The systolic reduction in cross-sectional area also is likely responsible, at least in part, for the attenuated systolic flow as recorded by intracoronary Doppler flow velocity. The angiographic appearance of myocardial bridging may depend on several factors as noted by Angelini et al. [6]. These factors include thickness and length of the muscle bridge, orientation of the artery to muscle fibers, amount of looser connective tissue, aortic outflow obstruction, coronary focus, and degree of atherosclerotic involvement.

The unique coronary physiologic findings were similar in the two patients presented here. Myocardial muscle bridging produced characteristic phasic flow alterations which included enhanced early diastolic flow, depressed systolic flow, altered systolic-to-diastolic flow ratio, and preserved CFR (Table I). The cause of the early notch of accelerated diastolic flow velocity is unknown, since some flow does occur normally in systole in human coronary arteries. These findings were unchanged by nitroglycerin and intracoronary adenosine, suggesting a strongly mechanical component to the flow disturbances.

Clinical Implications of Myocardial Bridging

Although chest pain syndromes are often present in patients with myocardial bridging, reports of significant clinical consequences or association with documented ischemia, arrhythmia, or infarction are rare. Angelini et al. [6] note that neither symptoms, stress electrocardiography, nuclear testing, nor myocardial metabolic testing reliably elicit ischemic responses in these patients. The clinical course, in general, depends on the extent of coronary artery disease and left ventricular function independent of the finding of myocardial bridge.

It can be hypothesized that the rapid normal diastolic predominant flow pattern is contributed to, in part, by systolic myocardial compression resulting in beat-to-beat coronary flow impairment with single beat hyperemia as part of normal diastolic flow. When the systolic flow is further compromised by muscle bridging, this beat-to-beat hyperemia produces a rapid and transient higher initial diastolic flow on release of the vessel narrowing immediately after muscle bridge relaxation. Whether sustained narrowing due to the bridge results in the consistent but increased early diastolic velocity pattern also remains under study [7–9].

Conclusion

Intramyocardial muscle bridging exhibits characteristic two-dimensional and coronary flow velocity patterns which are important adjunctive data to differentiate these anomalies physiologically from coronary vasospasm and obstructive coronary artery disease.

ACKNOWLEDGMENTS

The authors thank the J.G. Mudd Cardiac Catheterization Laboratory team and Donna Sander for manuscript preparation.

REFERENCES

1. Noble J, Bourassa MG, Petitclerc R, Dyrda I: Myocardial bridging and milking effect of the left anterior descending coronary artery: Normal variant or obstruction? Am J Cardiol 37:993–999, 1976.
2. Angelini P: Normal and anomalous coronary arteries: Definitions and classification. Am Heart J 117:418–434, 1989.
3. Roberts WC, Silver MA, Sapala JC: Intussusception of a coronary artery associated with sudden death in a college football player. Am J Cardiol 57:179–180, 1986.
4. Jain SP, White CJ, Ventura HO: De novo appearance of a myocardial bridge in heart transplant: Assessment by intravascular ultrasonography, Doppler, and angioscopy. Am Heart J 126:453–456, 1993.
5. Ofili EO, Kern MJ, Labovitz AJ, St. Vrain JA, Segal J, Aguirre F, Castello R: Analysis of coronary blood flow velocity dynamics in angiographically normal and stenosed arteries before and after endolumen enlargement by angioplasty. J Am Coll Cardiol 21:308–316, 1993.
6. Angelini P, Trivellato M, Donis J, Leachman RD: Myocardial bridges: A review. Prog Cardiovasc Dis 25:75–88, 1983.
7. Lee SS, Wu TI: The role of mural coronary artery in prevention of coronary atherosclerosis. Arch Pathol 93:32, 1972.
8. Benchimol A, Matsuo S, Wanj TF, et al.: Phasic coronary arterial flow velocity during arrhythmias in man. Am J Cardiol 29:604, 1972.
9. Polacek P, Zechmeister A: The occurrence and significance of myocardial bridges and loops on coronary arteries. Opusc Cardiol. Acta Fac Med Univ Brun, 1968.

Chapter 25

Dynamic Systolic Coronary Flow Reversal and Hyperemia in Left Anterior Descending Coronary Blood Flow Velocity During Valsalva Maneuver in a Patient With Hypertropic Cardiomyopathy

Richard G. Bach, MD, Morton J. Kern, MD, Thomas J. Donohue, MD,
Eugene A. Caracciolo, MD, Frank V. Aguirre, MD, and Joseph A. Moore, MD

INTRODUCTION

The phasic pattern of blood flow in normal coronary arteries supplying normal left ventricular myocardium shows diastolic predominance which is reflected in the Doppler spectrum of flow velocity. The responses of coronary flow to a variety of respiratory maneuvers have been described both in animal experiments and in patients during cardiac catheterization [1–4]. In response to the increased intraventricular and intrathoracic pressure and diminished arterial pressure during the strain phase of the Valsalva maneuver, previous studies using intracoronary Doppler in normal coronary arteries have shown a mild to moderate decline in mean flow velocity averaging 30–45%, with little reported effect on phasic pattern [2–4]. The effect of the Valsalva maneuver on coronary blood flow in normal hearts may be minimized by autoregulatory mechanisms which compensate to maintain adequate myocardial oxygen supply. Coronary hyperemia after release of the strain phase of the Valsalva maneuver has not been reported. Compensatory coronary hyperemia resulting from myocardial stress is not normally observed, despite the increased left ventricular pressure, probably due to offsetting effects of reduced left ventricular filling during the Valsalva maneu-

ver and reduced myocardial oxygen demands [1]. Respiratory maneuvers, such as cough, can decrease coronary blood flow transiently during vigorous compression of myocardium, but are also not associated with post-tussive hyperemia [4]. There are limited studies of the coronary circulatory responses in patients with hypertrophic cardiomyopathy. In the course of assessing an intermediate coronary stenosis in a patient with hypertrophic cardiomyopathy, we observed unusual alterations in coronary blood flow during a Valsalva maneuver which provoked a significant intraventricular pressure gradient. During normal sinus rhythm, resting coronary flow velocity had a normal phasic pattern and mean velocity. However, during the Valsalva maneuver, systolic flow reversal and, following release, a hyperemic response of the flow velocity were observed. This combined response in coronary blood flow velocity has not been previously described for this condition.

Valsalva Maneuver in a Patient With Hypertrophic Cardiomyopathy

A 63-year-old man had a 3-week history of syncopal episodes preceded by chest heaviness. The two-dimensional echocardiogram showed features of asymmetric septal hypertrophy without an intraventricular pressure

TABLE I. Hemodynamic and Flow Velocity Data During Valsalva Maneuvers*

	Pressure (mm Hg)				Velocity				
	Aortic	LV systolic	LVED	RR	APV	MPV	DSVR	Di	Si
Base	150/80	150	10	400	27	43	2.0	22	5
Valsalva strain	90/70	230	22	380	18	32	10.0	13	−3
Release	150/80	150	10	410	43	85	3.9	30	5

*APV = average peak velocity (cm/sec); Di,Si = diastolic, systolic flow velocity integrals (units); DSVR = diastolic/systolic velocity ratio; LVED = left venricular end-diastolic pressure; MPV = maximal peak velocity (cm/sec); RR = R-R interval (m/sec).

gradient at rest. Normal left ventricular contraction with impaired diastolic function, mild mitral regurgitation, left atrial enlargement, a calcified aortic root, and mitral annular calcification were also reported. Because of the syncopal episodes, a stress dobutamine echocardiogram was performed which provoked a 45 mm Hg pressure gradient assessed by Doppler echocardiography across the left ventricular outflow tract. An exercise thallium stress test was also performed. After 9 METS of exertion, the patient stopped due to fatigue. Although the thallium perfusion images remained normal, a cardiac catheterization was recommended for the evaluation of coronary artery disease and a chest pain syndrome. The patient received aspirin, Zantac, and Colace as his only prior medications. He also chewed tobacco. Before cardiac catheterization, Verapamil 80 mg po tid had been added to his regimen.

Physical examination at the time of cardiac catheterization revealed a well-developed man with a blood pressure of 110/68 mm Hg, pulse 56/min and regular, and normal respirations. There was no jugular venous distension. The lungs were clear to auscultation. The heart sounds were normal without murmurs. The peripheral arterial pulses were equal bilaterally. The remainder of the examination was unremarkable. The resting electrocardiogram demonstrated sinus bradycardia, but was in other respects normal.

In the cardiac catheterization laboratory, left ventriculography demonstrated hyper-dynamic systolic function with a CASS left ventricular score of 5 and an ejection fraction of 77% without angiographic evidence of mitral regurgitation. Selective coronary arteriography revealed a normal left coronary artery. The right coronary artery had a 60% proximal stenosis. Flow velocity and translesional hemodynamics were measured across the proximal right coronary lesion. The method and validation for use of coronary flow velocity measurements with a Doppler-tipped angioplasty guidewire and the techniques of translesional pressure measurement with a 2.2F tracking catheter have been previously reported [5,6]. There was a resting 5 mm Hg pressure gradient which increased to 30 mm Hg during intracoronary adenosine. Basal flow velocity increased 3-fold during hyperemia in both proximal and distal locations relative to the coronary lesion.

In view of the normal translesional hemodynamics of the right coronary artery and the negative thallium study in this zone, angioplasty was deferred.

In the course of assessing coronary physiology, hemodynamics and flow velocity were then measured in the left anterior descending coronary artery during Valsalva maneuver.

To assess the hemodynamic impact of the left ventricular outflow tract obstruction, left ventricular and aortic pressures were obtained at baseline and during Valsalva maneuver. The results are shown in Table I and Figures 1 and 2. The left ventricular catheter was then withdrawn and a 6F Judkins diagnostic left coronary angiographic catheter was situated in the left coronary ostium. The 0.018 in. flowire was then placed in the left anterior descending artery. Coronary flow velocity was recorded in the proximal region of the left anterior descending artery after the first septal perforator at rest during normal sinus rhythm. The flow velocity demonstrated a normal diastolic/systolic velocity ratio (DSVR ≥ 2.0) with an average peak velocity of 27 cm/sec. These flow findings occurred with normal left ventricular and aortic pressures at rest (Fig. 1). The Valsalva maneuver was repeated while measuring coronary flow velocity. Arterial pressure was continuously recorded through the side arm of the femoral sheath for both Valsalva maneuvers. The Valsalva maneuver provoked a large left ventricular-aortic pressure gradient. During the maximal strain phase, the aortic pressure declined from 150/80 to 90/70 mm Hg. Peak left ventricular diastolic pressure increased to 230 mm Hg with an end-diastolic pressure of 22 mm Hg (Table I). The normal aortic and left ventricular pressures were restored on release of Valsalva maneuver. During Valsalva, the flow velocity pattern was altered in a unique manner with a blunting of the peak diastolic flow velocity and moderate decrease in the diastolic flow velocity integral (from 22 to 13 units). Of note, the systolic flow velocity integral was markedly reduced with evidence of systolic flow reversal during the strain phase of the Valsalva maneuver (Fig. 2). Immediately on release of the Valsalva maneuver (Fig. 2), the flow velocity pattern normalized with a striking but transient hyperemic period lasting < 10 sec.

To assess the magnitude and time course of coronary

Proximal LAD

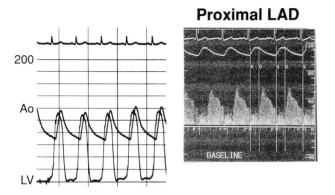

Fig. 1. Left panel: Left ventricular (LV) and aortic (Ao) pressures (0–200 mm Hg scale; time lines are 1 sec; electrocardiogram shown at the top) with left anterior descending flow velocity spectral Doppler signal (right panel). Note the deformed diastolic filling phase of the left ventricular pressure. There is no systolic left ventricular-aortic pressure gradient at rest. Coronary flow velocity is measured in the proximal portion of the left anterior descending artery at rest (0–200 cm/sec flow velocity scale). Systolic and diastolic periods are demarcated by the vertical lines labelled S and D. The electrocardiogram and aortic pressure are shown as the top 2 tracings. There is a normal coronary flow pattern with a diastolic to systolic velocity ratio (DSVR) of >2.0. The average peak velocity is 27 cm/sec with a systolic velocity integral of 5 units, and a diastolic velocity integral of 22 units.

Valsalva

During Valsalva   Release of Valsalva

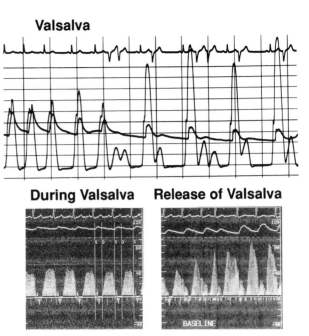

Fig. 2. Top: Aortic (Ao) and left ventricular (LV) blood pressure (0–200 mm Hg scale) during Valsalva maneuver with premature ventricular contractions. Bottom: Flow velocity during strain phase of Valsalva maneuver (left panel) and during release of Valsalva maneuver (right panel). During the Valsalva maneuver, the aortic pressure is reduced, the left ventricular pressure increased, and the rapid upstroke of diastolic flow velocity is blunted. The systolic portion of flow velocity is reduced and early systolic flow reversal is evident (S-D period). The average peak flow velocity is moderately reduced compared to baseline. During release of Valsalva maneuver (right panel), the flow velocity is seen to transiently increase above basal values with a peak flow velocity of 85 cm/sec, and there is a restoration of the inverted systolic flow velocity to its normal upright configuration (far right hand beats). Format as in Figure 1.

flow velocity during Valsalva maneuver compared to the maximal hyperemic response with intracoronary adenosine, the continuous trend of the average peak velocity was recorded during intracoronary adenosine (12 μg) and 3 serial Valsalva maneuvers (Fig. 3). The average peak flow velocity demonstrated normal pharmacologic hyperemic responses with coronary flow reserve (hyperemic/basal average peak flow velocity ratio) in the right coronary artery of 3.0, and in the left coronary artery of 3.2. As this trend plot shows, average peak flow velocity declined at peak strain of each Valsalva, with a brief hyperemic response to release. The maximal hyperemic flow responses on release of the Valsalva maneuvers are < 50% of the maximal hyperemia achieved with intracoronary adenosine.

For comparison, a flow velocity recording in the left anterior descending in a normal patient performing Valsalva maneuver is shown in Figure 4. During Valsalva, coronary flow velocity maintains the normal diastolic predominant phasic flow velocity relationship with a minor reduction in the diastolic velocity integral (area of flow) due to the shortening of the diastolic period with a decrease in the R-R interval during peak strain. On strain phase release, there is a restoration of the normal flow velocity pattern without hyperemia. Note that the sys-

tolic component of flow is not significantly reduced and remains antegrade throughout the entire Valsalva maneuver. This series of findings are in distinction to the systolic flow velocity reversal and post-strain hyperemia seen during Valsalva maneuver in the patient with hypertrophic obstructive cardiomyopathy.

DISCUSSION

The coronary flow responses in this patient are remarkable for several reasons. Phasic flow velocity at rest in a normal left anterior descending coronary artery supplying normally contracting hypertrophied left ventricular muscle had a normal pattern with a normal coronary vasodilatory reserve. During Valsalva maneuver in which intrathoracic pressure increases, venous return decreases, left ventricular chamber dimension decreases,

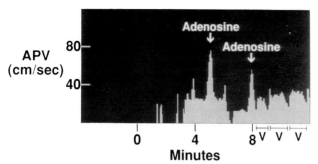

Fig. 3. Continuous trend plot of average peak velocity (APV) over 4 min in which Valsalva maneuver is performed 3 times (indicated by Vs). Intracoronary adenosine produces maximal hyperemia responses in both the right coronary artery (first peak), as well as in the left coronary artery (second peak) (arrows).

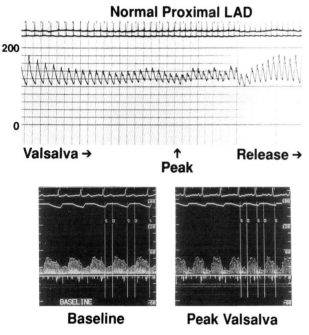

Fig. 4. Aortic (Ao) pressure during Valsalva maneuver in a patient with normal left ventricular myocardium and function and normal left anterior descending coronary artery. Flow velocity in the lower two panels demonstrates normal features at baseline and during peak Valsalva maneuver. Notice that the diastolic flow velocity integral is somewhat abbreviated due to a slight decrease R-R interval. Format for flow velocity as in Figure 1.

and left ventricular wall compression occurs, there is a blunting of the diastolic peak velocity with moderate decrease in the average peak velocity and, more interestingly, systolic flow velocity reversal. This systolic flow reversal may be due to the development of markedly increased left ventricular pressure and relatively decreased aortic driving pressure during systolic ejections forcing flow backwards out of the septum and left anterior descending, and limiting antegrade systolic flow. The force of contraction in this patient appears sufficient to stop, and even reverse systolic flow. Others have described angiographic evidence of septal perforator artery compression in hypertrophic cardiomyopathy [7], which could potentially reverse systolic blood flow proximally. On review of the coronary angiogram, this finding was not readily appreciated at baseline in our patient. The release phase of the Valsalva maneuver was associated with return of the left ventricular pressure to basal levels, abolition of the left ventricular-aortic gradient, and normalization of the phasic coronary flow velocity pattern.

Another unusual finding was the transient hyperemic response on release of the Valsalva strain phase. Coronary hyperemia has not been described after Valsalva in other patient groups, and one might speculate on the possible causes in this patient. Post-strain phase hyperemia may be the response to transient subendocardial ischemia from the very high left ventricular systolic pressure and reduced perfusion pressure. The left ventricular end-diastolic pressure had only a moderate increase during Valsalva from 10 to 22 mm Hg. It can be postulated that cessation of the antegrade systolic flow component through the penetrating left ventricular branches may elicit a transient ischemic hyperemic response. Other possible causes of hyperemia could include reduced global coronary blood flow to regions beyond the left anterior descending region measured or in remote zones not evaluated. A previous analysis of coronary blood flow in patients with hypertrophic cardiomyopathy has implicated reduced flow reserve as potentially causing myocardial ischemia despite normal epicardial arteries [8]. This was not specifically documented in our patient. These studies further revealed that, indeed, lactate production could be generated at maximal pacing stress in patients with hypertrophic cardiomyopathy, but that resting blood flow was not affected [8]. Of note, previous necropsy studies have documented transmural myocardial infarction in patients with hypertrophic cardiomyopathy without obstructive coronary artery narrowings [9], highlighting the potentially deleterious effects of this pathologic physiology. The unusual response documented by transient hyperemia in our patient suggests that flow change may be an early indicator of the ischemic potential of hypertrophic myocardium.

Coronary vasodilatory reserve may be impaired in hypertrophied or ''hypertrophic'' myocardial regions [8]. It is interesting that resting coronary flow reserve was normal in both the distribution of right and left coronary arteries in this patient. Finally, hyperemic flow velocity following Valsalva maneuver in this patient was < 50% of the intracoronary adenosine hyperemic reserve calculated to be approximately 3. Transient ischemic hyperemia after balloon deflation during angioplasty is generally 2–3 times basal flow.

In two recently reported series of patients with hypertrophic cardiomyopathy in which coronary blood flow velocity was analyzed by transesophageal Doppler echocardiography, heterogenous patterns of flow velocity were described [11,12]. In both studies, a small number of patients (4/25 total) had systolic flow reversal in the left anterior descending artery at baseline evaluation. In addition, angiographic evidence of coronary flow velocity reversal has been reported in other patients with left ventricular hypertrophy and aortic valve stenosis or insufficiency [10]. No provocative maneuvers, such as Valsalva, were performed in any of these studies. Our data showing the dynamic reversal of systolic flow during peak Valsalva strain may indicate a correlation between the magnitude of the outflow gradient and resultant ventricular wall tension and the pattern of coronary flow generated. We speculate that the Valsalva maneuver can cause a ventricular-to-aortic pressure differential with potentially marked compression of the intramyocardial arteries. This may cause impairment of antegrade flow during systole and flow reversal during maximal intraventricular gradient production. The attenuation of coronary flow, even if only the systolic component, is associated with post-Valsalva hyperemia which may be a reflection of myocardial ischemia induced by this benign physiologic maneuver in this patient with hypertrophic cardiomyopathy.

Investigation into coronary circulatory alterations in this interesting patient group may lead to better understanding of mechanisms of chest pain syndromes in such patients with normal coronary arteries.

ACKNOWLEDGMENTS

The authors thank the J.G. Mudd Cardiac Catheterization Laboratory Team and Donna Sander for manuscript preparation.

REFERENCES

1. Pepine CJ: Coronary circulatory effects of increased intrathoracic pressure in intact dogs. Chest 72:72–78, 1977.
2. Wilson RF, Marcus ML, White CW: Pulmonary inflation reflex: Its lack of physiological significance in coronary circulation of humans. Am J Physiol 255 (Heart Circ Physiol 24):H866–H871, 1988.
3. Benchimol A, Wang TF, Desser KB, Gartlan JL, Jr: The Valsalva maneuver and coronary arterial blood flow velocity. Ann Intern Med 77:357–360, 1972.
4. Kern MJ, Gudipati C, Tatineni S, Aguirre F, Serota H, Deligonul U: Effect of abruptly increased intrathoracic pressure on coronary blood flow velocity in patients. Am Heart J 119:863–870, 1990.
5. Donohue TJ, Kern MJ, Aguirre FV, Bach RG, Wolford T, Bell CA, Segal J: Assessing the hemodynamic significance of coronary artery stenoses: Analysis of translesional pressure-flow velocity relations in patients. J Am Coll Cardiol 22:449–458, 1993.
6. Kern MJ, Aguirre FV, Bach RG, Caracciolo EA, Donohue TJ: Interventional physiology, Part I: Translesional pressure-flow velocity assessment in patients. Cathet Cardiovasc Diagn 31:49–60, 1994.
7. Pichard AD, Meller J, Teichholz LE, Lipnik S, Gorlin R, Herman MV: Septal perforator compression (narrowing) in idiopathic hypertrophic subaortic stenosis. Am J Cardiol 40:310–314, 1977.
8. Cannon RO III, Rosing DR, Maron BJ, Leon MB, Bonow RO, Watson RM, Epstein SE: Myocardial ischemia in patients with hypertrophic cardiomyopathy: Contribution of inadequate vasodilator reserve and elevated left ventricular filling pressures. Circulation 71:234–243, 1985.
9. Maron BJ, Epstein SE, Roberts WC: Hypertrophic cardiomyopathy and transmural myocardial infarction without significant atherosclerosis of the extramural coronary arteries. Am J Cardiol 43:1086–1102, 1979.
10. Carroll RJ, Falsetti HL: Retrograde coronary artery flow in aortic valve disease. Circulation 54:494–499, 1976.
11. Memmola C, Iliceto S, Carella L, Napoli VF, de Martino G, Marangelli V, Rizzon P: Transesophageal Doppler evaluation of coronary blood flow velocity in hypertrophic obstructive cardiomyopathy (abstr). J Am Coll Cardiol 19:323A, 1992.
12. Tomochika Y, Tanaka N, Wasaki Y, Shimizu H, Hiro J, Takahashi T, Tone T, Matsuzaki H, Okada K, Matsuzaki M: Assessment of flow profile of left anterior descending coronary artery in hypertrophic cardiomyopathy by transesophageal pulsed Doppler echocardiography. Am J Cardiol 72:1425–1430, 1993.

Chapter 26

Blood Flow Velocity Alterations During Coronary Vasospasm

Morton J. Kern, MD, Thomas J. Donohue, MD, Richard G. Bach, MD, and Joseph A. Moore MD

INTRODUCTION

Ever since the introduction of selective coronary arteriography, accurate assessment of the severity of coronary stenoses has been a major concern. For many years, visual estimation of percent diameter stenosis was the only available tool, but this practice has been shown to be neither reproducible nor accurate [1–10]. Therefore, over recent years several computer-assisted systems for quantitative coronary analysis (QCA) have been developed. With regard to their precision and accuracy, some of these QCA systems have been compared in phantom studies [11,12]. It remains, however, uncertain to what extent data obtained by different QCA systems in patients can directly be compared. This issue relates directly to the question of whether angiographic data from trials studying the evolution of coronary stenoses during and after intervention or from atherosclerosis progression/regression trials can reliably be compared or used in meta-analyses without additional precautions.

These questions led us to perform a comparison of the coronary arterial measurements obtained in patients by means of three different algorithms routinely used for QCA before and immediately after coronary angioplasty (PTCA), as well as at follow-up coronary angiography.

MATERIALS AND METHODS
Patients and Image Acquisition

Images of 126 coronary artery lesions in 109 patients were studied before and after PTCA, and for 105 of these lesions a follow-up angiogram was also available at 6 months or earlier if clinically indicated. All patients were exclusively selected using clinical criteria for a pharmacological restenosis prevention study. Since there were no angiographic exclusion criteria, lesion characteristics and image quality were representative of routine inter-

43 yr old Male, LAD, Pre PTCA

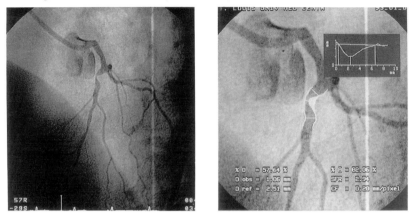

43 yr old Male, LAD, Post PTCA

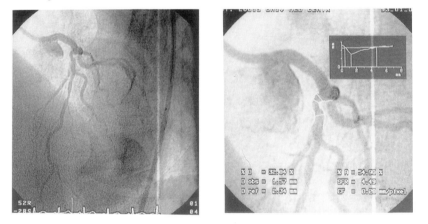

Fig. 1.   Coronary angiograms before (*Top*) and after (*Bottom*) coronary angioplasty in a 43-year-old man. The left anterior descending artery lesion is eccentric with a 58% diameter stenosis by quantitative coronary angiography (QCA). Flow velocity during the procedure is shown in Figure 2.

CASE REPORT 2: CORONARY VASOSPASM IN A TRANSPLANT EPICARDIAL ARTERY: EXAMINATION BY PRESSURE AND FLOW

A 55-year-old woman, 5½ years after cardiac transplant, had frequent episodes of chest pressure at rest associated with fatigue and dyspnea [5]. Treatment with nitrates provided initial symptomatic relief, but chest pressure periodically recurred. In the coronary care unit (CCU), a prolonged episode of chest pressure responded to intravenous nitroglycerin without electrocardiographic (ECG) evidence of myocardial infarction or ischemia.

Coronary arteriography revealed 50% concentric stenosis of the left anterior descending coronary artery, a totally occluded marginal branch, and minimal disease in an intermediate ramus artery (Fig. 3, top).

To assess the functional significance of the mid-left anterior descending artery lesion, an 0.018-inch Doppler flowire was advanced into the proximal and distal portions of the artery. Intracoronary adenosine (12 μg) was administered to assess hyperemic flow velocity. On translesional velocity assessment, the proximal and distal flow velocities were normal in both the phasic pattern, average peak velocity, and proximal-to-distal velocity

Coronary Spasm Post PTCA

Before NTG   After NTG

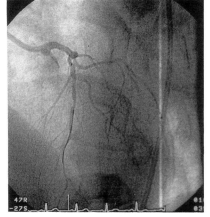 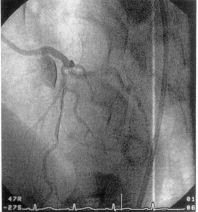

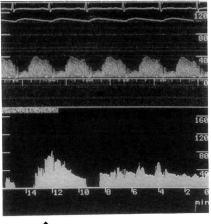

NTG

Fig. 2. *Top:* Coronary angiogram before (*left*) and after (*right*) the administration of intracoronary nitroglycerin demonstrating change in vessel caliber due to diffuse coronary vasoconstriction. *Bottom:* Flow velocity trend plot shows the continuous average peak velocity (0–200-cm/sec scale). Time intervals are 2 min. Immediately on balloon deflation (far left, at 14-min mark), flow velocity shows postocclusive hyperemia, which starts to decrease and then abruptly increases to a velocity of nearly 80 cm/sec. Intracoronary nitroglycerin (NTG) was instilled. Over the next 2.5 min, flow velocity decreases as the vessel lumen enlarges.

ratio, consistent with a gradient of <30 mm Hg across such stenoses [6]. Intracoronary adenosine produced hyperemia in both proximal and distal regions (CVR 3.4, 2.2, respectively).

To assess the translesional pressure gradient, a 2.2 French Tracker (Target Therapeutics) catheter was advanced into the distal vessel. A significant 50 mm Hg translesional gradient was demonstrated despite satisfactory catheter flushing and repositioning (Fig. 4). This severe gradient was out of proportion to the initially obtained flow velocity data. However, simultaneously acquired distal flow velocity recordings showed velocities higher than the baseline velocity (Fig. 4, upper left vs. Fig. 3, lower left, respectively). An angiogram was per-

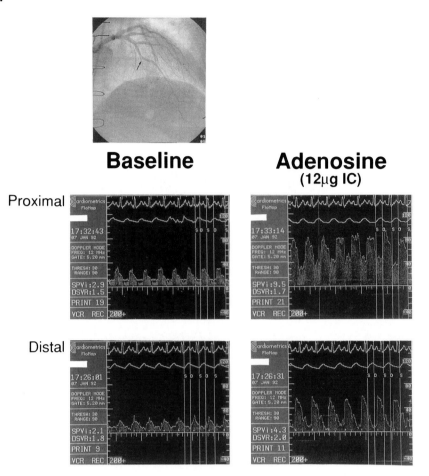

Fig. 3. *Top:* Baseline angiogram of the left coronary artery with a 50% concentric narrowing in the mid-left anterior descending artery (*arrow*). *Bottom:* Coronary flow velocity measurements proximal and distal to the mid-left anterior descending lesion at baseline and after intracoronary adenosine (12 μg intracoro-nary). Velocity scale is 0–200 cm/sec. Note similarities in prox-imal and distal flow velocity and hyperemic responses. S and D indicate the onset of systole and diastole, respectively, from the electrocardiogram. (From Donohue et al. [5], with permission.)

formed that revealed a new region of 70% diameter nar-rowing in the mid-left anterior descending artery consis-tent with epicardial spasm. While measuring distal flow and pressure, 150 μg of intracoronary nitroglycerin was administered. Within 10 sec, there was a decrease in the translesional pressure gradient from 50 mm Hg to <12 mm Hg, coincident with a decline in coronary blood flow velocity from 32 cm/sec to 17 cm/sec (Fig. 4). The decrease in blood flow velocity was coincident with ves-sel dilation and accompanied the reduction in the trans-lesional pressure demonstrated by continuous gradient measurements. Thus, the spontaneous epicardial narrow-ing created a significant but transient pressure gradient across the vessel associated with findings of increased coronary flow velocity. Nitroglycerin dilated the vessel to the preconstricted state and allowed velocity to return

to near-normal levels, as well as reducing the transle-sional pressure gradient. These changes occurred within 15 sec after drug administration, an important response time during ischemic episodes.

CASE REPORT 3: ATYPICAL CHEST PAIN SYNDROME, CORONARY SPASM, AND INTRACORONARY ACETYLCHOLINE

A 44-year-old man with atypical chest pain syndrome, treated hypertension, and mild hypercholesterolemia (205 mg/dl) had coronary angiography, which revealed normal coronary arteries. Because of the chest pain syn-drome at rest despite the absence of ECG changes during pain, provocation of coronary spasm was undertaken with the intracoronary acetylcholine method as described

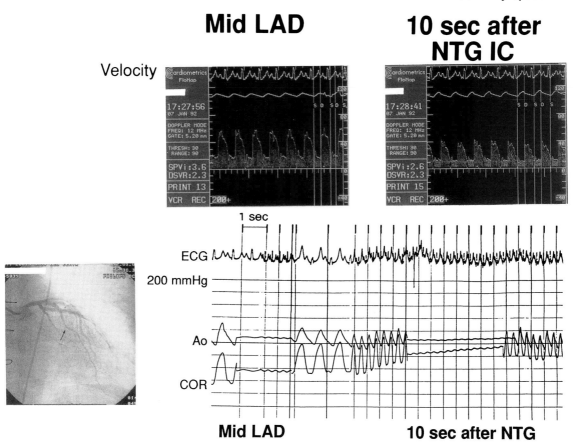

Fig. 4. *Left:* Cineangiogram of the left coronary artery in the right anterior oblique projection demonstrating epicardial spasm with a decrease in the diameter stenosis from 50–70% diameter narrowing (*arrow*). Bottom, *right:* Translesional pressure gradient is continuously recorded as nitroglycerin is administered. Ten seconds after nitroglycerin (bottom right side of tracing), vasoconstriction diminishes and translesional pressure gradient is reduced from 50 mm Hg to 12 mm Hg. Ao, aortic pressure; COR, distal coronary pressure, pressure 0–200 mm Hg. Top, *left:* Flow velocity measured in region of coronary narrowing before and during nitroglycerin. Flow velocity falls coincident with the decrease in pressure gradient and increase in vessel cross-sectional area. Velocity format as in Figure 3. (From Donohue et al. [5], with permission.)

by Horio et al. [7,8]. Coronary flow velocity was assessed with an 0.018-inch Doppler guidewire positioned through the 6 French diagnostic catheter. Before drug testing, a 5 French balloon-tipped pacing catheter was inserted into the right ventricle. Serial coronary angiography was performed before and after bolus administration of intracoronary acetylcholine (20 μg over 30–60 sec) and again after the administration of nitroglycerin (200-μg bolus over 5–10 sec). At baseline, the right coronary artery was of normal caliber without any focal luminal narrowing (Fig. 5). Coronary vasodilatory reserve was assessed by intracoronary adenosine (8-μg bolus over 5 sec). Adenosine produced a threefold increase in basal coronary flow velocity without any change in arterial caliber. Intracoronary acetylcholine produced severe, diffuse coronary vasoconstriction throughout

course of the right coronary artery, including the posterolateral and posterior descending branches (Fig. 5, top left) associated with a marked abrupt increase in flow velocity (Fig. 5, bottom trend plot). Intracoronary nitroglycerin (2 doses of 200 μg) immediately reversed the acetylcholine-induced vasoconstrictor effects. The high flow velocity values during vasoconstriction decreased after nitroglycerin-induced vasodilation with a return of coronary flow velocity to basal levels. Radiographic contrast administration within the artery produced transient hyperemia, peaking at ≤30% of the intracoronary adenosine response.

The vasoreactivity of the left coronary artery was also examined. The flow velocity guidewire was positioned in the mid left anterior descending artery (Fig. 6, top left). After 20-μg bolus of acetylcholine, there was dif-

Atypical chest pain
Normal coronary arteries

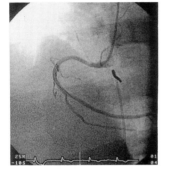 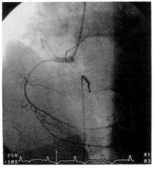 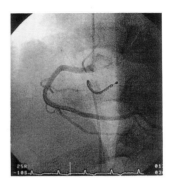

RCA Control   RCA Ach 20   RCA After
NTG 400

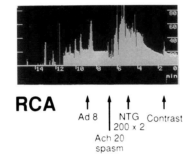

RCA

Ad 8   NTG   Contrast
200 × 2
Ach 20
spasm

Fig. 5. *Top:* Angiograms of the right coronary artery in a patient with atypical chest pain syndrome at baseline (*left*), after 20-μg bolus of acetylcholine (ACH, *middle*), and after 400 μg of intracoronary nitroglycerin (*right*). A temporary pacing wire is positioned in the right ventricle. *Bottom:* Mean coronary flow velocity trend plot demonstrating the hyperemic effect of 8 μg of adenosine (AD), acetylcholine during diffuse vasoconstriction, and nitroglycerin (200-μg bolus × 2). Contrast hyperemia is seen at the far right. The velocity scale is 0–100 cm/sec. Time intervals are 2-min markers.

fuse vasoconstriction. Intracoronary nitroglycerin rapidly reserved this vasoconstriction. These luminal changes were associated with patterns of flow velocity similar to those observed in the right coronary artery during vasospasm induced by intracoronary acetylcholine and reversed with nitroglycerin (Fig. 6, bottom).

CASE REPORT 4: ATYPICAL CHEST PAIN SYNDROME, CORONARY SPASM, AND INTRACORONARY ACETYLCHOLINE

In contrast to patient #3, a 63-year-old woman with an atypical chest pain syndrome had coronary angiography that revealed mild evidence of atherosclerotic right coronary artery disease. Coronary spasm provocation with bolus acetylcholine testing was performed in a manner similar to that used in patient #3. It is known that in patients with atherosclerotic irregularities of the coronary artery without significant narrowing, acetylcholine may produce profound vasoconstriction [9]. A Flowire was positioned in the proximal portion of the right coronary artery through a 6 French diagnostic catheter and a pacemaker was placed into the right ventricle before the administration of intracoronary acetylcholine in 20- and 50-μg boluses. Acetylcholine produced severe focal vasoconstriction in the mid-right coronary artery and proximal posterolateral and posterior descending branches (Fig. 7) without chest pain, but with significant bradycardia requiring temporary pacing. Intracoronary nitroglycerin was given. Vasoconstriction persisted in the posterolateral and posterior descending branches after administration of 200 μg of intracoronary nitroglycerin and required and additional 400-μg bolus for relief.

Coronary flow velocity in the proximal right coronary artery at baseline and after acetylcholine (50 μg) is shown in Figure 8. The phasic pattern of flow in the right coronary artery demonstrated equal systolic and diastolic flow velocity (37 cm/sec). During acetylcholine, bradycardia occurred with activation of demand pacing. Phasic flow velocity then demonstrated a systolic predominance (Fig. 8, top right). The trend plot of average peak velocity (Fig. 8, bottom) during the administration of aden-

Atypical chest pain
Normal coronary arteries

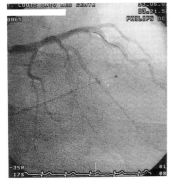

LCA Control

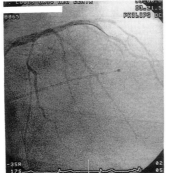

**Spasm After
Ach 20**

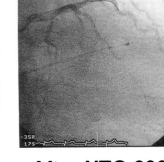

After NTG 200

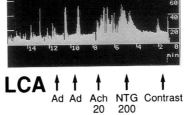

LCA ↑ ↑ ↑ ↑ ↑
Ad Ad Ach NTG Contrast
       20 200

Fig. 6. *Top:* Left coronary artery (LCA) (right anterior oblique projection) in the same patient as Figure 5. Left coronary artery vasoreactivity was assessed in a similar manner. Acetylcholine (20 μg) produces diffuse vasospasm. Nitroglycerin (200 μg) dilates the constricted vessel. Intracoronary adenosine (AD, 12 μg) indicated on the trend plot (*bottom*) elicits reproducible hyperemia approximately 2.5 times basal flow. Acetylcholine increases flow velocity due to vasoconstriction. Nitroglycerin produces a decline in this peak flow velocity due to vasodilation. Contrast hyperemia is shown at the far right of this average peak velocity trend plot. Velocity trend format as in Figure 5.

osine (8 μg), acetylcholine (20 μg, 50 μg), and nitroglycerin (200 μg, 400 μg) documents the changes in flow velocity during coronary narrowing occurring with acetylcholine. Vasodilation after intracoronary nitroglycerin restored flow to basal levels. Evidence of endothelial dysfunction can be demonstrated by acetylcholine in this method [7–9].

CASE REPORT 5: ACETYLCHOLINE BOLUS VS CONTINUOUS INFUSION METHODS

Continuous intracoronary infusion of $10^{-8}M$ to $10^{-5}M$ acetylcholine have been used to assess coronary endothelial function [9]. Comparison of intracoronary infusion to bolus administration of acetylcholine in our laboratory has suggested some variance of these methods, likely due to concentration effects, producing significant differences in coronary vasoconstriction. Patient #5 had an atypical chest pain syndrome with angiographically normal coronary arteries and underwent a serial bolus administration of acetylcholine (20, 50, and 100 μg) into the left coronary artery, followed by serial 2-min continuous infusions of acetylcholine ($10^{-8}M$, $10^{-7}M$, and $10^{-6}M$). Angiograms of the left coronary artery (Fig. 10) demonstrated minimal to mild coronary narrowing with bolus intracoronary acetylcholine administration up to 100 μg. Measurement of flow velocity with each bolus of acetylcholine demonstrated that transient hyperemia was induced, nearly equivalent to that obtained with intracoronary adenosine, representing resistance-vessel vasorelaxation (Fig. 11). Compared to bolus technique, the continuous infusion method at $10^{-8}M$ and $10^{-7}M$ of acetylcholine also produced minimal angiographic narrowing of the left anterior descending artery (Fig. 10). However, at $10^{-6}M$ acetylcholine, total left anterior descending occlusion due to severe vasoconstriction occurred, and 3 boluses of intracoronary nitroglycerin (200 μg) were required to restore the cali-

Resting Angina

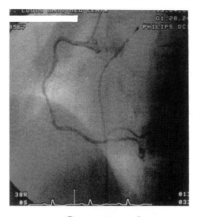

Control

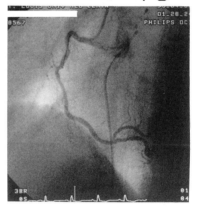

IC Ach 50μg

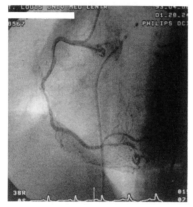

IC NTG 200μg

IC NTG 400μg

Fig. 7. *Top, left:* Control angiogram showing minimal disease in the mid- and distal portion of the right coronary artery in the left anterior oblique projection. *Arrow* notes diffuse disease at the posterolateral and posterior descending bifurcation. *Top, right:* Diffuse severe vasoconstriction with focal narrowing at the posterolateral and posterior descending takeoff. *Bottom, left:* Marked bradycardia and temporary pacing was a result of 50-μg intracoronary bolus of acetylcholine. *Bottom, right:* Intracoronary nitroglycerin (200-μg) bolus restored the proximal and midportion of the right coronary artery but did not relieve the vasoconstriction occurring at the posterior descending/posterolateral bifurcation. After 400 μg, the bifurcation coronary spasm has been relieved.

ber of the vessel to its basal diameter (Fig. 10, middle, bottom right). The coronary flow velocity response during 10^{-8}M intracoronary infusion was similar to that produced by the 100-μg bolus dose of acetylcholine. However, as the infusion dose was increased, flow velocity responded with difficulty, failing to increase to the previous peak with 10^{-7}M and falling to 0 with 10^{-6}M infusion during distally occlusive coronary spasm. Thus, in contrast to the accelerated flow velocity observed with subocclusive coronary spasm at the wire tip, epicardial occlusion due to spasm can produce a striking decrease in coronary flow velocity. Notably, if the distal lumen area at the flowire tip remains unchanged, significant focal proximal coronary vasospasm will decrease blood flow and, thus, register a decreasing velocity signal.

DISCUSSION

Unexplained increases in coronary flow velocity can occur due to guidewire malpositioning in a small septal or diagonal branch and/or coronary vasospasm. As shown in case #1, these flow changes may occur before the onset of symptoms or ischemic events. Detection of coronary spasm based on flow velocity, rather than on symptoms, may be useful in providing more rapid treat-

Resting Angina

RCA Baseline	Acetylcholine (ACh) 50 μg

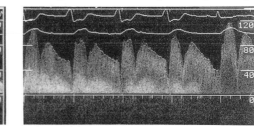

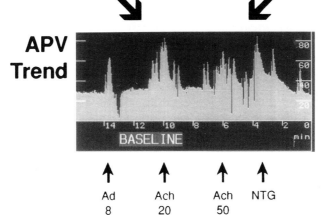

APV Trend

Ad 8 Ach 20 Ach 50 NTG

Fig. 8. Flow velocity changes accompanying acetylcholine (ACH), adenosine (AD), and nitroglycerin (NTG). *Top, left:* Phasic coronary flow velocity spectra in the proximal portion of the right coronary artery. Note equal phasic systolic and diastolic components demarcated by the S and D, respectively. Mean velocity is 38 cm/sec. *Top, right:* Flow velocity during 50-μg bolus of intracoronary adenosine. Flow velocity increases during vasoconstriction and a systolic predominant phasic pattern emerges with transient complete heart block and temporary pacing. *Bottom:* The average velocity trend plot demonstrates changes in flow velocity during intracoronary adenosine (AD), which produces a doubling of coronary flow velocity. The vasoconstriction of acetylcholine (20 μg) increases flow velocity markedly. Acetylcholine (50 μg) produces an initial increase, followed by a decrease in flow velocity as temporary pacing, bradycardia, and hypotension occur. Nitroglycerin is administered, relieving the effects of vasoconstriction and returning sinus rhythm and decreasing hyperemia to control levels. Flow velocity scale for the phasic tracings (*top*) is 0–160 cm/sec. Flow velocity scale for the average velocity trend (APV) is 0–100 cm/sec. Time markers are 2 min.

Resting Angina

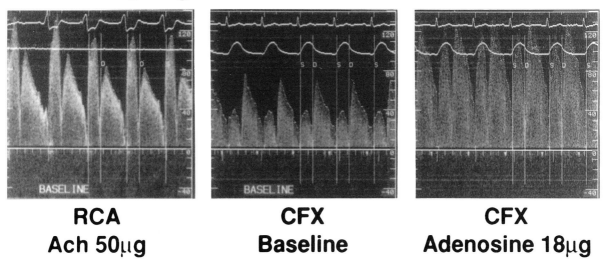

RCA	CFX	CFX
Ach 50μg	Baseline	Adenosine 18μg

Fig. 9. Comparison of flow velocity signals obtained in the proximal right coronary artery during acetylcholine (50-μg) bolus (*left*) and in the circumflex artery at baseline (*middle*) and during maximal hyperemia produced with adenosine (*right*). Note the systolic predominant pattern of the right coronary artery, possibly due to right coronary outflow limitations and/or ischemia. Velocity scale is 0–160 cm/sec. S and D represent systolic and diastolic periods, respectively.

Atypical CP

Control

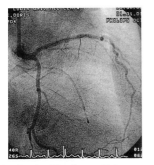

IC Ach 10⁻⁷

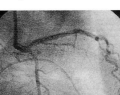

IC Ach Bolus 50 μg

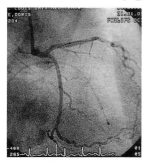

IC Ach 10⁻⁶

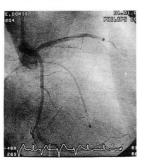

IC Ach Bolus 100 μg   IC NTG 400 μg

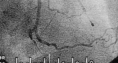

Fig. 10. Coronary angiograms demonstrating changes occurring with intracoronary bolus and intracoronary continuous infusions of acetylcholine. *Left, top to bottom:* Angiograms after control, 50-μg, and 100-μg bolus infusions. The flowire is located in the proximal mid left anterior descending artery. Minimal changes in vessel diameter occur with the bolus administrations. *Right, top to bottom:* Angiograms obtained during 10⁻⁷M acetylcholine and 10⁻⁶M acetylcholine and after 400 μg of nitroglycerin. Note the complete occlusion of the left anterior descending artery after 10⁻⁶M infusion.

ment to prevent myocardial ischemia and its sequelae during interventional procedures.

Diffuse vasoconstriction with luminal reduction around the velocity guidewire tip produces the markedly increased flow velocity which, on vessel dilation, returned toward basal values as demonstrated by acetyl-

choline stimulation in cases 3–5. Since acetylcholine has effects at both the epicardial and microvessel levels, coincident acetylcholine-induced dilation of resistance vessels cannot be discounted as contributing to augmented flow [10–12]. Abrupt increases in flow during spontaneous vessel spasm correspond to velocity changes observed in patients 1 and 2. Intracoronary acetylcholine-induced diffuse hyperresponsiveness with vasoconstriction consistent with abnormal endothelium-dependent responses in several patients. Whether this represented a clinically equivalent response to focal spasm of Prinzmetal's variant is uncertain. In our experience, ergonovine administered to similar patients has not consistently produced focal narrowings of the coronary vessels.

In response to various stimuli, both epicardial conduit vessels and microvascular resistance vessels may vasoconstrict. Provided volumetric flow remains constant, epicardial coronary spasm at the site of Doppler signal acquisition produces a characteristic increase in flow velocity in proportion to cross-sectional luminal narrowing. Spasm occurring proximal to the Doppler sample volume may reduce volumetric conduit flow and thus reduce distal flow velocity. Variability in vasomotion of resistance channels, inapparent by angiography, may confound the interpretation of flow velocity responses to vasoactive agents. The use of direct flow-pressure measurements in these situations will enhance our understanding of the pathophysiologic responses to coronary vasospasm and appropriate therapeutic maneuvers.

ACKNOWLEDGMENTS

The authors thank the J.G. Mudd Cardiac Catheterization Laboratory team and Donna Sander for manuscript preparation.

REFERENCES

1. Maseri A: Role of coronary artery spasm in symptomatic and silent myocardial ischemia. J Am Coll Cardiol 9:249–262, 1987.
2. Conti CR: Large vessel coronary vasospasm: Diagnosis, natural history and treatment. Am J Cardiol 55:41B–49B, 1985.
3. Miller DD, Waters DD, Szlachcic J, Theroux E: Clinical characteristics associated with sudden death in patients with variant angina. Circulation 66:588–592, 1982.
4. Hillis LD, Braunwald E: Coronary-artery spasm. N Engl J Med 299:695–701, 1978.
5. Donohue T, Kern MJ, Wolford T, Bach R, Aguirre F, Miller L: The effects of epicardial coronary spasm on intracoronary flow velocity and pressure gradient in a patient after cardiac transplantation. Am Heart J 124:1645–1648, 1992.
6. Donohue TJ, Kern MJ, AGuirre FV, Bach RG, Wolford T, Bell CA, Segal J: Assessing the hemodynamic significance of coronary artery stenoses: Analysis of translesional pressure-flow velocity relations in patients. J Am Coll Cardiol 22:449–458, 1993.

Atypical CP

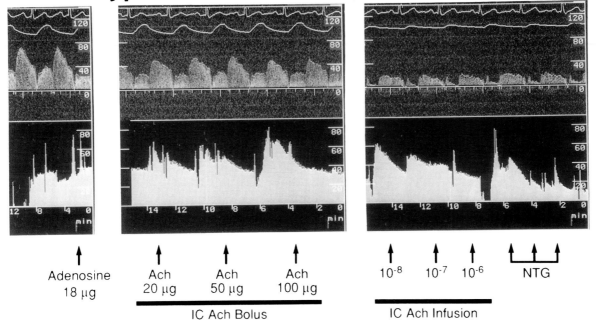

Fig. 11. Flow velocity during the study shown in Figure 10.
Top, left: Phasic flow velocity demonstrating normal left anterior descending phasic flow with a mean velocity of 42 cm/sec and normal diastolic-to-systolic velocity ratio (DSVR) *Bottom, left:* Intracoronary adenosine increases flow velocity 2× basal values. *Top, middle:* Phasic flow velocity during acetylcholine (100 µg) shows reduction in DSVR. *Bottom, middle:* Mean flow velocity responses to 20, 50, and 100 µg demonstrate nearly equivalent increases in coronary flow velocity. (*Arrows* are shifted to peak response. Infusions begin 30 sec earlier.) *Top and bottom, right:* After an equilibration period, flow velocity during continuous infusion is compared to that of intracoronary bolus. Continuous infusions produce less hyperemia than does bolus acetylcholine. At 10^{-6}M infusion, coronary occlusion occurs and flow stops (*bottom right*) at the blank space immediately after 10^{-6}M infusion. Three boluses of intracoronary nitroglycerin are administered with return of the flow velocity during dilation. Vasodilation reduces flow velocity to 20 cm/sec. (Top phasic velocity scales are 0–160 cm/sec; bottom average velocity trend scales are 0–100 cm/sec. Average peak velocity trend, *far left,* is 4-min intervals. The remaining flow velocity time intervals are 2-min intervals).

7. Horio Y, Yasue H, Okumura K, Takaoka K, Matsuyama K, Got K, Minoda K: Effects of intracoronary injection of acetylcholine on coronary arterial hemodynamics and diameter. Am J Cardiol 62:887–891, 1988.

8. Horio Y, Yasue H, Rokutanda M, Nakamura N, Ogawa H, Takaoka K, Matsuyama K, Kimura T: Effects of intracoronary injection of acetylcholine on coronary arterial diameter. Am J Cardiol 57:984–989, 1986.

9. Ludmer PL, Selwyn AP, Shook TL, Wayne RR, Mudge GH, Alexander RW, Ganz P: Paradoxical vasoconstriction induced by acetylcholine in atherosclerotic coronary arteries. N Engl J Med 315:1046–1051, 1986.

10. Kushwaha SS, Crossman DC, Bustami M, Davies GJ, Mitchell AG, Maseri A, Yacoub MH: Substance P for evaluation of coronary endothelial function after cardiac transplantation. J Am Coll Cardiol 17:1537–1544, 1991.

11. Egashira K, Inou T, Hirooka Y, Kai H, Sugimachi M, Suzuki S, Kuga T, Urabe Y, Takeshita A: Effects of age on endothelium-dependent vasodilation of resistance coronary artery by acetylcholine in humans. Circulation 88:77–81, 1993.

12. Brush JE Jr, Faxon DP, Salmon S, Jacobs AK, Ryan TJ: Abnormal endothelium-dependent coronary vasomotion in hypertensive patients. J Am Coll Cardiol 19:809–815, 1992.

Chapter 27

Quantitative Demonstration of Dipyridamole-Induced Coronary Steal and Alteration by Angioplasty in Man:
Analysis by Simultaneous, Continous Dual Doppler Spectral Flow Velocity

Morton J. Kern, MD, Thomas Wolford, MD, Thomas J. Donohue, MD,
Richard G. Bach, MD, Frank V. Aguirre, MD,
Eugene A. Caracciolo, MD, and Michael S. Flynn, MD

INTRODUCTION

The postulated mechanisms by which pharmacologic hyperemic stress testing produces ischemic ventricular dysfunction or scintigraphic malperfusion patterns include horizontal coronary steal from one epicardial zone to another or vertical coronary steal via shunting from the endocardial to epicardial regions [1–4]. Both postulated mechanisms may be operative in a given patient depending on the extent and severity of the coronary artery obstructions [5–7]. Experimental animal models using stenotic coronary artery preparations often demonstrate vertical redistribution and reversal of the endocardial/epicardial flow ratio [8,9]. Despite the technical limitations in patients using relative rather than absolute coronary flow quantitation, noninvasive methods have been highly consistent with a horizontal redistribution of epicardial blood flow [10]. A quantitative demonstration of horizontal steal has remained unproven due, in large part, to indirect methodologies of coronary blood flow measurements such as radionuclide methods [10] and regional venous efflux (coronary sinus thermodilution technique) [11] in patients. Direct Doppler catheter flow velocity techniques do not permit determination of distal blood flow during hyperemia [12]. With the advent of a Doppler-tipped angioplasty guidewire (Flowire™, Cardiometrics, Mountain View, CA), spectral flow velocity beyond a stenosis can be continuously quantitated during various mechanical and pharmacologic perturbations (13–15).

CASE EXAMPLE

A 48-year-old man recently hospitalized for a non-Q wave myocardial infarction continued to have mild angina with at least 2 episodes occurring at rest. The patient was stabilized with intravenous heparin, nitrates, oral calcium channel blockers, and aspirin. For risk stratification, a dipyridamole stress thallium perfusion study was performed and showed reversible ischemia in the distribution of the lateral ventricular wall.

Coronary angiography revealed moderately severe (57% diameter narrowing) single vessel disease of a large first marginal branch originating from a nondominant circumflex coronary artery. The left ventriculogram was normal with an ejection fraction of 0.54. Coronary angioplasty was to be performed with a 0.018″ Doppler flowire. The validation and methods of use of the Doppler flowire have been previously reported [13,14].

Prior to angioplasty, one Doppler flowire was advanced into the first obtuse marginal beyond the lesion (Fig. 1). Distal flow velocity was unaffected by the wire and maintained stable for at least 5 min by continuous mean velocity trend plotting. At 1–2 min after inserting the first flowire distal to the stenosis, a second flowire was introduced into the proximal circumflex artery, reading flow velocity proximal to the marginal branch origin. Simultaneous continuous dual location coronary flow velocity was thus quantitated during the following interventions: pre-angioplasty intracoronary adenosine-induced hyperemia (12–18 mcg) [16], intravenous dipyridamole (peak 4-min response after 0.14 mg/kg × 4 min) [17], aminophylline (125 mg intravenous × 2 min)

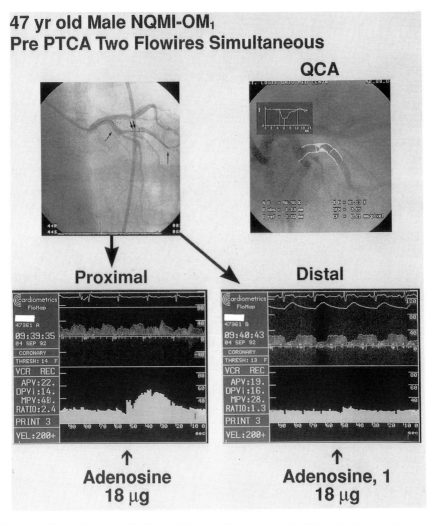

47 yr old Male NQMI-OM₁
Pre PTCA Two Flowires Simultaneous

Fig. 1. Before angioplasty: first obtuse marginal branch is instrumented with one flowire positioned distal to the lesion and a second one proximal (top cineangiogram, left side, single arrows). By quantitative coronary angiography (right side cineangiogram), the lesion (left side cineangiogram, double arrows) is 57% diameter narrowed. The lower 2 panels show the trend plots of mean velocity over 90 sec during adenosine (18 mcg intracoronary). The velocity panels are divided into a phasic display (with electrocardiogram and aortic pressure) on top and mean velocity plot beneath. The velocity scale is 0–100 cm/sec. The time of events is located on left border. Adenosine injection causes a notch in the trend plot of mean velocity (arrow, at 50 sec) on both tracings. Proximal but not distal hyperemia is evident after adenosine.

[18] and after angioplasty, repeated intracoronary adenosine-induced hyperemia (18 mcg). The diastolic flow velocity integral (area under the peak instantaneous velocity envelope), mean velocity, calculated coronary vasodilatory reserve (hyperemia/basal mean velocity) in the proximal and distal locations for each intervention are summarized on Table I.

Impaired Distal Coronary Reserve Before Angioplasty

Prior to angioplasty, maximal coronary hyperemia induced by intracoronary adenosine (18 mcg) was evident proximal but not distal to the marginal branch stenosis. Proximal mean velocities increased from 22 to 53 cm/

sec, whereas distal flow increased from 16 to 18 cm/sec. Coronary vasodilatory reserve was 2.4 proximally and only 1.1 distally (Fig. 1).

Evidence for Coronary Steal

After returning to baseline flow values, intravenous dipyridamole was infused (0.14 mg/kg) for 4 min (Fig. 2). In the proximal but not distal region, maximal coronary hyperemia was achieved by 3 min. Proximal mean velocity was 51 cm/sec. Distal to the stenosis, the mean velocity decreased to 8 cm/sec, a value lower than baseline. As shown on Figure 2 (right panel), the distal flow velocity declined over the same period of proximal hyperemia with nearly zero flow by min 5. This low flow

TABLE I. Simultaneous Coronary Flow Velocity Data Proximal and Distal to Coronary Stenosis*

| | Proximal | | | Distal | | | Blood pressure | |
	DFVi	MV	CVR	DFVi	MV	CVR	(mmHg)	HR
Pre-PTCA (QCA: % Diameter = 57; % Area = 81; Absolute diameter = 1.13 mm)								
Base	14	22	—	13	16	—	130/70	63
Adenosine	30	53	2.4	14	18	1.1	130/70	63
Dipyridamole	27	51	2.3	4	8	0.5	92/56	80
Aminophylline	13	22	—	8	18	—	95/62	70
Post-PTCA (QCA: % Diameter = 24; % Area = 42; Absolute diameter = 2.33 mm)								
Base	17	26	—	16	25	—	120/79	62
Adenosine	26	50	1.9	22	38	1.5	122/79	62

*Abbreviations: DFVi = diastolic flow velocity integral (units); MV = mean velocity (cm/sec); CVR = coronary vasodilatory reserve (hyperemic/basal mean velocity); PTCA = coronary angioplasty; QCA = quantitative coronary angiography; % Diameter = percent diameter stenosis; % area = percent area stenosis.

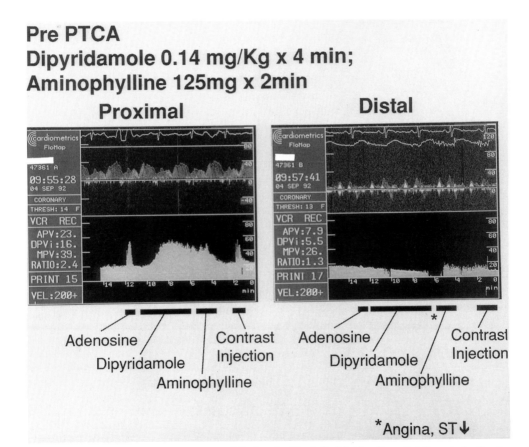

Fig. 2.   Evidence for dipyridamole-induced coronary steal (Left side). Proximal mean velocity trend plot and corresponding distal coronary velocity (right side). Format as in Figure 1. Velocity trend is now plotted over a 15-min period. Note the brief (30 sec) adenosine hyperemia of proximal but not distal flow velocity. Dipyridamole produced hyperemia proximally and co-incident diminishing flow distally culminating in angina and ST segment depression. Intravenous aminophylline reversed dipyridamole hyperemia and augmented distal flow with improved in ischemia. Contrast angiography to examine vessel dimensions produced transient hyperemia again only proximally.

state was associated with the development of anginal-like chest pain and ST segment depression (Fig. 2, right panel, asterisk). Aminophylline (125 mg intravenously) was infused over the next 2 min with marked and imme-diate reversal of proximal flow hyperemia and, importantly, restoration of diminished distal flow with resolution of ischemic symptoms and electrocardiographic changes.

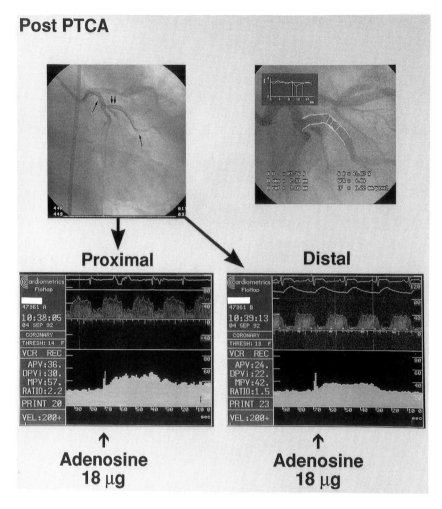

Fig. 3. Angiographic and flow velocity responses after angioplasty. Distal flow is increased and hyperemia occurs in parallel with proximal flow augmentation with adenosine. Format as in Figure 1.

Effect of Angioplasty on Distal Coronary Flow and Hyperemia

Coronary angioplasty was then performed using the distally positioned flowire without complications. Distal basal coronary flow was increased from 16 to 25 cm/sec coincident with quantitative angiographic improvement from 57% to 24% diameter narrowing (Fig. 3).

After angioplasty, intracoronary adenosine (12–18 mcg) induced hyperemia was re-examined with the flowires in the same proximal and distal locations as before coronary angioplasty (Fig. 3). Proximal hyperemia produced a lower coronary vasodilatory reserve (1.9 units) due, at least in part, to increased basal (mean velocity 26 cm/sec) and diminished hyperemic flow (50 cm/sec). Importantly, distal coronary vasodilatory reserve was improved (from 1.1 to 1.5) but not normalized, despite an excellent angiographically successful coronary angio-

plasty result. Due to clinical considerations, a second dipyridamole infusion was not performed.

DISCUSSION

The physiology of coronary steal requires a redistribution of blood flow away from a myocardial zone of potential ischemia associated with a coronary stenosis. Blood may preferentially flow to adjacent zones supplied by arteries with lesser resistance or to zones supplied by collateral channels of lower regional resistance. The quantitative flow velocity measurements in this patient are both unique and compelling in their support of a flow redistribution away from a zone supplied by a stenotic vessel while simultaneously increasing flow to the zones of lower resistance. Both the brief and sustained hyperemia induced by intracoronary adenosine and intravenous dipyridamole demonstrated impaired distal coronary vasodilatory reserve. More interesting, the distal flow decrease during sustained dipyridamole hyperemia was associated with a critical flow reduction sufficient to produce ischemic symptoms and new electrocardiographic abnormalities.

An alternative mechanism to distal flow reduction during dipyridamole hyperemia is the effect of arterial vasodilation producing passive collapse with distal pressure reduction in conjunction with altered stenosis geometry. This change in the arterial and stenosis configuration due to vasodilators has been reported in experimental animal models [19], but only postulated in humans receiving agents such as nitroglycerin and dipyridamole.

Also unique to this demonstration was the effect of aminophylline on dipyridamole hyperemia and coronary steal. Within 2 min of aminophylline, a phosphodiesterase inhibitor, proximal hyperemia returned to basal levels and distal diminished flow was improved with resolution of ischemia. The resolution of ischemic symptoms with restoration of distal flow after aminophylline also supports the mechanism of vasodilator-induced distal vessel pressure loss or exacerbation of lesion significance. Aminophylline could raise distal pressure and ameliorate vasospasm [20], thus restoring stenosis geometry and promote antegrade flow. This mechanism remains only a postulate since angiography and distal pressure were not measured during ischemia. Although aminophylline is routinely used for treatment of side effects of dipyridamole stress testing, the precise dose-related effects on coronary flow responses have not been convincingly demonstrated [18] and never before identified using a dual coronary flow velocity technique.

The clinical significance of the angiographically moderate stenosis was evidenced by an impaired distal hyperemic flow response. Although no translesional pressure gradient was measured, flow velocity data from prior studies [21] comparing the ratio of proximal and distal flow velocity to translesional gradients would suggest only a moderate hemodynamically significant lesion (< 30 mmHg gradient). The phasic nature of the distal flow is also consistent with only a moderate flow limiting lesion. Angioplasty increased distal flow mean velocity, distal hyperemia, and the diastolic-predominant phasic flow pattern, all criteria indicative of a successful result. Coronary vasodilatory reserve obtained from the calculation of coronary basal and hyperemic flow was not normalized, a common finding occurring in at least 50% of postangioplasty patients in similar studies [22,23]. Since both basal and hyperemic flow alterations may occur after interventions, it is not surprising that the coronary vasodilatory reserve values are not reproducible enough to be used in clinical decision making following interventions.

Limitations

Technical factors related to obtaining dependable flow velocity measurements have been discussed in detail elsewhere [13–15]. The use of 2 flowires, both producing identical signals, was satisfactory in this patient but may be complicated by signal interference, transient loss of signal due to motion artifact or wire rotation, and in more critical lesions, reduction of cross-sectional area by guidewire size producing a lower distal flow velocity, an artifact of the measuring system. In our patient, velocity signals remained satisfactory during the preangioplasty hyperemia interventions with stability of both proximal and distal flow signals demonstrated by continuous velocity monitoring. After angioplasty, the proximal flow velocity sample location may not have been in the exact preangioplasty position, but provided similar basal velocity signals with nearly equal hyperemia.

As an alternative to implicating coronary steal as the cause of diminishing distal flow during proximal hyperemia, one might postulate coronary vasoconstriction and/or thrombus accumulation at the lesion site producing ischemia. Both mechanisms might have participated in producing ischemia, but it would be unusual to have such events respond to aminophylline alone. Coronary angiography after aminophylline did not show significant intraluminal filling defects. Also, marked coronary cross-sectional area increase with constant volumetric flow would result in diminished flow velocity. Angiography immediately after ischemia did not support this mechanism.

CONCLUSION

Using a new method of dual intracoronary Doppler guidewire flow velocity monitoring, the physiology of coronary blood flow and distribution was observed during brief and sustained hyperemia before and after angioplasty of a symptom-producing lesion. Intracoronary flow velocity determinations beyond lesions in question will provide new insights into pharmacologic and mechanical interventions in patients with atherosclerotic coronary artery disease.

ACKNOWLEDGMENTS

The authors thank the J.G. Mudd Cardiac Catheterization Laboratory team and Donna Sander for manuscript preparation.

REFERENCES

1. Fam WM, McGregor M: Effect of coronary vasodilator drugs on retrograde flow in areas of chronic myocardial ischemia. Circ Res 15:355, 1964.

2. Fam WM, McGregor M: Effect of nitroglycerin and dipyridamole on regional coronary resistance. Circ Res 22:649, 1968.

3. Marshall RJ, Parratt JR: The effect of dipyridamole on blood flow and oxygen handling in the acutely ischaemic and normal canine myocardium. Br J Pharmac 49:391–399, 1973.

4. Gallagher KP, Folts JD, Shebuski RJ, Ranklin JHG, Rowe GG: Subepicardial vasodilator reserve in the presence of critical coronary stenosis in dogs. Am J Cardiol 46:67–73, 1980.

5. Befeler B, Wells DE, Machado H, Thurer RJ, Castellanos A, Myerburg R: Intercoronary steal syndrome resulting from aortocoronary bypass surgery. Am Heart J 51:610–612, 1983.

6. Winbury MM, Howe BB, Hefner MA: Effect of nitrates and other coronary dilators on large and small coronary vessels: An hypothesis for the mechanism of action of nitrates. J Pharmacol Exp Ther 168(1):70–95, 1969.

7. Marchant E, Pichard AD, Cassanegra P, Lindsay J: Effect of intracoronary dipyridamole on regional coronary blood flow with 1-vessel coronary artery disease: Evidence against coronary steal. Am J Cardiol 53:718–721, 1984.

8. Gross GJ, Warltier DC: Coronary steal in four models of single or multiple vessel obstruction in dogs. Am J Cardiol 48:84–92, 1981.

9. Patterson RE, Kirk ES: Coronary steal mechanisms in dogs with one-vessel occlusion and other arteries normal. Circulation 67:1009–1015, 1983.

10. Bodenheimer MM, Banka VS, Helfant RH: Nuclear Cardiology II. The role of myocardial perfusion imaging using thallium-201 in diagnosis of coronary artery disease. Am J Cardiol 45:674–684, 1980.

11. Ganz W, Marcus H: Failure of intracoronary nitroglycerin to alleviate pacing induced angina. Circulation 46:880–889, 1972.

12. Wilson RF, Laughlin DE, Ackell PH, et al: Transluminal subselective measurement of coronary artery blood flow velocity and vasodilator reserve in man. Circulation 72:82–92, 1985.

13. Doucette JW, Corl PD, Payne HM, et al: Validation of a Doppler guidewire for intravascular measurement of coronary artery flow velocity. Circulation 85:1899–1911, 1992.

14. Segal J, Kern MJ, Scott NA, King SB III, Doucette JW, Heuser RR, Ofili E, Siegel R: Alterations of phasic coronary artery flow velocity in humans during percutaneous coronary angioplasty. J Am Coll Cardiol 20:276–286, 1992.

15. Ofili EO, Kern MJ, Labovitz AJ, St. Vrain JA, Segal J, Aguirre F, Castello R: Analysis of coronary blood flow velocity dynamics in angiographically normal and stenosed arteries before and after endoluminal enlargement by angioplasty. J Am Coll Cardiol 21:308–316, 1993.

16. Wilson RF, Wyche K, Christensen BV, Zimmer S, Laxson DD: Effects of adenosine on human coronary arterial circulation. Circulation 82:1595–1606, 1990.

17. Francisco DA, Collins SM, Go RT, Ehrhardt JC, Van Kirk OC, Marcus ML: Tomographic thallium-201 myocardial perfusion scintigrams after maximal coronary artery vasodilation with intravenous dipyridamole: Comparison of qualitative and quantitative approaches. Circulation 66:370–379, 1982.

18. Brown BG, Josephson MA, Petersen RB, Pierce CD, Wong M, Hecht HS, Bolson E, Dodge HT: Intravenous dipyridamole combined with isometric handgrip for near maximal acute increase in coronary flow in patients with coronary artery disease. Am J Cardiol 48:1077–1085, 1981.

19. Goldstein RA, Kirkeeide RL, Demer LL, Merhige M, Nishikawa A, Smalling RW, Mullani NA, Gould KL: Relation between geometric dimensions of coronary artery stenoses and myocardial perfusion reserve in man. J Clin Invest 79:1473–1478, 1987.

20. Picano E, Lattanzi F, Masini M, Distant A, L'Abbate A: Aminophylline termination of dipyridamole stress as a trigger of coronary vasospasm in variant angina. Am J Cardiol 62:694–697, 1988.

21. Donohue TJ, Kern MJ, Aguirre FV, Bell C, Penick D, Segal J, Ofili E, Heuser R: Determination of the hemodynamic significance of angiographically intermediate coronary stenoses by intracoronary doppler flow velocity. J Am Coll Cardiol 19:242A, 1992.

22. Wilson RF, Johnson MJ, Talman CL, et al: The effect of coronary angioplasty on coronary flow reserve. Circulation 76:873–885, 1988.

23. Kern MJ, Deligonul U, Vandormael M, Labovitz A, Gudipati R, Gabliani G, Bodet J, Shah Y, Kennedy HL. Impaired coronary vasodilatory reserve in the immediate postcoronary angioplasty period: Analysis of coronary arterial velocity flow indices and regional cardiac venous efflux. J Am Coll Cardiol 13:860–872, 1989.

Chapter 28

Characterization of Intra-Arterial Flow Velocity Within Left Coronary to Pulmonary Artery Fistula

Saad R. Bitar, MD, Frank V. Aguirre, MD, Lawrence McBride, MD, Courtland Munroe, MD, and Morton J. Kern, MD

INTRODUCTION

Congenital coronary artery fistulae were first described by Krause in 1865 [1]. Fistulae can connect any coronary artery with any formative structure, including the four cardiac chambers, pulmonary artery, vena cavae, pulmonary veins, or coronary sinus [2–4]. The first presentation of such fistulas may be either in childhood or adulthood with the most common symptoms being angina and exertional dyspnea [4–7]. Because of limited methodologies, the only reported physiologic assessment of coronary artery fistulas in awake patients was performed indirectly using treadmill exercise with or without radionuclide thallium-201 perfusion imaging [7,8]. Direct intraoperative flow measurement of a giant fistula tract using electromagnetic flow meter was made by Dedichen and colleagues in 1966 [9]. To our knowledge, no description of the flow velocity characteristics of coronary fistulas has been reported in awake patients. In this case report, we identified bilateral coronary-to-pulmonary artery fistulas and measured intra-arterial flow velocity within the largest fistula branch. The flow velocity pattern of coronary fistula supports the hypothesis that flow is predominantly continuous without a phasic coronary flow pattern that might be anticipated from connections between high and low pressure sources across the heart.

CASE HISTORY

A 45-year-old woman experienced anterior chest tightness at rest, radiating to the left arm and associated with dyspnea 2 d prior to admission. Risk factors for atherosclerotic coronary artery disease include current smoking and family history of premature coronary artery disease. The electrocardiogram showed T wave inversion in the anterolateral leads. Chest pain continued despite heparin and nitroglycerin infusions. Serial electrocardiograms and enzymatic assays showed no evolutionary changes of myocardial infarction.

The blood pressure was 110/80 mm Hg; pulse was 80/min and regular. Cardiac examination revealed regular rate and rhythm, normal heart sounds, and no murmurs were appreciated. The remainder of the physical examination was unremarkable.

At catheterization, left ventriculography revealed normal systolic wall motion with an ejection fraction of 77%. However, upon review of the left ventriculogram, a large fistulous connection and opacification of the pulmonary artery could be seen (Fig. 1). Intracardiac or intra-arterial shunting was suspected as a possible etiology. Selective coronary arteriography showed a large fistulous connection originating from the left anterior descending artery at the origin of the first diagonal artery (Fig. 2, top). The fistula drained into the main pulmonary artery just above the pulmonic valve. The left coronary artery system was free of atherosclerotic luminal irregularities. Right coronary arteriography demonstrated a second separate fistula arising from the proximal right coronary artery which also drained into the main pulmonary artery (Fig. 2, bottom). Again, there was no evidence of atherosclerotic disease in the right coronary artery. Right heart catheterization was performed. The mean right atrial pressure was 8 mm Hg, pulmonary artery pressure was 22/10 mm Hg with a mean of 16 mm Hg, and the mean pulmonary wedge pressure was 10 mm Hg. Blood sampling for

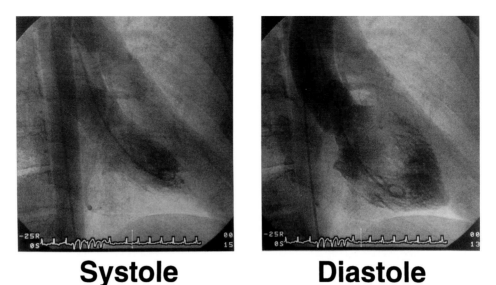

Systole   **Diastole**

Fig. 1.   Cineangiographic frames from left ventriculography in systole and diastole demonstrating opacification of the pulmonary artery and fistulous-like appearance of the coronary arising from the left coronary artery.

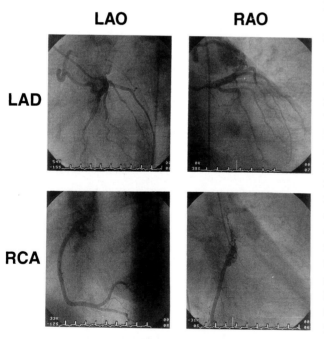

Fig. 2.   Cineangiographic frames of the left anterior descending coronary artery (LAD) (top). Left panel: Left anterior oblique (LAO). Right panel: Right anterior oblique (RAO). Lower panels: Right coronary artery (RCA). The fistulous connection can be seen arising anterior and lateral to the left anterior descending artery connecting to the pulmonary artery in multiple connections. The fistula arising from the right coronary artery emanates superiorly and anteriorly.

oxygen saturation obtained from the inferior vena cava (81%), right atrium (75%), right ventricle (74%), main pulmonary artery (76%), and right pulmonary artery (76%) failed to show any oximetric evidence of left-to-right shunt.

To determine whether the fistula might be impairing coronary blood flow and reserve, an 0.018-in. Doppler-tipped flowire (Cardiometrics, Mountain View, CA) was inserted into the mid left anterior descending artery distal to the origin of the fistula and beyond the origin of the first diagonal. Measurements were then made in the first diagonal and into the fistula itself from its origin near the first diagonal branch. Flow velocity was measured both at rest and during hyperemia induced by 18 μg of intracoronary adenosine. Coronary flow velocity in the left anterior descending artery at rest showed an average peak velocity of 20 cm/sec and normal phasic pattern with predominantly diastolic flow (diastolic-to-systolic velocity ratio = 2.5; normal > 1.8) (Fig. 3, top). After intracoronary adenosine, the coronary flow velocity reserve (hyperemic/basal flow mean flow velocity) was normal at 3.1. Coronary blood flow velocity was then measured in the fistula (Fig. 3, bottom). At rest, the flow pattern was a continuous systolic/diastolic flow with slightly higher velocity in systole than diastole. After adenosine, both systolic and diastolic flow increased with a flow reserve ratio of 1.2. Flow velocity was then measured in the diagonal artery adjacent to the fistula (Fig. 3, middle) which showed a pattern of flow intermediate between that noted in the left anterior descending artery and the fistula

Base   Hyperemia

LAD

D_1

Fistula

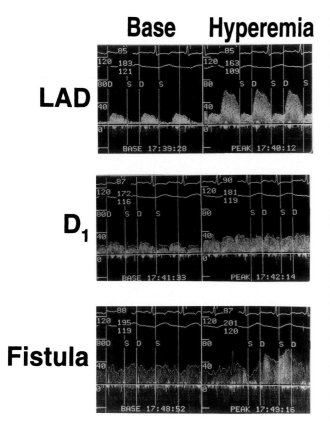

Fig. 3. Coronary flow velocity data at baseline and hyperemia in the left anterior descending (LAD), first diagonal (D1), and fistulous track. The phasic pattern of flow in the left anterior descending is normal at rest and at hyperemia. The phasic pattern of flow in the first diagonal is somewhat attenuated due to the connection to the fistula and hyperemia is also blunted due to flow diversion. In the fistulous track, the phasic pattern of coronary flow is abnormal with predominant systolic flow and hyperemia limited. Velocity scale is 0–120 cm/sec. EKG and arterial pressure are shown at the top tracings above the spectral flow velocity signal. S and D = systole and diastole, respectively, according to the EKG.

TABLE I. Flow Velocity Data*

	LAD	D_1	Fistula
APV			
Base	20	18	36
Hyperemia	62	40	40
CVR	3.1	2.2	1.2
DSVR	2.5	1.5	0.8

*APV, average peak velocity (cm/sec); CVR, coronary vasodilatory reserve; D_1, first diagonal artery; DSVR, basal diastolic/systolic velocity ratio; LAD, left anterior descending artery.

track. Coronary flow reserve was not measured in the right coronary artery fistula. The flow velocity data are summarized in Table I.

Although there was no evidence of coronary obstruction or steal, resting and exertional chest pain recurred in the hospital. During stress testing, she exercised for 16 min, 30 sec using a manual protocol, achieving 86% of maximum predicted heart rate with an estimated peak work load of 5 METS without chest pain. There were no significant arrhythmias and only a maximum of 1 mV horizontal ST depression in the inferior leads at peak exercise which resolved early into the recovery phase. Radionuclide (cardiolite) images revealed decreased activity in the distal anterolateral wall which was felt to represent breast attenuation. No definitive reversible defects were seen.

However, because of recurrent chest pain and the presence of dyspnea and to prevent possible long-term complications such as bacterial endocarditis, heart failure, myocardial infarction, or rupture of aneurysmal fistula [3,6,10,11], the patient underwent surgical ligation of both coronary fistulas using extracorporeal circulation. Intraoperatively, a large tortuous vessel was found coursing from the area of the right coronary artery across the base of the pulmonary artery (Fig. 4). In addition, there was a network of small arteries at the base of the pulmonary artery and at the level of the pulmonary artery bifurcation near the pericardial reflection. The main pulmonary artery was opened and the orifice of both fistulas was identified within the sinuses of the pulmonic valve leaflets. The fistula track from the right coronary artery was located anteriorly while the other fistula opened posteriorly. All fistula tracks were ligated and the pulmonary artery was closed using a pericardial patch. The patient did well post-operatively and discharged home three days later. At 3 mo of follow-up, she is asymptomatic.

DISCUSSION

The overall incidence of coronary fistulas is reported to be 0.11% in an adult population primarily referred to cardiac catheterization for angina [7]. Coronary fistulas are the second most common congenital malformation of coronary arteries after anomalous origins of the coronary arteries [12]. Krause reported the pathoanatomic description in 1865 [1] and the increased frequency reported in the past 40 yr reflects the angiographic description with the advent of cardiac catheterization [4]. The first surgical intervention was reported by Bjork and Crafoord [13] in 1947. In our catheterization laboratory, the overall incidence is 0.01% in over 35,000 catheterizations.

Although some fistulas are acquired secondary to trauma after coronary angioplasty or bypass surgery [14], the vast majority are due to embryological variations of coronary veins starting as an endothelial outgrowth that penetrates the myocardium to form intratrabecular spaces terminating in the epicardial surface and eventually forming a capillary network [3]. The coronary arteries originate as an outgrowth from the base of the aorta and branch to join the venous capillary network. Normally, the intramyocardial trabecular spaces narrow separating the epicardial network. The remnant of the coronary veins form Thebesian veins in adulthood. Persistence of the sinusoidal spaces (i.e., fistulous connections) is usually followed by aneurysmal dilatation of the fistula due to gradual weakening of the walls from increased blood pressure and flow [4,15–18]. In previous pathological reports, the walls of the fistula track contain mainly an endothelial layer surrounded by fibrous tissue with fragmented elastic fibers and lipid accumulations [4,15,19,20]. Multiple fistulas may be present and each fistula may terminate in a unique network rather than a single opening [21,22].

This case is unique in two respects: 1) The presence of multiple and bilateral coronary to pulmonary artery fistulas, and 2) the in vivo measurement of coronary flow velocity within a fistula. The blood flow pattern in a coronary fistula was measured directly for the first time preoperatively, demonstrating that, in contrast to normal phasic coronary flow, the velocity pattern is generally continuous with a higher velocity in systole than diastole.

A similar observation was made by Dedichen et al. in 1966 [9] during intraoperative flow measurements of a right coronary to a pulmonary vein fistula using an electromagnetic flow meter when they noted near continuous flow with a distinct systolic increase. Houghton et al. [23] measured coronary flow velocity and reserve in the proximal left anterior descending artery in a patient with left anterior descending to pulmonary artery fistula using an intracoronary Doppler catheter and found diminished coronary flow reserve (<1.1) during both nitroglycerin and papaverine-induced hyperemia. However, flow velocities were not measured in the fistula itself.

Although angina is a commonly reported symptom in patients with coronary fistulas, we found no evidence of inducible myocardial ischemia. Moreover, several investigators have postulated that ischemic pain might be attributed to a "coronary steal" phenomenon [3,18]. Although medical therapy is occasionally helpful in minimizing symptoms, the surgical ligation of the fistula tracks remains the standard of therapy [4,5,6,21]. Transcatheter approaches for closure of coronary fistulas have also been reported and are often successful [24]. In this case, because of the location and multiple fistula tracks, definitive surgical closure was selected. The blood flow measurements in the native left anterior descending artery distal to the fistula track did not support the steal hypothesis, but coronary flow reserve in the first diagonal was reduced relative to the left anterior descending, a response which correlated with the exercise perfusion

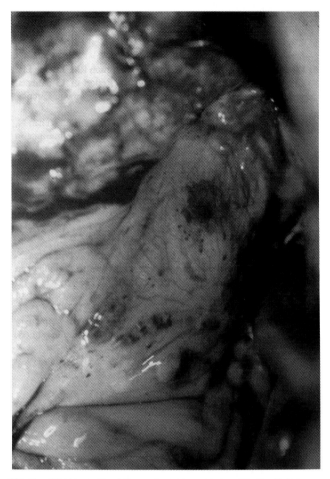

Fig. 4. Photograph of the pulmonary artery with the fistulous connection arising from the right coronary artery.

scintigraphic data. The exact pathophysiology of chest pain in patients with coronary fistulas is not yet fully understood.

ACKNOWLEDGMENTS

The authors wish to thank the J.G. Mudd Cardiac Catheterization Laboratory and Donna Sander for manuscript preparation.

REFERENCES

1. Krause W: Uber derr Ursprung einer akzessorischen a. coronaria aus der a. pulmonalis. Ztschr ratl med 24:225, 1865.
2. Eguchi S, Nitta H, Asano K, Tanaka M, Hoshino K: Congenital fistula of the right coronary artery to the left ventricle: The third case in the literature. Am Heart J 80:242–246, 1970.
3. McNamara JJ, Gross RE: Congenital coronary artery fistula. Surgery 65:59–69, 1969.
4. Rittenhouse EA, Doty DB, Ehrenhaft JL: Congenital coronary

artery-cardiac chamber fistula. Ann Thorac Surg 20:468–485, 1975.

5. Klingman R, Peetz D, Rothberg M: Congenital coronary artery fistula. Surg Rounds December 68–72, 1988.

6. Liberthson RR, Sagar K, Berkoben JP, Weintraub RM, Levine FH: Congenital coronary arteriovenous fistula: Report of 13 patients, review of the literature and delineation of management. Circulation 59:849–854, 1979.

7. Bhandari S, Kanojia A, Kasliwal RR, Kler TS, Seth A, Trehan N, Bhatia ML: Coronary artery fistulae without audible murmur in adults. Cardiovasc Intervent Radio 16:219–223, 1993.

8. Gupta NC, Beauvais J: Physiologic assessment of coronary artery fistula. Clin Nucl Med 16:40–42, 1991.

9. Dedichen H, Skalleberg L, Chappellen C Jr.: Congenital coronary artery fistula. Thorax 21:121, 1966.

10. Alkhulaifi AM, Horner SM, Pugsley WB, Swanton RH: Coronary artery fistula presenting with bacterial endocarditis. Ann Thorac Surg 60:202, 1995.

11. Shirai K, Ogawa M, Kawaguchi H, Kawano T, Nakashima Y, Arakawa K: Acute myocardial infarction due to thrombus in congenital artery fistula. Eur Heart J 15(4);577, 1994.

12. Lowe JE, Oldham HN, Sabiston DC: Surgical management of congenital coronary artery fistulas. Ann Surg 194:373–380, 1981.

13. Bjork G, Grafoord C: Arteriovenous aneurysm on the pulmonary artery simulating patent ductus arteriosus. J Thorac Surg 2:65, 1947.

14. Blanche C, Chaux A, Buchbinder N, O'Connor L: Acquired left coronary artery to left atrium fistula: Unusual complication of aortocoronary bypass. J Cardiovasc Surg 27:231, 1987.

15. Edwards JE: Anomalous coronary arteries with special reference to arteriovenous like communications. Circulation 17:1001, 1958.

16. Edwards JE, Gladding TC, Weir AB Jr.: Congenital communication between the right coronary artery and right atrium. J Thoracic Surg 35:662, 1956.

17. Grant RT: Development of the cardiac coronary vessel in the rabbit. Heart 13:126, 1926.

18. Black IW, Loo C, Allan RM: Multiple coronary artery-left ventricular fistula. Cathet Cardiovasc Diagn 23:133–135, 1991.

19. Hudspeth AS, Linder JH: Congenital coronary arteriovenous fistula. Arch Surg 96:832–835, 1968.

20. Ueno T, Nakayama Y, Yoshikai M, Watanabe Y, Minato N, Natsuaki M, Itoh T: Unique manifestations of congenital coronary artery fistulas. Am Heart J 124:1388–1391, 1992.

21. Blanche C, Chaux A: Long-term results of surgery for coronary artery fistulas. Int Surg 75:238–239, 1990.

22. Ogden JA: Congenital variation of coronary arteries. Thesis. New Haven, CT: Yale University School of Medicine, 1968.

23. Houghton JL, Saxena R, Frank MJ: Angina and ischemia electrocardiographic changes secondary to coronary arteriovenous fistula with abnormal basal and reserve coronary blood flow. Am Heart J 125:886–889, 1993.

24. Perry SB, Rome J, Keane JF, Baim DS, Lock JE: Transcatheter closure of coronary artery fistulas. J Am Coll Cardiol 20:205–209, 1992.

Index